500

15-Minute

Low Sodium
Recipes

500
15-Minute
Low Sodium
Recipes

FAST AND FLAVORFUL LOW-SALT RECIPES
THAT SAVE YOU TIME, KEEP YOU ON TRACK,
AND TASTE DELICIOUS

DICK LOGUE

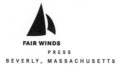

FAIR WINDS
PRESS
BEVERLY, MASSACHUSETTS

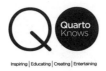

Brimming with creative inspiration, how-to projects, and useful information to enrich your everyday life, Quarto Knows is a favorite destination for those pursuing their interests and passions. Visit our site and dig deeper with our books into your area of interest: Quarto Creates, Quarto Cooks, Quarto Homes, Quarto Lives, Quarto Drives, Quarto Explores, Quarto Gifts, or Quarto Kids.

© 2012 Fair Winds Press
Text © 2012 Dick Logue

First published in 2012 by Fair Winds Press,
an imprint of The Quarto Group,
100 Cummings Center, Suite 265-D,
Beverly, MA 01915, USA.
T (978) 282-9590 F (978) 283-2742
www.QuartoKnows.com

Fair Winds Press titles are also available at discount for retail, wholesale, promotional, and bulk purchase. For details, contact the Special Sales Manager by email at specialsales@quarto.com or by mail at The Quarto Group, Attn: Special Sales Manager, 401 Second Avenue North, Suite 310, Minneapolis, MN 55401, USA.

19 18 17   10 11 12 13

ISBN: 978-1-59233-501-5

Digital edition published in 2012
eISBN: 978-1-61058-402-9

Library of Congress Cataloging-in-Publication Data available

Printed and bound in USA

SUSTAINABLE FORESTRY INITIATIVE
Certified Chain of Custody
Promoting Sustainable Forestry
www.sfiprogram.org
SFI-01268
SFI label applies to the text stock

The information in this book is for educational purposes only. It is not intended to replace the advice of a physician or medical practitioner. Please see your health care provider before beginning any new health program.

Dedication:

*To everyone whose support and encouraging words
have kept me doing new recipes for all these years,
family, friends and newsletter subscribers who have
told me that it made living a low-sodium lifestyle easier.*

Contents

Why Another Low-Sodium Cookbook?

Some of you may be wondering why there is a need for another low-sodium cookbook. If you stop in at your local bookstore or visit an online bookseller, you'll see that there are already a number of books on the subject. And a quick search online will reveal a number of websites focusing on low-sodium cooking. I've contributed to this existing information myself. I have a website at www.lowsodiumcooking.com, and in 2007 I wrote *500 Low-Sodium Recipes*. So what made me think that there was a need for another low-sodium book? The main reason was what I hear from people who have visited my website or who are readers of my email newsletter. They tell me that they know they would be healthier if they lowered the amount of sodium in their diet, but it's not as easy as it sounds.

In listening to people, I have found there are a couple of recurring themes that seem to be the most common reasons why people find it difficult to stick to a low-sodium diet. And as I thought about my previous books and other low-sodium books that I have collected, it became more obvious that no one has really tried to specifically address these difficulties. The more I thought about it, the more it seemed like a new book might be what was needed.

What Makes Low-Sodium Cooking Difficult?

The reasons people identified seemed to group into a few key areas.

- Low-sodium food doesn't taste as good. There is a pretty much widely accepted belief that low-sodium food has no taste, or at least very inferior taste.

- Low-sodium cooking costs too much. People believe that because they need to buy ingredients that they haven't bought before and that may only be available online, low-sodium cooking is going to be more expensive.

- Low-sodium cooking is difficult. The main complaints here are that people don't know where to find low-sodium ingredients or how to make food that tastes good without using high-sodium ingredients.

And the big one . . .

- Low-sodium cooking takes too much time. Everyone is busy these days. There is work, family commitments, and generally busier-than-ever lives. People don't want to spend a lot of their precious time preparing food, so fast food restaurants and convenience foods fill that need, but at the cost of high sodium levels.

How Can We Solve Those Problems?

The purpose of this book is to help people overcome these difficulties and find a way to make the transition to a lower sodium diet easier. Let's take a quick look at how we'll do that.

- Taste. While it's true that it does take some time to get used to the taste of food without added salt and high-sodium ingredients, I have heard from a number of people how surprised they were at the taste of the recipes in my first book. But to get to that point does sometimes require being creative, experimenting and tweaking recipes until they taste the way you'd like. Many people don't have the time or the desire to do that, so I've done it for you.

- Cost. This is one of the areas where being informed and making smart choices makes all the difference. Yes, it's true that you may need to buy some ingredients that you didn't buy before, but you also can make a lot of meals for a lot less money than buying prepared dinners. Instead of spending fifteen dollars for a delivery pizza, you can make one that is healthier, tastes just as good, and costs maybe half that.

- Difficulty. There are several keys here. One is knowing which ingredients are available and where to find them. That's something that has changed a lot since I started my low-sodium diet in 1999. And it has even changed since my first book came out. So it's time for an update. The other key here is knowing how to easily make the things you can't readily buy. I've included a chapter here on make-ahead items that you can just pull off the shelf and use. And that helps to solve . . .

- Time. There's no way around it—you are going to have to cook more things from scratch to maintain a low-sodium diet. Not as many as in 1999, when I was making my own mustard and ketchup, but it's still difficult to find really low-sodium versions of a lot of things, which is where my make-aheads chapter comes in. You will no longer be able to stop at the fast food place or microwave a frozen entrée. And *that* is the real focus of this book. It is filled with 15-minute recipes: main dishes, side dishes, and desserts that you can have on the table in about a quarter of an hour. There's also a section of recipes that you can prepare in 15 minutes and then let them cook on their own. Many of these involve appliances such as slow cookers and bread machines.

So the bottom line is that you can have tasty, inexpensive, easy, low-sodium meals without spending your life in the kitchen. And that is what people tell me they need in order to successfully transition to a low-sodium diet.

A Little Bit about Me

Some of you may already know me from my Low-Sodium Cooking website and newsletter or from my other books focused on low-sodium and other heart-healthy recipes. For those who don't, perhaps a little background information might be useful.

I started thinking about heart-healthy cooking after being diagnosed with congestive heart failure in 1999. One of the first, and biggest, things I had to deal with was the doctor's insistence that I follow a low-sodium diet . . . 1,200 mg a day or less. At first, like many people, I found it easiest to just avoid the things that had a lot of sodium in them. But I was bored. And I was convinced that there had to be a way to create low-sodium versions of the foods I missed. So I learned all kinds of *new* cooking things. I researched where to get low-sodium substitutes for the things that I couldn't have anymore, bought cookbooks, and basically redid my whole diet. And I decided to share this information with others who may be in the same position I had been in. I started a website, www.lowsodiumcooking.com, to share recipes and information. I sent out an email newsletter with recipes that now has more than 20,000 subscribers. And I wrote my first book, *500 Low Sodium Recipes*.

Perhaps the best way to start in telling you who I am is by telling you who I'm not. I'm not a doctor. I'm not a dietician. I'm not a professional chef. What I *am* is an ordinary person just like you who has some special dietary needs. I have enjoyed cooking most of my life. I guess I started it seriously about the time my mother went back to work when I was twelve or so. In those days, it was simple stuff such as burgers and hot dogs and spaghetti. But the interest stayed. After I married my wife, we got pretty involved in some food-related pursuits—growing vegetables in our garden, making bread and other baked goods, canning and jelly making, that kind of thing. She always said that my "mad chemist" cooking was an outgrowth of the time I spent in college as a chemistry major, and she might be right. So creating the kind of food that people said couldn't be done, low in sodium and high in taste, was a fun challenge for me.

Along the way, I also learned about other things that make a diet heart healthy. I became more aware of cholesterol, fiber, and the glycemic index and began incorporating what we learned into the recipes. So you will find that the recipes here are not only low in sodium, but they also tend to be low in saturated fat, contain whole grains and other high-fiber foods, and tend to focus on fresh ingredients. This all actually comes together nicely, because in many cases the same foods that fit those requirements are also low in sodium and taste better than the less healthy alternatives.

How Is the Nutritional Information Calculated?

The nutritional information included with these recipes was calculated using the AccuChef program. It calculates the values using the latest U.S. Department of Agriculture National Nutrient Database for Standard Reference. I've been using this program since I first started trying to figure out how much sodium was in the recipes I've created. It's inexpensive, is easy to use, and has a number of really handy features. For instance, if I go in and change the nutrition figures for an ingredient, it remembers those figures whenever I use that ingredient. AccuChef is available online from www.accuchef.com. They offer a free trial version if you want to try it out and the full version costs less than twenty dollars.

Of course, this implies that these figures are estimates. Every brand of tomatoes, or any other product, is a little different in nutritional content. These figures were calculated using products that I buy here in southern Maryland. If you use a different brand, your nutrition figures may be different. Use the nutritional analysis as a guideline in determining whether a recipe is right for your diet.

1

The Keys to Fast, Great-Tasting, Low-Sodium Meals

Perhaps the first questions I need to answer are why we should be interested in following a low-sodium diet and what I mean by one. Even if your doctor hasn't specifically told you to lower your sodium intake, there is a lot of research and recommendations that says it's a good idea.

- The U.S. Food and Drug Administration recommends 2,300 milligrams (mg) of sodium daily for healthy adults.

- The U.S. Department of Agriculture recommends that individuals with hypertension, African Americans, and adults fifty years old and above should consume no more than 1,500 mg of sodium per day.

- The United Kingdom's Reference Nutrient Intake (RNI) is 1,600 mg daily.

- The National Research Council of the National Academy of Sciences recommends 1,100 to 1,500 mg daily for adults.

- Studies have shown that many people in the United States and Canada routinely consume two to three times these amounts daily.

Given these figures, it's pretty safe to say that many of us consume more sodium than is good for us. If you already have a history of heart disease, or have a family history of it, it's even worse. I know I sound a bit like a zealot in this, but I can honestly say that I felt much better when I first started my low-sodium diet more than ten years ago. And I'm probably in a better position now medically than I was then. All I can say is, it's worked for me and lots of other people I've talked to.

As I said in the introduction, I started off being interested in low-sodium meals that I wanted to eat every night. There is only one recipe in this book with more than 300 mg of sodium (the pork fajitas have 314, and that's basically a whole meal). I later became interested in other things that contribute to heart health. There are a couple of general principles that I have come to believe are important in maintaining a heart-healthy diet.

- Eat foods low in sodium. We've already talked about this.

- Eat foods low in saturated fat. Fats such as those found in olive and canola oils do have some health benefits and you will see them specified whenever a recipe uses oil. Generally, most studies seem to support the idea that both saturated and trans fats represent health risks, so I have tried to limit them as much as possible. I feel that trans fats are the bigger hazard, and so I use butter whenever solid fat is called for. It just seems to me that the more we eliminate manufactured and highly processed foods the better.

- Eat foods high in fiber. Eating foods high in fiber is another of those things that has multiple positive effects. I haven't always specified ingredients such as whole-grain pasta and brown rice here, but that is what I usually eat. If nothing else, I think it has more flavor.

- Focus on fresh, minimally processed foods. There has been an increased focus on avoiding processed foods in recent years. The Canyon Ranch spa cookbook I own suggests, "Don't eat anything your great-grandmother didn't," and that seems like a reasonable approach to me. In general, raw is better than cooked and fresh is better than frozen, which is better than canned.

Tip and Tricks

So, given that information from abundant sources suggests that we need to eat healthier, low-sodium meals, my goal is to show you how to get one on the table in 15 minutes. We need to be conscious of a few things to make that happen. In the next few paragraphs, we'll look at how things such as being careful in your choice of ingredients, planning, and buying or making the things you are going to need ahead of time can have a big impact on how long it takes to prepare a low-sodium meal.

- Ingredient choices. The ingredients we choose are important for several reasons. First of all, as obvious as it seems, if we choose high-sodium ingredients, we are not going to end up with a low-sodium meal. So no matter how quick it is to prepare, it's not going to be as healthy as we might want. It's easy to prepare quick meals using canned, frozen, and boxed products that are meant to save you time, but from a sodium standpoint, you might as well just stop at McDonalds. The next chapter will give you a lot more information on finding and selecting low-sodium ingredients. Ingredients are also important in terms of how long they take to cook. This is probably also obvious, but it does require a different way of thinking about meal preparation. If you have a really busy evening and it's important to get a meal ready in 15 minutes, there are some choices that just aren't going to work. You'll notice that the pasta recipes in this book call for angel hair pasta or spaghetti. Now I happen to love fettuccini and linguini, and from the standpoint of the recipe, they would work just as well. The problem is that they can take 14 to 16 minutes to cook, and that's after you get the water boiling. So I save that for days when I have more time. There are a number of things that fall into that category: rice that takes 20 minutes or more to cook (although the "Instant" Rice recipe in chapter 14 solves that problem); vegetables or meats that must be braised; roasts and baked items; and so on. But that doesn't mean you can't still have a wide variety of great-tasting meals. The notes at the beginning of each chapter will help steer you in the right direction. And there are almost 400 recipes that can be on the table within 15 minutes of the time you walk into the kitchen.

- Substitutions. There are some decisions you can make about substituting one ingredient for another that affect both the speed of preparation and the sodium content. Some are the kinds of things we talked about in the last section, such as substituting thin spaghetti for thick, instant rice for long-cooking rice, and so on. But there are also a lot of choices you make that, more importantly, affect the sodium content. If there were one piece of advice I could give people who are trying to reduce the amount of sodium in their diets, it would be this: Become a label reader. If you just pick a few categories and look at the options in your favorite store you will quickly see why I say this. Canned tomatoes may have as little as

20 mg per serving or as much as 200 mg. The last time I bought bacon, I found a brand with 120 mg of sodium per two slices right next to a brand with almost three times as much. Chicken, turkey, and pork often come "enhanced" with broth to make them juicier—and with three to four times the sodium. If you are aware of these things when you are buying your groceries, you can either make it easier to produce fast, healthy meals or set yourself up for failure.

- Planning ahead. How many times have you thought of the perfect idea for dinner only to find that you don't have the ingredients on hand? I know it has happened to me. Or do you arrive home and have no idea what you are going to fix? The way to avoid that is planning ahead. This becomes especially important if you are trying to make quick meals. If you look at your upcoming week, you'll often see that there are nights when things are going to be especially hectic. Maybe it's a night when you have activities with the children or you know you are going to be late getting home from work. That's the night you want to know ahead of time what you are fixing and not end up staring into the freezer wondering what you can thaw in time or whether you just need to order pizza delivery. I've learned to look at my upcoming week on the weekend when I have more time (and more energy than in the evening). Then I can plan what each night's dinner is going to be and see whether I need a trip to the grocery store in order to have everything I need.

- Make ahead. I have two chapters in this book of make-ahead recipes because I've found that to be key in getting healthy meals on the table fast. There are some things that you really need to have available when you start. Many of these are the kinds of things you would normally just buy in a can or bottle. Salad dressings are a good example of this. Other than a few fruit-flavored dressings, it's really difficult to find any in a regular grocery store that are low in sodium. They typically run from about 250 mg per serving up to almost 400 mg. That means you could end up with a third of the sodium you'd like to have for the day in just one serving of salad dressing. You know you can make dressing, but sometimes you don't want to spend that extra 5 or 10 minutes to do it. So I've included a number of low-sodium ones that you can make ahead of time and have ready to use in the refrigerator. Half an hour when you have the time will get you a good assortment that you can just pull out and use. That's true of many of the recipes in chapter 3, which include things such as low-sodium soy sauce and salad dressings that are used in other recipes later in the book.

Chapter 14 addresses a little different situation. If you look at books and websites with quick meals, they often rely on meat or rotisserie chicken from the deli section. But those items also contain a lot of sodium. The solution? On the weekend, while you are running errands or doing chores around the house, take a few minutes to put a chicken, turkey breast, or beef roast in the oven. It doesn't really take much, if any, attention, and it gives you that head start on 15-minute meals. One other recipe in chapter 14 has become a real favorite of ours. We like rice with a lot of meals, but steaming it takes 45 minutes. There are a couple of ways around that. You can buy instant rice like Minute Rice that cooks in 5 minutes, but I'm not really as fond of the flavor and texture as I am of long-cooked rice. You can buy the little microwavable bags of precooked white or brown rice that cook in 90 seconds. I like those; they are easy, quick, and taste great. The only problem is they cost two to three dollars for two servings. Or you can buy a 5-pound bag of long-cooking rice and get fifty servings for about the same price as three of the microwave bags. But now we're back to the 45-minute problem. So I steam a batch as big as my steamer will hold when I have the time, pack it 2 cups at a time in freezer bags, and when I want some I pop it in the microwave and have the taste and convenience of the microwave bags without the cost. This same technique works well with some vegetables. Things such as broccoli, cauliflower, and green beans can be bought in quantity when they are cheap and fresh, steamed for a few minutes, plunged into cold water to keep them from cooking further, and packed in freezer bags to be microwaved later. You have frozen veggies with all the taste and nutrition of fresh ones, and all you have to do is punch a little hole in the top with the point of a knife and you have the convenience of the microwave bags at a fraction of the cost.

- Cooking techniques. I should probably include just a couple of comments about some of the cooking techniques used in this book to speed the process of making healthy meals. One that is sometimes overlooked is the microwave. I've included a number of microwave recipes here. Some are the kinds of things people have gotten used to microwaving all the time, such as hot breakfast cereal and fruit desserts. Others are ones that people tend to shy away from. However, I've found that if you are careful to cook things until they are just done and not overcooked, you can successfully microwave a number of chicken, beef, and fish dishes. It's the *only* way I know that you are going to get a meatloaf for a family on the table in 15 minutes. The other technique that I discovered (at least I've never seen it anywhere else) is what I call mock kabobs. You'll find these recipes scattered throughout many of the 15-minute chapters. The idea is this: Kabobs are in many ways a great way to get the meat and/or vegetables for a meal cooked quickly, because everything is cut up into small pieces. The only problem is the preparation time tends to be a bit long. Not only do you have to cut them up, but then there's also that tedious job of threading them onto skewers. However, I've found that you can eliminate the second step. Instead of skewering them and putting them on the grill, cut them up and stick them under the broiler or in a heavy frying pan for a few minutes.

2

Ingredients and Sources

The following are general guidelines for reducing the amount of sodium in your diet. Bear in mind that just following these guidelines may not be enough depending on how low the amount of sodium you are targeting. You may also find that you need to pick and choose, eating some higher sodium items that you can't find an easy replacement for. You also still need to be a careful label reader; there are big variations within some categories, with specific products being either better or worse than the average.

- Breads
  - Better: Homemade, English muffins, white, wheat, pumpernickel, other types of regular or unsalted breads and rolls
  - Avoid: Sweet rolls, breads or rolls with salted tops, packaged cracker or bread crumb coatings unless unsalted, packaged stuffing mixes, biscuits, cornbread

- Cereals
  - Better: Regular cooked cereals such as oats, cream of wheat, rice, or farina; puffed wheat; puffed rice; shredded wheat
  - Avoid: Instant hot cereals, any other regular ready-to-eat cereals

- Crackers and snack foods
  - Better: All unsalted crackers and snack foods, unsalted peanut butter
  - Avoid: Salted crackers and snack items, regular peanut butter, prepared spreads and dips

- Pasta and carbohydrates
  - Better: All types of pastas such as macaroni, spaghetti, rigatoni, ziti; potatoes; rice
  - Avoid: Macaroni and cheese mix; seasoned rice, noodle, and spaghetti mixes; canned spaghetti; frozen lasagna, macaroni and cheese, rice, and pasta dishes; instant potatoes unless unsalted; seasoned potato mixes

- Dried beans and peas
  - Better: Pinto beans, Great Northern beans, black-eyed peas, lima beans, lentils, split peas, and so on.
  - Avoid: Any beans or peas prepared with ham, bacon, salt pork, or bacon grease; all canned beans unless no-salt-added

- Meat, poultry, and fish
  - Better: Fresh or frozen meat, poultry, and fish, unless they contain added higher sodium ingredients; low-sodium canned tuna and salmon; eggs
  - Avoid: Salted, smoked, canned, spiced, and pickled meats, poultry, and fish; bacon; ham; sausage; scrapple; regular canned tuna or salmon; cold cuts; luncheon meats; hot dogs; breaded frozen meats, fish, and poultry; TV dinners; meat pies; kosher meats

- Fruits and vegetables
  - Better: Fresh, frozen, or low-sodium canned vegetables or vegetable juices; low-sodium tomato products; fresh, canned, or frozen fruits and juices
  - Avoid: Regular canned vegetables and vegetable juices, regular tomato sauce and tomato paste, olives, pickles, relishes, sauerkraut or vegetables packed in brine, frozen vegetables in butter or sauces, frozen peas or lima beans with added salt, crystallized and glazed fruit, maraschino cherries, fruit dried with sodium sulfite

- Dairy products
  - Better: Milk, cream, sour cream, nondairy creamer, yogurt, low-sodium cottage cheese, low-sodium cheese

- Avoid: Buttermilk, Dutch-processed chocolate milk, processed cheese slices and spreads, regular cheese, cottage cheese

- Fats and oils
  - Better: Unsalted butter or margarine; cooking oils; salt-free gravies, cream sauces, and salad dressings
  - Avoid: Bacon grease; salt pork; commercially prepared sauces, gravies, and salad dressings

- Soups
  - Better: Salt-free soups and low-sodium bouillon cubes
  - Avoid: Regular commercially canned or prepared soups, stews, broths, or bouillon; packaged and frozen soups

- Desserts
  - Better: Gelatin, sherbet, fruit ices, pudding and ice cream as part of milk allowance, angel food cake, salt-free baked goods, sugar, honey, jam, jelly, marmalade, syrup
  - Avoid: Regular commercially prepared and packaged baked goods, chocolate candy

- Condiments
  - Better: Fresh and dried herbs; lemon juice; low-sodium mustard, vinegar, and hot pepper sauce; low-sodium or no-salt-added ketchup; extracts (almond, lemon, vanilla); baking chocolate and cocoa; seasoning blends that do not contain salt
  - Avoid: Table salt, lite salt, meat extract, Worcestershire sauce, tartar sauce, ketchup, chili sauce, cooking wines, onion salt, prepared mustard, garlic salt, meat flavorings, meat tenderizers, steak and barbecue sauce, seasoned salt, monosodium glutamate (MSG), Dutch-processed cocoa

Comments on a Few Specific Ingredients

- Eggs. The recipes call for egg substitute rather than eggs. I started this as a way to reduce the amount of cholesterol I was taking in, especially since I have eggs for breakfast fairly often. The brand I use does have 25 mg more sodium than whole eggs, so there is a tradeoff. If cholesterol isn't an issue for you, it's cheaper and easier to just use whole eggs.

- Milk. Although the recipes call for skim milk, to keep down the amount of fat, there are some lower sodium alternatives, such as low-sodium soymilk products.

- Baking powder and baking soda. In my humble opinion, this is a no-brainer. If you bake anything that uses baking powder with the regular stuff off your grocer's shelves you are eating sodium that can easily be avoided. Given the amount of sodium in standard baking powder, it's likely to be 100 to 200 mg per serving. Some doctors also believe the aluminum in regular baking powder is bad for you. The simple solution is sodium-free, aluminum-free baking powder. There are several brands available, but they have been difficult to find locally. I've found the Featherweight brand at a health food store. It's also available online at Healthy Heart Market. The price is comparable to regular baking powder. Recently Clabber Girl released a reduced sodium version of their Rumford baking powder. It's not sodium-free like the Featherweight, but it does contain significantly less sodium than regular baking powder and is widely available at many grocery chains. Like baking powder, regular baking soda is unnecessary sodium intake. The only brand of sodium-free baking soda I'm familiar with is Ener-G and the only place I've seen it is online at Healthy Heart Market. The manufacturer does recommend doubling the amount of baking soda called for in your favorite recipes when using this product. The recipes in this book already have the amount doubled. I've used both products for more than eleven years. The baking powder has never failed to produce the desired results. The baking soda sometimes doesn't seem to rise as much as I would have expected. I don't know whether that's because mine has gotten old or whether it has to do with particular recipes, but it's something to be aware of.

- Seasoning blends. You'll likely be able to find some salt-free versions of these on your regular grocer's shelves. Mrs. Dash makes a number of different blends that are widely available, and major spice manufacturers such as McCormick do also. Many spices come in bottles small enough to be exempt from the usual labeling requirements in the United States, so you'll need to read the ingredient list and look for added salt. Health food stores often stock salt-free spice blends, and there are a number of places to get them online. You'll also find recipes for making some of your own in chapter 3.

- Sauces and condiments. In looking at products like barbecue sauce, Asian sauces, ketchup, mustard, and salsa, you'll find a wide range of sodium levels. Most of the low-sodium varieties are made by companies in the organic and specialty foods area, so you'll have a better chance of finding them in health food stores or markets with large organic food sections. Many of the products you'll find on regular grocery shelves contain high amounts of sodium. Low-sodium varieties are also available for sale online, or you can make your own using the recipes in chapters 3 and 14.

- Canned tomato products, vegetables, and beans. In the United States, most of the large food companies such as Hunt's and Del Monte make salf-free versions of these products. I have no trouble finding a good selection of no-salt-added tomato products and a more limited selection of other no-salt-added vegetables in any large supermarket. Beans are less common and are another area where organic food producers are leading the way. With a little more effort you can cook your own dried beans without salt for a fraction of the cost of the canned ones. I usually cook a 1-pound (455 g) bag at a time and freeze what I don't need for future use.

- Soups, broths, and bouillon. Like other products, low-sodium versions of these are available, but not as widely as we might like. Again, organic food producers are the best bet for finding a truly low-sodium item. There are recipes in chapter 14 for making your own stock to use in place of canned broth. There are also some very low-sodium soup bases from companies such as Redi-Base available online. These come in a variety of flavors and have a much more natural taste than the sodium-free bouillon cubes.

- Bread. Low-sodium bread is hard to find in many places. I highly recommend a bread machine so you can make your own. The notes in chapter 23 go into this in detail, and the chapter contains a number of recipes to get you started.

- Meats. These days, many fresh meats are "enhanced" by injecting them with a broth solution to make them juicer. Unfortunately, it also increases the sodium level from 75 to 80 mg per serving to more than 300 mg. This is especially true of chicken and turkey and increasingly true of pork. There is still unadulterated meat around, but you have to be careful and look for it. I've also seen several instances of pork that was marked as being "enhanced" but that didn't contain a nutrition label to let you know how much sodium had been added.

- Salt substitutes. You won't find any salt substitutes listed in the ingredients in this book. I know that some people really like them as a way to get that salty flavor without the sodium, but I'm not fond of them myself. There are two reasons. One is that the potassium chloride they contain tends to have a metallic aftertaste. The other is that I'm concerned that using the substitute will make it harder for your body to adjust to the taste of food without salt. If you are considering using one you should check with your doctor first to make sure the increased potassium will not be an issue.

Where Do I Find These Ingredients?

The first place to look for low-sodium ingredients is in your local grocery stores. I can't tell you what may be available at your local market, wherever in the world you may be, but I find a number of low-sodium ingredients locally. And at least here in southern Maryland, it's gotten easier to find products since I first started this diet twelve years ago. At that time, there were a lot of things I couldn't find. I spent quite a bit of time trying to come up with a good low-sodium recipe for ketchup. Now Hunt's and Heinz both market it nationally. I shop at several of the large supermarket chains, a couple of discount clubs, and one local store. I buy many of the items I use at one of these places. They all carry different things, but between them I find quite a few low-sodium items. I also stop by my local health food store occasionally. Because many of the manufacturers that are involved in organic products also tend to make salt-free versions, you'll find health food stores to be a good source, especially for spices and canned products. Any of these stores, either grocery or health food ones, carry what they think will sell, and the store manager has some discretion in choosing those items. So letting your local store manager know that you want low-sodium items stocked *may* help. I've seen cases where managers will order something new if asked and ones where they won't, because they feel the space could be used for something that more people want. It never hurts to ask.

Another great source for low-sodium foods is stores that specialize in organic and gourmet foods, such as Whole Foods and Trader Joe's. They are kind of like mainstream health food stores. If you live near one of these, or a similar store, you should definitely check them out. You can get a list of locations from their websites. Be on the lookout for local stores that cater to similar clientele. I have one that carries all the salt-free seasoning blends from several organic suppliers.

There are online sources that specialize in low-sodium products, but you need to be careful. Some just offer this as a sideline to another business and aren't as careful as they could be about what they label as low sodium. There is one online site that was founded by a heart transplant recipient and carries only low-sodium products: Healthy Heart Market at www .healthyheartmarket.com. They carry some things that you probably didn't even know came in low-sodium versions. Healthy Heart Market ships to the United States and Canada. The service is great, the prices and shipping costs are reasonable, and the selection is extensive. Besides that, it makes good sense to patronize places that are striving to make a living by providing the products that we all need but often find difficult to locate. It's a win for both sides.

Portion Control

One final comment that I want to make is that you need to be careful about portion sizes. I know that's something everyone thinks goes without saying. But I know that I sometimes struggle with it, so I just thought I would mention it. I find it particularly an issue with things such as dairy products. If you carefully read the label and it says there are 100 mg of sodium in a cup of milk and you fill a 12-ounce glass, that is 150 mg, not 100.

3

5-Minute Make-Aheads that Make 15-Minute Meals Easy

Because some things are difficult (or impossible) to find in low-sodium versions, the easiest way to obtain them is to make them yourself. These are quick recipes that you can make in a few minutes in quantities that will allow you to make multiple meals. Having these kinds of items on hand is one of the keys to making the other recipes in 15 minutes or less. Some of them, such as the soy and teriyaki sauces and the soup and dressing mixes, are used in a number of recipes throughout the book to boost flavor without adding sodium. Others, such as the salad dressings, are simply good things to have in the refrigerator so you have a low-sodium option available when you want it.

Buttermilk Baking Mix

Use this baking mix in any recipe that calls for Bisquick. It's a lot lower in sodium than even their heart-healthy version.

10½ cups (1260 g) all-purpose flour

¼ cup (60 g) sodium-free baking powder

½ cup (100 g) sugar

1 cup (120 g) buttermilk powder

1½ teaspoons sodium-free baking soda

2 cups (400 g) shortening

In a large bowl, mix all the ingredients with an electric mixer or pastry blender until pieces are small and uniform in size. Store on a shelf in a tightly covered container for up to 1 year.

Yield: About 14 cups, ½ cup per serving

Per serving: 358 calories (41% from fat, 8% from protein, 51% from carbohydrate); 7 g protein; 17 g total fat; 4 g saturated fat; 7 g monounsaturated fat; 4 g polyunsaturated fat; 46 g carbohydrate; 1 g fiber; 6 g sugar; 256 mg phosphorus; 162 mg calcium; 27 mg sodium; 361 mg potassium; 8 IU vitamin A; 2 mg ATE vitamin E; 0 mg vitamin C; 3 mg cholesterol

Salt-Free Seasoning

This blend comes close to approximating the flavors in the typical seasoned salt blends like Lawry's, without the sodium. Use it anywhere seasoned salt is called for or when you want to give food a little extra flavor. I like it in soups and egg dishes.

1 teaspoon chili powder

¼ teaspoon celery seed

½ teaspoon nutmeg

½ teaspoon coriander

1 teaspoon onion powder

1 teaspoon paprika

¼ teaspoon garlic powder

1 teaspoon turmeric

Mix all the ingredients well and store in an airtight container. Will keep indefinitely, but the flavor will be best if used within 6 months.

Yield: 5½ teaspoons, ¼ teaspoon per serving

Per serving: 2 calories (28% from fat, 11% from protein, 60% from carbohydrate); 0 g protein; 0 g total fat; 0 g saturated fat; 0 g monounsaturated fat; 0 g polyunsaturated fat; 0 g carbohydrate; 0 g fiber; 0 g sugar; 2 mg phosphorus; 2 mg calcium; 1 mg sodium; 9 mg potassium; 82 IU vitamin A; 0 mg ATE vitamin E; 0 mg vitamin C; 0 mg cholesterol

Salt-Free Mexican Seasoning

Add to chili, beans, or other Mexican dishes or sprinkle on grilled vegetables such as potatoes or onions.

1 tablespoon (6 g) ground chile pepper

2 teaspoons garlic powder

2 teaspoons onion powder

1 teaspoon paprika

1½ teaspoons ground cumin

(continued on page 28)

1 teaspoon celery seed

1 teaspoon dried oregano

¼ teaspoon cayenne pepper

¼ teaspoon ground bay leaf

Mix all the ingredients well and store in an airtight container. Will keep indefinitely, but the flavor will be best if used within 6 months.

Yield: 11 teaspoons, 1 teaspoon per serving

Per serving: 7 calories (20% from fat, 14% from protein, 65% from carbohydrate); 0 g protein; 0 g total fat; 0 g saturated fat; 0 g monounsaturated fat; 0 g polyunsaturated fat; 1 g carbohydrate; 0 g fiber; 0 g sugar; 7 mg phosphorus; 10 mg calcium; 1 mg sodium; 28 mg potassium; 193 IU vitamin A; 0 mg ATE vitamin E; 1 mg vitamin C; 0 mg cholesterol

Salt-Free Taco Seasoning

Use to flavor meat for tacos and fajitas or to add Mexican flavor to soups and other Mexican dishes.

2 tablespoons (16 g) chili powder

2 tablespoons (16 g) all-purpose flour

2 teaspoons ground cumin

2 teaspoons dried oregano

½ teaspoon onion powder

½ teaspoon garlic powder

½ teaspoon cayenne pepper

Mix all the ingredients well and store in an airtight container. Will keep indefinitely, but the flavor will be best if used within 6 months. Add entire recipe to browned ground beef along with ½ to ¾ cup (120 to 180 ml) water and cook until reduced to the desired consistency.

Yield: About 6 tablespoons, 1 tablespoon per serving

Per serving: 23 calories (23% from fat, 12% from protein, 65% from carbohydrate); 1 g protein; 1 g total fat; 0 g saturated fat; 0 g monounsaturated fat; 0 g polyunsaturated fat; 4 g carbohydrate; 1 g fiber; 0 g sugar; 16 mg phosphorus; 20 mg calcium; 27 mg sodium; 76 mg potassium; 834 IU vitamin A; 0 mg ATE vitamin E; 2 mg vitamin C; 0 mg cholesterol

Salt-Free Seafood Seasoning

Here in Maryland, summer means crabs and other seafood. And seafood means steamed, with Old Bay Seasoning or the locally produced equivalent from the seafood market. Only trouble is, Old Bay contains 330 mg of sodium per ½ teaspoon. So next time you want some steamed seafood, or just to add flavor to a dish, try this low-sodium taste-alike substitute.

1 tablespoon celery seed

1 tablespoon (6 g) freshly ground black pepper

6 bay leaves, ground

½ teaspoon cardamom

½ teaspoon dry mustard powder

⅛ teaspoon ground cloves

1 teaspoon paprika

¼ teaspoon mace

Mix all the ingredients well and store in an airtight container. Will keep indefinitely, but the flavor will be best if used within 6 months.

Yield: About 8 teaspoons, ½ teaspoon per serving

Per serving: 4 calories (33% from fat, 14% from protein, 53% from carbohydrate); 0 g protein; 0 g total fat; 0 g saturated fat; 0 g monounsaturated fat; 0 g polyunsaturated fat; 1 g carbohydrate; 0 g fiber; 0 g sugar; 4 mg phosphorus; 10 mg calcium; 1 mg sodium; 15 mg potassium; 78 IU vitamin A; 0 mg ATE vitamin E; 0 mg vitamin C; 0 mg cholesterol

Salt-Free Cajun Seasoning

Add a little Cajun flavor to your favorite dishes. Similar in spices and flavor to Emeril's Creole seasoning, but without the salt.

1 tablespoon paprika

2½ teaspoons dried onion flakes

2 teaspoons minced garlic

1½ teaspoons dried thyme

1 teaspoon dried marjoram

½ teaspoon fennel

1 teaspoon ground cumin

½ teaspoon cayenne pepper

Mix all the ingredients well and store in an airtight container. Will keep indefinitely, but the flavor will be best if used within 6 months.

Yield: 4 tablespoons, ½ teaspoon per serving

Per serving: 3 calories (22% from fat, 13% from protein, 65% from carbohydrate); 0 g protein; 0 g total fat; 0 g saturated fat; 0 g monounsaturated fat; 0 g polyunsaturated fat; 1 g carbohydrate; 0 g fiber; 0 g sugar; 3 mg phosphorus; 4 mg calcium; 0 mg sodium; 14 mg potassium; 172 IU vitamin A; 0 mg ATE vitamin E; 0 mg vitamin C; 0 mg cholesterol

Low-Sodium Soy Sauce

Soy sauce, even the reduced-sodium kinds, contains more sodium than many people's diet can stand. A teaspoon often contains at least a quarter of the amount of sodium that is recommended for a healthy adult. This sauce gives you real soy sauce flavor while holding the sodium to a level that should fit in most people's diets.

¼ cup (60 g) sodium-free beef bouillon powder

¼ cup (60 ml) cider vinegar

2 tablespoons (40 g) molasses

1½ cups (355 ml) boiling water

⅛ teaspoon freshly ground black pepper

⅛ teaspoon ground ginger

¼ teaspoon garlic powder

¼ cup (60 ml) reduced-sodium soy sauce

(continued on page 30)

Combine all the ingredients, stirring to blend thoroughly. Pour into jars. Cover and seal tightly. May be kept refrigerated indefinitely.

Yield: About 1½ cups, ½ tablespoon per serving

Per serving: 6 calories (13% from fat, 9% from protein, 78% from carbohydrate); 0 g protein; 0 g total fat; 0 g saturated fat; 0 g monounsaturated fat; 0 g polyunsaturated fat; 1 g carbohydrate; 0 g fiber; 1 g sugar; 3 mg phosphorus; 3 mg calcium; 35 mg sodium; 19 mg potassium; 3 IU vitamin A; 0 mg ATE vitamin E; 0 mg vitamin C; 0 mg cholesterol

Low-Sodium Teriyaki Sauce

The story on this recipe is the same as the soy sauce. In this case, you can sometimes find some commercial teriyaki sauces that aren't *really* high in sodium. But this one is much lower and to my palate tastes just as good, if not better.

1 cup (235 ml) Low-Sodium Soy Sauce (page 29)

1 tablespoon (15 ml) sesame oil

2 tablespoons (30 ml) mirin wine

½ cup (100 g) sugar

3 cloves garlic, crushed

½ teaspoon fresh ginger, grated

Pinch of freshly ground black pepper

Combine all the ingredients in a saucepan over medium heat and heat until the sugar is

dissolved, about 3 to 4 minutes. Will keep indefinitely stored in the refrigerator in an airtight container.

Yield: About 10 tablespoons, ½ tablespoon per serving

Per serving: 35 calories (18% from fat, 8% from protein, 74% from carbohydrate); 1 g protein; 1 g total fat; 0 g saturated fat; 0 g monounsaturated fat; 0 g polyunsaturated fat; 6 g carbohydrate; 0 g fiber; 5 g sugar; 14 mg phosphorus; 2 mg calcium; 32 mg sodium; 24 mg potassium; 0 IU vitamin A; 0 mg ATE vitamin E; 0 mg vitamin C; 0 mg cholesterol

Tip: You can substitute sherry or saki for the mirin, a sweet Japanese rice wine.

Better-than-Bottled Barbecue Sauce

This is a quick to make barbecue sauce that starts with low-sodium ketchup. It is tomatoey and relatively sweet, and the spices have a basic chili flavor. In other words, it's not too different than most bottled sauces, except in the amount of sodium.

½ cup (120 g) no-salt-added ketchup

½ cup (120 ml) vinegar

½ cup (170 g) honey

¼ cup (85 g) molasses

1 tablespoon (8 g) chili powder

1 tablespoon (9 g) onion powder

½ teaspoon garlic powder

1 tablespoon (9 g) dry mustard powder

¼ teaspoon cayenne pepper

Mix all the ingredients well and store in an airtight container in the refrigerator. Best if used within 6 months.

Yield: About 2 cups, 2 tablespoons per serving

Per serving: 61 calories (2% from fat, 2% from protein, 96% from carbohydrate); 0 g protein; 0 g total fat; 0 g saturated fat; 0 g monounsaturated fat; 0 g polyunsaturated fat; 16 g carbohydrate; 1 g fiber; 14 g sugar; 9 mg phosphorus; 17 mg calcium; 9 mg sodium; 143 mg potassium; 229 IU vitamin A; 0 mg ATE vitamin E; 2 mg vitamin C; 0 mg cholesterol

Sweet and Savory Barbecue Sauce

This sauce has layers of flavor and takes only a few minutes to make. The flavor will improve overnight, so plan on making it before the day you need to use it.

⅓ cup (55 g) chopped onion

3 tablespoon (42 g) unsalted butter

1 cup (240 g) no-salt-added ketchup

⅓ cup (80 ml) vinegar

2 tablespoons (30 g) packed brown sugar

½ cup (120 ml) water

2 teaspoons mustard

1 tablespoon (15 ml) Worcestershire sauce

⅛ teaspoon freshly ground black pepper

Slowly cook the onion in the butter in a saucepan over medium heat until the onion is tender, about 5 minutes. Add all the remaining ingredients. Cover and simmer for about 10 minutes. Store in an airtight container in the refrigerator. Best if used within 6 months.

Yield: 12 servings or about 2 cups, 2 tablespoons per serving

Per serving: 45 calories (42% from fat, 3% from protein, 55% from carbohydrate); 0 g protein; 4 g total fat; 1 g saturated fat; 1 g monounsaturated fat; 0 g polyunsaturated fat; 7 g carbohydrate; 0 g fiber; 6 g sugar; 9 mg phosphorus; 7 mg calcium; 13 mg sodium; 97 mg potassium; 225 IU vitamin A; 18 mg ATE vitamin E; 4 mg vitamin C; 6 mg cholesterol

Condensed Cream of Mushroom Soup

Ever come across one of those recipes that calls for condensed soup? Have you checked how much sodium is in there? And even though there are some low-sodium varieties available, they are ready to eat, rather than condensed, which can throw off the amount of moisture in a recipe. The solution? Make your own. It's a lot easier than you think. This was developed from a soup recipe in an old cookbook, with the broth and milk quantities halved. You can substitute celery, broccoli, or other veggies for the mushrooms. I prefer using evaporated milk for this because it makes a thicker, creamier soup than regular milk does. This makes approximately as much as a 10¾-ounce (300-g) can of condensed cream of mushroom soup and can be used in

(continued on page 32)

any recipe that calls for one. It can also be made in larger quantities and freezes well. If you use homemade chicken broth, the amount of sodium would be even less. To make uncondensed cream of mushroom soup, just double the chicken broth and the milk.

1 cup (70 g) sliced mushrooms

½ cup (80 g) chopped onion

½ cup (120 ml) Low-Sodium Chicken Broth (page 231)

1 tablespoon (0.4 g) dried parsley

¼ teaspoon garlic powder

⅔ cup (155 ml) nonfat evaporated milk

2 tablespoons (16 g) cornstarch

Cook the mushrooms, onion, chicken broth, and spices in a saucepan over medium heat until soft, about 5 minutes. Process in a blender or food processor until well puréed. In a jar with a lid, shake together the evaporated milk and cornstarch until dissolved. Pour into the saucepan and cook, stirring, until thick, 3 to 4 minutes. Stir in the veggie mixture. Pour into an airtight container and store in the refrigerator for up to a week. May also be frozen for up to 6 months.

Yield: About 1½ cups, ¼ cup per serving

Per serving: 41 calories (2% from fat, 26% from protein, 72% from carbohydrate); 3 g protein; 0 g total fat; 0 g saturated fat; 0 g monounsaturated fat; 0 g polyunsaturated fat; 8 g carbohydrate; 0 g fiber; 4 g sugar; 70 mg phosphorus; 87 mg calcium; 34 mg sodium; 155 mg potassium; 165 IU vitamin A; 34 mg ATE vitamin E; 2 mg vitamin C; 1 mg cholesterol

Southern-Style Bread Crumbs

This is a basic breading mix for pork chops, fish, or chicken. It has sort of a Southern flavor, but you could just as easily make it Mexican, barbecue, or whatever you want by varying the seasonings.

½ cup (55 g) low-sodium bread crumbs

1 tablespoon (0.4 g) dried parsley

½ teaspoon crumbled sage

½ teaspoon dried thyme

1 teaspoon white pepper

1 teaspoon onion powder

1 teaspoon dried basil

¼ teaspoon cayenne pepper

Mix all the ingredients well and store in an airtight container. Will keep for several weeks if refrigerated or may be frozen for up to 6 months.

Yield: About 8 tablespoons, 2 tablespoons per serving

Per serving: 59 calories (12% from fat, 14% from protein, 74% from carbohydrate); 2 g protein; 1 g total fat; 0 g saturated fat; 0 g monounsaturated fat; 0 g polyunsaturated fat; 11 g carbohydrate; 1 g fiber; 1 g sugar; 27 mg phosphorus; 37 mg calcium; 1 mg sodium; 48 mg potassium; 151 IU vitamin A; 0 mg ATE vitamin E; 2 mg vitamin C; 0 mg cholesterol

Italian-Style Bread Crumbs

Next time you are looking for a low-sodium topping to add a little crunch and flavor to a casserole or some veggies, give this a try. It can be made in bigger batches and stored indefinitely in the freezer.

½ cup (55 g) Southern-Style Bread Crumbs (page 32)

1 teaspoon packed brown sugar

½ teaspoon sesame seeds

1 tablespoon (7 g) wheat germ

½ teaspoon celery seed

½ teaspoon dried oregano

¼ teaspoon garlic powder

1 teaspoon dried minced onion

½ teaspoon dried parsley

1 teaspoon Italian seasoning

1½ teaspoons buttermilk powder

Combine all the ingredients in a blender or food processor and mix well. Store in an airtight container. Will keep for several weeks if refrigerated or may be frozen for longer periods.

Yield: About 8 tablespoons, 2 tablespoons per serving

Per serving: 19 calories (15% from fat, 18% from protein, 67% from carbohydrate); 1 g protein; 0 g total fat; 0 g saturated fat; 0 g monounsaturated fat; 0 g polyunsaturated fat; 3 g carbohydrate; 0 g fiber; 2 g sugar; 28 mg phosphorus; 25 mg calcium; 6 mg sodium; 55 mg potassium; 41 IU vitamin A; 0 mg ATE vitamin E; 1 mg vitamin C; 1 mg cholesterol

All-Purpose Coating Mix

Ever get a craving for the good old days of Shake 'n Bake chicken? Actually, neither do I. But I think you'll find the flavor of this mix an improvement on the original.

½ cup (60 g) all-purpose flour

½ cup (70 g) cornmeal

2 tablespoons (16 g) cornstarch

2 teaspoons sugar

2 teaspoons poultry seasoning

2 teaspoons paprika

1 teaspoon onion powder

½ teaspoon garlic powder

½ teaspoon dried thyme

Mix all the ingredients well and store in an airtight container. Will keep for up to 6 months.

Yield: About 1¼ cups, 3 tablespoons per serving

Per serving: 76 calories (4% from fat, 9% from protein, 87% from carbohydrate); 2 g protein; 0 g total fat; 0 g saturated fat; 0 g monounsaturated fat; 0 g polyunsaturated fat; 16 g carbohydrate; 1 g fiber; 1 g sugar; 20 mg phosphorus; 8 mg calcium; 1 mg sodium; 43 mg potassium; 332 IU vitamin A; 0 mg ATE vitamin E; 1 mg vitamin C; 0 mg cholesterol

Onion Soup Mix

I've used Goodman's Low Sodium Onion Soup Mix in the past, which I found in the kosher foods section of my local Safeway. However, it can be hard to locate. You can easily make your own mix that is even lower in sodium. You can use this the same as you would a one-serving envelope of one of the commercial brands (some brands make multiple servings per envelope).

1 tablespoon dried minced onion

1 teaspoon sodium-free beef bouillon

½ teaspoon onion powder

⅛ teaspoon freshly ground black pepper

⅛ teaspoon paprika

Mix all the ingredients well and store in an airtight container. Will keep indefinitely, but the flavor will be best if used within 6 months.

Yield: 1 serving

Per serving: 23 calories (3% from fat, 10% from protein, 86% from carbohydrate); 1 g protein; 0 g total fat; 0 g saturated fat; 0 g monounsaturated fat; 0 g polyunsaturated fat; 5 g carbohydrate; 1 g fiber; 2 g sugar; 21 mg phosphorus; 19 mg calcium; 2 mg sodium; 103 mg potassium; 153 IU vitamin A; 0 mg ATE vitamin E; 4 mg vitamin C; 0 mg cholesterol

Tip: Mixed with a pint of sour cream, this makes a good dip.

Ranch Dressing Mix

Like the Italian dressing mix on page 35, this one is handy for a lot of recipes. Keep in mind that if you're making salad dressing, the milk and mayonnaise add sodium to the final dressing.

½ cup (60 g) buttermilk powder

1 tablespoon (0.4 g) dried parsley, crushed

1 teaspoon dried dillweed

1 teaspoon onion powder

1 teaspoon dried minced onion

¼ teaspoon freshly ground black pepper

½ teaspoon garlic powder

Combine all the ingredients in a food processor or blender and process on high speed until well blended and powdery smooth. Store in an airtight container for up to 1 year.

To make salad dressing, combine 2 tablespoons (15 g) dry mix with 1 cup (235 ml) milk and 1 cup (225 g) mayonnaise. Mix well.

Yield: About 10 tablespoons, serving size ⅛ tablespoon when prepared as directed

Per serving: 3 calories (13% from fat, 33% from protein, 54% from carbohydrate); 0 g protein; 0 g total fat; 0 g saturated fat; 0 g monounsaturated fat; 0 g polyunsaturated fat; 0 g carbohydrate; 0 g fiber; 0 g sugar; 7 mg phosphorus; 9 mg calcium; 4 mg sodium; 14 mg potassium; 6 IU vitamin A; 0 mg ATE vitamin E; 0 mg vitamin C; 1 mg cholesterol

Italian Dressing Mix

Occasionally, you'll come across a recipe that calls for a package of Italian dressing mix. Unfortunately, those mixes are high in sodium. The solution is to make your own.

2 teaspoons dried oregano

1 teaspoon onion powder

2 teaspoons dried basil

2 teaspoons paprika

1½ teaspoons freshly ground black pepper

2 tablespoons (18 g) garlic powder

6 tablespoons (75 g) sugar

Mix all the ingredients well and store in an airtight container for up to 1 year.

To make salad dressing, combine 1½ tablespoons (12 g) dry mix with ¾ cup (180 ml) olive oil and ¼ cup (60 ml) white wine vinegar and mix well.

Yield: About 1 cup, serving size about ½ teaspoon when prepared as directed

Per serving: 12 calories (2% from fat, 4% from protein, 93% from carbohydrate); 0 g protein; 0 g total fat; 0 g saturated fat; 0 g monounsaturated fat; 0 g polyunsaturated fat; 3 g carbohydrate; 0 g fiber; 3 g sugar; 3 mg phosphorus; 3 mg calcium; 0 mg sodium; 14 mg potassium; 85 IU vitamin A; 0 mg ATE vitamin E; 0 mg vitamin C; 0 mg cholesterol

Peppercorn Ranch Dressing

This has been far and away the most popular low-sodium dressing in our family.

1 cup (225 g) mayonnaise

1 cup (235 ml) buttermilk

2 teaspoons dried parsley

1 teaspoon onion powder

¼ teaspoon garlic powder

¼ teaspoon dried dillweed

1 teaspoon black peppercorns, coarsely cracked

Mix all the ingredients well and store in an airtight container. Refrigerate overnight before using. Best flavor if used within 6 months.

Yield: 2 cups, 2 tablespoons per serving

Per serving: 106 calories (92% from fat, 3% from protein, 5% from carbohydrate); 1 g protein; 11 g total fat; 2 g saturated fat; 3 g monounsaturated fat; 5 g polyunsaturated fat; 1 g carbohydrate; 0 g fiber; 1 g sugar; 19 mg phosphorus; 22 mg calcium; 20 mg sodium; 33 mg potassium; 57 IU vitamin A; 13 mg ATE vitamin E; 0 mg vitamin C; 9 mg cholesterol

Tip: You can crack the peppercorns by putting them in a plastic bag and beating on them with a mallet or rolling pin, so you might want to try this recipe on a day when you are feeling a need to release some frustration.

Italian Dressing

Here's a simple Italian vinaigrette dressing.

¼ cup (60 ml) olive oil

½ cup (120 ml) cider vinegar

2 tablespoons (22 g) Dijon mustard

½ teaspoon garlic powder

½ teaspoon freshly ground black pepper

½ teaspoon sugar

1 teaspoon dried basil

1 teaspoon dried oregano

½ teaspoon dried rosemary

Combine all the ingredients in a jar with a tight-fitting lid. Shake well. Store in the refrigerator. Best flavor if used within 6 months.

Yield: ¾ cup, 2 tablespoons per serving

Per serving: 90 calories (89% from fat, 1% from protein, 10% from carbohydrate); 0 g protein; 9 g total fat; 1 g saturated fat; 2 g monounsaturated fat; 5 g polyunsaturated fat; 2 g carbohydrate; 0 g fiber; 2 g sugar; 9 mg phosphorus; 12 mg calcium; 59 mg sodium; 40 mg potassium; 31 IU vitamin A; 0 mg ATE vitamin E; 0 mg vitamin C; 0 mg cholesterol

Tip: A nice addition to this is a couple of tablespoons of chopped sun-dried tomatoes packed in oil.

Caesar Salad Dressing

This easy dressing makes quick work of turning some romaine lettuce into a great Caesar salad. And that is definitely a good thing.

1 tablespoon (14 g) mayonnaise

½ teaspoon minced garlic

⅓ cup (80 ml) red wine vinegar

½ cup (120 ml) olive oil

¼ cup (25 g) grated Parmesan cheese

Mix all the ingredients well and store in an airtight container in the refrigerator. Best flavor if used within 6 months.

Yield: About 1 cup, 2 tablespoons per serving

Per serving: 146 calories (94% from fat, 3% from protein, 2% from carbohydrate); 1 g protein; 16 g total fat; 3 g saturated fat; 11 g monounsaturated fat; 2 g polyunsaturated fat; 1 g carbohydrate; 0 g fiber; 1 g sugar; 24 mg phosphorus; 36 mg calcium; 58 mg sodium; 15 mg potassium; 19 IU vitamin A; 5 mg ATE vitamin E; 0 mg vitamin C; 3 mg cholesterol

Dijon Vinaigrette

Dijon mustard adds a little spark to this dressing. And while it also adds a little sodium, the total amount per serving is still much less than any commercial dressing.

⅔ cup (160 ml) olive oil

⅓ cup (80 ml) red wine vinegar

2 tablespoons (22 g) Dijon mustard

¼ teaspoon freshly ground black pepper

¼ teaspoon sugar

Combine all the ingredients in a jar with a tight-fitting lid; shake until blended. Store in the refrigerator. Best flavor if used within 6 months.

Yield: 1 cup, 2 tablespoons per serving

Per serving: 164 calories (97% from fat, 0% from protein, 2% from carbohydrate); 0 g protein; 18 g total fat; 2 g saturated fat; 13 g monounsaturated fat; 2 g polyunsaturated fat; 1 g carbohydrate; 0 g fiber; 1 g sugar; 4 mg phosphorus; 4 mg calcium; 44 mg sodium; 16 mg potassium; 8 IU vitamin A; 0 mg ATE vitamin E; 0 mg vitamin C; 0 mg cholesterol

Tip: Use as a substitute wherever Italian dressing is called for.

Raspberry Vinaigrette

Slightly sweet salad dressing is great on salads containing fruit or just plain greens.

12 ounces (340 g) raspberry preserves

½ cup (100 g) sugar

½ cup (120 ml) water

¼ cup (40 g) chopped onion

2 tablespoons (30 ml) balsamic vinegar

1 teaspoon dried tarragon

1 teaspoon curry powder

1 teaspoon white pepper

½ teaspoon freshly ground black pepper

½ cup (120 ml) olive oil

In a large saucepan, bring the preserves and sugar to a boil over medium heat. Remove from the heat; let cool slightly. Transfer to a blender. Add the water, onion, vinegar, tarragon, curry powder, white pepper, and black pepper; cover and process until smooth. With the motor running, gradually add the oil in a steady stream and process to emulsify. Store in the refrigerator. Best flavor if used within 6 months.

Yield: About 2½ cups, 2 tablespoons per serving

Per serving: 116 calories (41% from fat, 0% from protein, 58% from carbohydrate); 0 g protein; 5 g total fat; 1 g saturated fat; 4 g monounsaturated fat; 1 g polyunsaturated fat; 17 g carbohydrate; 0 g fiber; 13 g sugar; 5 mg phosphorus; 6 mg calcium; 6 mg sodium; 21 mg potassium; 2 IU vitamin A; 0 mg ATE vitamin E; 2 mg vitamin C; 0 mg cholesterol

Baked Tortilla Chips

These are just like you used to get at your favorite Mexican restaurant. I like these sprinkled with a little salt-free taco seasoning (page 28).

1 corn tortilla

Vegetable oil spray

(continued on page 38)

Preheat the oven to 350°F (180°C, or gas mark 4). Cut the tortilla into 6 wedges. Place the tortilla pieces on a baking sheet and coat with cooking spray. Turn over and spray the other side. Bake until crispy and browned on the edges, about 10 minutes.

Yield: 1 serving

Per serving: 58 calories (10% from fat, 10% from protein, 80% from carbohydrate); 1 g protein; 1 g total fat; 0 g saturated fat; 0 g monounsaturated fat; 0 g polyunsaturated fat; 12 g carbohydrate; 1 g fiber; 0 g sugar; 82 mg phosphorus; 46 mg calcium; 3 mg sodium; 40 mg potassium; 0 IU vitamin A; 0 mg ATE vitamin E; 0 mg vitamin C; 0 mg cholesterol

Part I

15-Minute Meals from Start to Finish

4

15-Minute Snacks, Appetizers, and Party Foods

Many snacks are notoriously high in sodium. If you are trying to prepare a healthy nibbler, either for your family or for a party, you don't want to spend hours in the kitchen. This chapter contains a number of recipes to solve that problem, none of which take longer than 15 minutes to fix (and some that take a lot less). It includes party foods such as shrimp and Buffalo wings, an assortment of dips, and sweet but healthy snacks that you can have available for times when your family (or you) just want a little something.

Boneless Buffalo Wings

Chicken wings tend to be fairly high in saturated fat, because it isn't easy to avoid eating the skin, where most of the fat is. But you can have that classic Buffalo wing taste with these low-fat, easy-to-make boneless wings from chicken breasts.

6 boneless chicken breasts

3 tablespoons (45 ml) hot pepper sauce

2 tablespoons (30 ml) white vinegar

Preheat the broiler and place the oven rack 6 inches (15 cm) below the heat source. Cut the breasts into strips, about 8 per breast. Spread on a baking sheet and broil until no longer pink, about 10 minutes. Mix the hot pepper sauce and white vinegar together in a bowl. Place the chicken pieces in a large bowl with a tight-sealing cover. Pour the mixture over the pieces and shake to coat. Transfer to a serving platter, allowing the extra sauce to drain back into the bowl.

Yield: 16 appetizer servings

Per serving: 30 calories (11% from fat, 87% from protein, 2% from carbohydrate); 6 g protein; 0 g total fat; 0 g saturated fat; 0 g monounsaturated fat; 0 g polyunsaturated fat; 0 g carbohydrate; 0 g fiber; 0 g sugar; 53 mg phosphorus; 3 mg calcium; 34 mg sodium; 73 mg potassium; 49 IU vitamin A; 2 mg ATE vitamin E; 0 mg vitamin C; 15 mg cholesterol

Curried Chicken Balls

Curried chicken balls are a great way to use leftover chicken (or turkey) in a very easy and quick appetizer your guests will love. The curry flavor is not overpowering, particularly if you use a mild curry powder, but enough to give some interest to what would otherwise be a bland result.

8 ounces (225 g) cream cheese, softened

¼ cup (75 g) mango chutney

2 teaspoons curry powder

2 cups (280 g) coarsely chopped cooked chicken breast

⅔ cup (96 g) finely chopped unsalted cashews

¼ cup (25 g) sliced scallion

In a large bowl with a mixer, beat the cream cheese until softened. Add the chutney and curry powder; beat until well mixed. Stir in the chicken, cashews, and scallion until well mixed. Form the mixture into 1-inch (2.5-cm) balls; you should get 48 balls.

Yield: 24 servings, 2 balls per serving

Per serving: 82 calories (60% from fat, 24% from protein, 16% from carbohydrate); 5 g protein; 6 g total fat; 3 g saturated fat; 2 g monounsaturated fat; 1 g polyunsaturated fat; 3 g carbohydrate; 0 g fiber; 0 g sugar; 56 mg phosphorus; 13 mg calcium; 38 mg sodium; 71 mg potassium; 165 IU vitamin A; 35 mg ATE vitamin E; 0 mg vitamin C; 20 mg cholesterol

Mini Pizzas

Want a quick pizza snack that doesn't take forever or completely blow your diet? Then these are just what you are looking for. You can add additional vegetables and meat as desired, but be aware that most meats traditionally used as pizza toppings such as pepperoni and sausage are high in sodium.

2 English muffins, split in half
½ cup (125 g) Low-Sodium Spaghetti Sauce (page 234)
1 cup (110 g) shredded Swiss cheese

Preheat the oven to 350°F (180°C, or gas mark 4).

Place the muffin halves on a cookie sheet. Divide the spaghetti sauce evenly among them and spread on the muffins. Sprinkle ¼ cup (25 g) of the cheese on top of each. Bake until the cheese is melted and the muffin is crispy, about 10 minutes.

Yield: 4 servings

Per serving: 224 calories (44% from fat, 22% from protein, 34% from carbohydrate); 12 g protein; 11 g total fat; 6 g saturated fat; 4 g monounsaturated fat; 1 g polyunsaturated fat; 19 g carbohydrate; 2 g fiber; 5 g sugar; 249 mg phosphorus; 375 mg calcium; 145 mg sodium; 194 mg potassium; 462 IU vitamin A; 70 mg ATE vitamin E; 4 mg vitamin C; 30 mg cholesterol

Tip: Try these with the fresh tomato sauce on page 171.

Sesame Fried Shrimp

Sweet Asian-flavored sesame shrimp cook in less than 2 minutes and make a great quick appetizer. Or steam some frozen broccoli and rice to have with them for a complete meal.

1 tablespoon (15 ml) Low-Sodium Soy Sauce (page 29)
2 tablespoons (40 g) honey
1 tablespoon (15 ml) olive oil
1 tablespoon (8 g) sesame seeds
1 pound (454 g) raw deveined shrimp

Mix the soy sauce and honey in a cup. Heat the oil in a pan or wok over medium heat until very hot. Add the sesame seeds. When they start to brown, add the shrimp and cook until pink, about 3 to 4 minutes. Pour in the honey–soy mixture, remove from the heat, and stir to coat. Serve immediately.

Yield: 4 servings

Per serving: 197 calories (30% from fat, 48% from protein, 22% from carbohydrate); 24 g protein; 6 g total fat; 1 g saturated fat; 3 g monounsaturated fat; 2 g polyunsaturated fat; 11 g carbohydrate; 0 g fiber; 9 g sugar; 251 mg phosphorus; 82 mg calcium; 179 mg sodium; 233 mg potassium; 204 IU vitamin A; 61 mg ATE vitamin E; 2 mg vitamin C; 172 mg cholesterol

Stuffed Jalapeños

These are as simple as an appetizer can be, with only 2 ingredients and very little preparation required. But they are really tasty (if you are the sort of person who like's jalapeños).

11 ounce can (308 g) whole jalapeño peppers, drained, about 20 peppers.
8 ounces (225 g) cream cheese, softened

Cut a slit along one side of each pepper. Remove the seeds; rinse and dry. Fill the inside of each with about 2 teaspoons of cream cheese.

Yield: 20 servings, 1 jalapeño per serving

Per serving: 44 calories (80% from fat, 9% from protein, 11% from carbohydrate); 1 g protein; 4 g total fat; 3 g saturated fat; 1 g monounsaturated fat; 0 g polyunsaturated fat; 1 g carbohydrate; 0 g fiber; 1 g sugar; 17 mg phosphorus; 11 mg calcium; 34 mg sodium; 47 mg potassium; 277 IU vitamin A; 41 mg ATE vitamin E; 7 mg vitamin C; 12 mg cholesterol

Tip: Wear latex gloves when handling the peppers to avoid burning your skin.

Beef and Cheese Ranch Salad Roll-Ups

These quick roll-ups are like a chef's salad with ranch dressing, except that you can eat them by hand. They make good use of leftover roast beef for a crowd-pleasing appetizer.

2 tablespoons (30 ml) Ranch Dressing (page 34)
2 flour tortillas
2 large romaine lettuce leaves
4 ounces (115 g) leftover roast beef, thinly sliced
3 ounces (85 g) Swiss cheese, sliced
2 teaspoons diced red onion

Spread 1 tablespoon (15 ml) dressing on each tortilla, covering the entire surface. Top each with a lettuce leaf and half of the beef, cheese, and onion. Roll up each tortilla tightly. Cut the roll-ups into eight 1-inch (2.5 cm) slices. Insert a cocktail toothpick into each to secure.

Yield: 16 servings

Per serving: 60 calories (48% from fat, 26% from protein, 26% from carbohydrate); 4 g protein; 3 g total fat; 1 g saturated fat; 1 g monounsaturated fat; 0 g polyunsaturated fat; 4 g carbohydrate; 0 g fiber; 0 g sugar; 51 mg phosphorus; 59 mg calcium; 31 mg sodium; 29 mg potassium; 48 IU vitamin A; 11 mg ATE vitamin E; 0 mg vitamin C; 13 mg cholesterol

Tip: Cut in half instead of into slices and make a lunch of it for 2 people.

Bruschetta

This is a fairly traditional brushcetta recipe, full of the flavors of fresh herbs and garlic. The thing that makes it healthier than usual is the use of the low-sodium bread. This recipe works best with very ripe tomatoes. Try it in late summer when vine-ripened tomatoes are abundant. I like it with the additional flavor that grilling imparts, but it's also very good when broiled.

4 large tomatoes

1 cup (150 g) fresh finely diced mozzarella

⅓ cup (13 g) fresh basil, chopped

3 cloves garlic, minced

2 tablespoons (8 g) chopped fresh parsley

2 tablespoons (30 ml) olive oil

½ teaspoon freshly ground black pepper

1 Loaf Low-Sodium Italian Bread (page 315)

3 cloves garlic

Prepare a grill for medium-high heat or preheat the broiler and place the oven rack 6 inches (15 cm) below the heat source. Cut the tomatoes in half through the equator and squeeze out the seeds. Cut into a very small dice. Transfer the tomatoes to a bowl and add the mozzarella, basil, garlic, parsley, olive oil, and pepper. Cut the bread into sixteen ½-inch (1.3-cm) slices. Lightly crush the whole garlic cloves with the side of a large knife or cleaver. Remove the peel. Rub the bread with the garlic and toast both sides on the grill or under the broiler. To serve, transfer the tomato mixture to a small bowl placed in the center of a platter, and surround with the toasted bread.

Yield: 16 servings

Per serving: 125 calories (30% from fat, 17% from protein, 53% from carbohydrate); 5 g protein; 4 g total fat; 1 g saturated fat; 2 g monounsaturated fat; 1 g polyunsaturated fat; 17 g carbohydrate; 1 g fiber; 1 g sugar; 83 mg phosphorus; 102 mg calcium; 35 mg sodium; 114 mg potassium; 303 IU vitamin A; 11 mg ATE vitamin E; 4 mg vitamin C; 4 mg cholesterol

Parmesan Cheese Toast Triangles

These appetizers look and taste fancy and are full of flavor from the Parmesan cheese. But they only contain 4 ingredients and are really quick to prepare.

2 tablespoons (28 g) mayonnaise

2 teaspoons mustard

6 Slices Low-Sodium Bread (pages 312 to 324), crusts removed

⅓ cup (33 g) grated Parmesan cheese

Preheat the broiler and place the oven rack 4 inches (10 cm) below the heat source. Lightly grease a baking sheet. Combine the mayonnaise and mustard in a small bowl; spread on one side of each slice of bread. Cut each slice into 4 triangles; place on the prepared baking sheet. Sprinkle with the cheese. Broil for 1 to 2 minutes, or until lightly browned.

Yield: 6 servings

Per serving: 101 calories (32% from fat, 18% from protein, 50% from carbohydrate); 5 g protein; 4 g total fat; 1 g saturated fat; 1 g monounsaturated fat; 1 g polyunsaturated fat; 13 g carbohydrate; 1 g fiber; 1 g sugar; 78 mg phosphorus; 89 mg calcium; 99 mg sodium; 61 mg potassium; 26 IU vitamin A; 7 mg ATE vitamin E; 0 mg vitamin C; 6 mg cholesterol

Easy Quesadillas

The trick here is to use Swiss cheese to hold down the sodium level while using Mexican spices to make it taste more traditional. And it's all done in a few minutes. If you have some leftover chicken you could add that for even more flavor.

4 tortillas

2 cups (220 g) shredded Swiss cheese

1 tablespoon (8 g) chili powder

1 tablespoon (7 g) ground cumin

½ teaspoon garlic powder

Heat the tortillas in a dry frying pan over medium-high heat for 10 seconds on each side. Transfer to a plate. Spread about ½ cup (55 g) of the grated cheese on each and sprinkle with one-fourth of the cumin and the chili and garlic powders. Fold the tortilla in half and return to the pan. Heat until both sides are browned and the cheese is melted, about 5 minutes per side. Cut in half and serve immediately.

Yield: 8 servings

Per serving: 151 calories (57% from fat, 27% from protein, 17% from carbohydrate); 10 g protein; 10 g total fat; 6 g saturated fat; 3 g

monounsaturated fat; 1 g polyunsaturated fat; 6 g carbohydrate; 1 g fiber; 1 g sugar; 236 mg phosphorus; 343 mg calcium; 30 mg sodium; 84 mg potassium; 558 IU vitamin A; 70 mg ATE vitamin E; 1 mg vitamin C; 30 mg cholesterol

Curried Cashews

These spicy little nibbles contain only 3 ingredients and take 10 minutes to prepare, but they are full of flavor and a nice change of pace from the more common spiced nuts using cinnamon and other sweeter spices. They store well in the refrigerator and will keep in an airtight container for several weeks with no loss of flavor.

¼ cup (55 g) unsalted butter

10 ounces (280 g) unsalted cashews

2 tablespoons (13 g) curry powder

In a skillet over medium heat, melt the butter. Add the cashews; cook and stir until lightly browned, about 10 minutes. Remove to paper towels to drain. Sprinkle with the curry powder.

Yield: 16 servings

Per serving: 130 calories (73% from fat, 8% from protein, 18% from carbohydrate); 3 g protein; 11 g total fat; 3 g saturated fat; 6 g monounsaturated fat; 2 g polyunsaturated fat; 6 g carbohydrate; 1 g fiber; 1 g sugar; 90 mg phosphorus; 13 mg calcium; 4 mg sodium; 113 mg potassium; 96 IU vitamin A; 24 mg ATE vitamin E; 0 mg vitamin C; 8 mg cholesterol

Tip: These cashews also make a great topping for curry dishes, salads, and more.

The World's Quickest Mexican Dip

Two ingredients, 2 minutes, refrigerator to table (I timed it). This is just the thing when you have hungry kids or unexpected guests or you just want a little something to snack on while fixing dinner. Serve with vegetable sticks or low-sodium crackers or baked tortilla chips (page 37).

8 ounces (225 g) cream cheese, softened
½ cup (130 g) Low-Sodium Salsa (page 232)

Combine the cream cheese and salsa in a small bowl.

Yield: 12 servings

Per serving: 69 calories (85% from fat, 9% from protein, 6% from carbohydrate); 2 g protein; 7 g total fat; 4 g saturated fat; 2 g monounsaturated fat; 0 g polyunsaturated fat; 1 g carbohydrate; 0 g fiber; 0 g sugar; 22 mg phosphorus; 18 mg calcium; 65 mg sodium; 43 mg potassium; 318 IU vitamin A; 68 mg ATE vitamin E; 1 mg vitamin C; 21 mg cholesterol

Corny In a Good Way Dip

This makes a creamy dip, moderately spicy with the flavors of Swiss and Cheddar cheeses. But the real surprise, and the thing that makes it special, is the added flavor of the corn. Serve with low-sodium chips.

2 ounces (55 g) shredded Cheddar cheese
4 ounces (115 g) shredded Swiss cheese
12 ounces (336 g) frozen corn, thawed
¼ cup (25 g) chopped scallion, plus more for garnish
4 ounces (115 g) chopped green chiles
1 jalapeño pepper, seeded and minced
¾ cup (175 g) mayonnaise
¾ cup (175 g) sour cream
⅛ teaspoon sugar

In a large bowl, combine the cheeses, corn, scallion, chiles, and jalapeño. In a small bowl, combine the mayonnaise, sour cream, and sugar; stir into the corn mixture. Cover and refrigerate overnight. Sprinkle with the remaining scallion just before serving.

Yield: 20 servings

Per serving: 78 calories (60% from fat, 15% from protein, 25% from carbohydrate); 3 g protein; 5 g total fat; 3 g saturated fat; 1 g monounsaturated fat; 1 g polyunsaturated fat; 5 g carbohydrate; 1 g fiber; 1 g sugar; 71 mg phosphorus; 88 mg calcium; 56 mg sodium; 71 mg potassium; 134 IU vitamin A; 28 mg ATE vitamin E; 4 mg vitamin C; 13 mg cholesterol

Tip: Too spicy? Leave out the jalapeño.

Super Dip for Veggies

Even though it contains only five ingredients this dip is not lacking in taste. The caraway seeds provide an unusual accent. The flavor combination is the perfect accompaniment to a platter of fresh vegetables.

8 ounces (225 g) cream cheese, softened

¼ cup (61 g) Chili Sauce (page 233)

¼ teaspoon garlic powder

½ teaspoon caraway seed

¼ teaspoon paprika

In a small bowl, combine all the ingredients.

Yield: 12 servings

Per serving: 69 calories (85% from fat, 9% from protein, 6% from carbohydrate); 2 g protein; 7 g total fat; 4 g saturated fat; 2 g monounsaturated fat; 0 g polyunsaturated fat; 1 g carbohydrate; 0 g fiber; 0 g sugar; 21 mg phosphorus; 18 mg calcium; 63 mg sodium; 26 mg potassium; 363 IU vitamin A; 68 mg ATE vitamin E; 1 mg vitamin C; 21 mg cholesterol

Edamame Hummus

Hummus is traditionally made with chickpeas, but this variation uses edamame, soybeans, giving it a little different flavor and added nutrition. The rest of the ingredients are similar to traditional hummus. If you enjoy serving things that leave people guessing about the ingredients, this is a good choice.

1 cup (250 g) edamame, cooked

½ teaspoon minced garlic

2 tablespoons (30 ml) lemon juice

2 tablespoons (30 g) tahini

1 teaspoon ground cumin

1 teaspoon sesame oil

Purée all the ingredients in a blender, adding water if needed to achieve a dip-able consistency.

Yield: 9 servings

Per serving: 68 calories (53% from fat, 24% from protein, 24% from carbohydrate); 4 g protein; 4 g total fat; 1 g saturated fat; 1 g monounsaturated fat; 2 g polyunsaturated fat; 4 g carbohydrate; 2 g fiber; 0 g sugar; 81 mg phosphorus; 73 mg calcium; 9 mg sodium; 199 mg potassium; 6 IU vitamin A; 0 mg ATE vitamin E; 10 mg vitamin C; 0 mg cholesterol

Tip: Look for edamame with the frozen vegetables at the grocery store.

Chocolate Cinnamon Spread

This chocolatey spread can be used on toast, as a frosting for cupcakes, or just as a dip with fruit or graham crackers. It has just a hint of cinnamon as an additional flavor note.

1 cup (225 g) unsalted butter, softened

2 cups (240 g) confectioners' sugar

2 tablespoons (16 g) cocoa

2 tablespoons (14 g) ground cinnamon

In a large bowl, beat the butter, sugar, cocoa, and cinnamon until smooth. Serve immediately. Store leftovers in an airtight container in the refrigerator.

Yield: 32 servings

(continued on page 48)

Per serving: 82 calories (62% from fat, 1% from protein, 38% from carbohydrate); 0 g protein; 6 g total fat; 4 g saturated fat; 2 g monounsaturated fat; 0 g polyunsaturated fat; 8 g carbohydrate; 0 g fiber; 7 g sugar; 4 mg phosphorus; 7 mg calcium; 1 mg sodium; 9 mg potassium; 178 IU vitamin A; 48 mg ATE vitamin E; 0 mg vitamin C; 15 mg cholesterol

Cheesy Snack Mix

This is a savory variation on the Chex Mix type of snack. Using unsalted pretzels and mini shredded wheat cereal keeps the sodium level down. The Parmesan cheese and goldfish cracker raise it beyond ordinary cereal snack mixes.

3 cups (142 g) mini shredded wheat cereal

4 ounces (115 g) unsalted pretzel sticks

1 cup (55 g) Goldfish crackers

¼ cup (25 g) grated Parmesan cheese

4 tablespoons (55 g) unsalted butter, melted

½ teaspoon garlic powder

Preheat the oven to 325°F (170°C, or gas mark 3). Toss all the ingredients together in a large bowl. Spread on a baking sheet and bake for 15 minutes, stirring occasionally, until toasted.

Yield: 24 servings

Per serving: 68 calories (32% from fat, 9% from protein, 59% from carbohydrate); 2 g protein; 3 g total fat; 1 g saturated fat; 1 g monounsaturated fat; 0 g polyunsaturated fat; 11 g carbohydrate; 1 g fiber; 2 g sugar; 39 mg phosphorus; 18 mg

calcium; 33 mg sodium; 38 mg potassium; 64 IU vitamin A; 17 mg ATE vitamin E; 0 mg vitamin C; 6 mg cholesterol

Curried Potato Chips

You can find unsalted potato chips, but they tend to be kind of bland in flavor. Or you can easily make your own with almost no sodium and lots of flavor. This method will work with other spice combinations too, but the curry powder gives this version a nice little flavor surprise. Use a mandoline, if you have one, for slicing the potatoes.

2 large Russet potatoes, very thinly sliced (Can use other types too)

2 tablespoons (30 ml) olive oil

1 tablespoon (6 g) curry powder

Preheat the oven and 2 baking sheets to 425°F (220°C, or gas mark 7). Toss the potatoes with the olive oil and curry powder. Spread on the hot baking sheets and bake for 10 minutes, until crispy.

Yield: 10 servings

Per serving: 84 calories (30% from fat, 8% from protein, 62% from carbohydrate); 2 g protein; 3 g total fat; 0 g saturated fat; 2 g monounsaturated fat; 0 g polyunsaturated fat; 13 g carbohydrate; 2 g fiber; 0 g sugar; 45 mg phosphorus; 14 mg calcium; 5 mg sodium; 339 mg potassium; 12 IU vitamin A; 0 mg ATE vitamin E; 8 mg vitamin C; 0 mg cholesterol

Tip: Vary the flavor by using chili powder or one of the spice blends in chapter 3.

Minute Mushroom Morsels

Baked mushrooms are probably not the first thing that comes to mind when you are thinking about appetizers. But you will change your mind when you've tried these great little snacks. They taste neither quick nor low in sodium. But they are in fact both. Feel free not to volunteer this information to the guests at your next party.

2 cups (240 g) all-purpose flour

½ cup (112 g) unsalted butter, softened

½ cup shredded Swiss cheese

2 Teaspoons Onion Soup Mix (page 34)

8 ounces (225 g) mushrooms

Preheat the oven to 350°F (180°C, or gas mark 4). Combine the flour, butter, cheese, and soup mix in a large mixing bowl. Mix together until a dough forms. Wrap each mushroom in about 1 teaspoon of dough. Shape into a firm ball, covering completely. Place on an ungreased baking sheet. Bake for 12 minutes, or until lightly browned.

Yield: 12 servings

Per serving: 168 calories (50% from fat, 10% from protein, 39% from carbohydrate); 4 g protein; 9 g total fat; 6 g saturated fat; 2 g monounsaturated fat; 0 g polyunsaturated fat; 17 g carbohydrate; 1 g fiber; 0 g sugar; 74 mg phosphorus; 59 mg calcium; 3 mg sodium; 90 mg potassium; 281 IU vitamin A; 75 mg ATE vitamin E; 0 mg vitamin C; 25 mg cholesterol

Spicy Banana Crackers

A little bit of hot pepper sauce raises these simple cracker above the ordinary. They are sweet and slightly spicy crackers and great with just about any kind of dip. They are also popular for just nibbling by themselves.

¼ cup (55 g) unsalted butter

½ cup (60 g) all-purpose flour

4 drops hot pepper sauce

1 banana, mashed

Preheat the oven to 450°F (230°C, or gas mark 8) and grease a 12 × 15-inch (30.5 × 38-cm) cookie sheet. In a medium bowl using a pastry blender, mix together the butter and flour until crumbly. Using a fork, stir in the hot pepper sauce and banana. On a floured surface, knead the mixture gently, adding a small amount of flour if necessary to make the dough firm. Roll out on a floured surface until thin enough to cover the prepared cookie sheet. Place the dough on the cookie sheet. Using a pastry cutter, cut the dough into 1-inch (2.5-cm) squares. Bake for 6 to 8 minutes, or until lightly browned.

Yield: 30 servings, 180 crackers

Per serving: 26 calories (54% from fat, 4% from protein, 42% from carbohydrate); 0 g protein; 2 g total fat; 1 g saturated fat; 0 g monounsaturated fat; 0 g polyunsaturated fat; 3 g carbohydrate; 0 g fiber; 1 g sugar; 4 mg phosphorus; 1 mg calcium; 11 mg sodium; 21 mg potassium; 50 IU vitamin A; 13 mg ATE vitamin E; 0 mg vitamin C; 4 mg cholesterol

(continued on page 50)

Tip: Use a cookie sheet without a lip and roll the dough out directly on the sheet to make it even easier.

Chocolate Chow Mein

This is a quick and easy sweet snack treat, loved by kids and grown-ups alike. And what's not to like about chocolate and peanut butter? But the best part is you can make it in about 5 minutes so if you have hungry children or unexpected guests it can be a real life-saver.

¼ cup (65 g) no-salt-added peanut butter

⅓ cup (60 g) chocolate chips

¼ cup (55 g) unsalted butter

3 cups (135 g) chow mein noodles

3 cups (142 g) mini shredded wheat cereal

½ cup (50 g) unsalted peanuts

½ cup (75 g) raisins

2 cups (240 g) confectioners' sugar

Combine the peanut butter, chocolate chips, and butter in a microwave-safe bowl and microwave until melted. Put the chow mien noodles, cereal, peanuts, and raisins in a resealable plastic bag; add the chocolate mixture and shake to coat. Add the confectioners' sugar and shake again.

Yield: 28 servings

Per serving: 134 calories (34% from fat, 6% from protein, 61% from carbohydrate); 2 g protein; 5 g total fat; 2 g saturated fat; 2 g monounsaturated fat; 1 g polyunsaturated fat; 21 g carbohydrate; 1 g fiber; 13 g sugar; 46 mg phosphorus; 12 mg calcium; 34 mg sodium; 80 mg potassium; 54 IU vitamin A; 15 mg ATE vitamin E; 0 mg vitamin C; 5 mg cholesterol

Peanut Butter Granola Balls

These tasty little nibbles with oatmeal and cereal are held together by peanut butter and honey. And to make it even better, they get both a flavor and nutrition boost from apples.

⅓ cup (115 g) honey

¼ cup (65 g) no-salt-added peanut butter

2 tablespoons (28 g) unsalted butter

1 cup (25 g) crispy rice cereal

1 cup (80 g) rolled oats

¼ cup (38 g) dried apples

In a small saucepan over medium heat, heat the honey, peanut butter, and butter. Stir until smooth, 1 to 2 minutes. Remove from the heat; stir in the cereal, oats, and dried apples. Drop the mixture by the tablespoon into 24 mini paper cupcake or candy liners. Place on a rimmed baking sheet, and refrigerate until set, about 10 minutes.

Yield: 24 servings

Per serving: 56 calories (38% from fat, 9% from protein, 53% from carbohydrate); 1 g protein; 3 g total fat; 1 g saturated fat; 1 g monounsaturated fat; 1 g polyunsaturated fat; 8 g carbohydrate; 1 g fiber; 4 g sugar; 27 mg phosphorus; 4 mg calcium; 12 mg sodium; 37 mg potassium; 47 IU vitamin A; 13 mg ATE vitamin E; 0 mg vitamin C; 3 mg cholesterol

Quick Chocolatey Nibblers

This makes a great after-school snack (or adult snack, for that matter). It has just enough chocolate to make everyone like it, but lots of good nutrition from the other ingredients.

12 ounces (340 g) chocolate chips

12 ounces (340 g) unsalted sunflower seeds

12 ounces (340 g) mini shredded wheat cereal

6 ounces (170 g) raisins

Mix all the ingredients together in a large bowl. Store in an airtight container.

Yield: 24 servings

Per serving: 227 calories (43% from fat, 9% from protein, 48% from carbohydrate); 5 g protein; 12 g total fat; 3 g saturated fat; 3 g monounsaturated fat; 5 g polyunsaturated fat; 29 g carbohydrate; 4 g fiber; 15 g sugar; 243 mg phosphorus; 47 mg calcium; 17 mg sodium; 275 mg potassium; 28 IU vitamin A; 7 mg ATE vitamin E; 0 mg vitamin C; 3 mg cholesterol

Chocolate Peanut Butter Energy Snacks

The taste of the chocolate and peanut butter will win you over. The protein from the milk and the peanut butter will help keep you going (and keep you coming back for more).

1 cup (120 g) confectioners' sugar

1 cup (260 g) no-salt-added peanut butter

1 cup (175 g) chocolate chips

½ cup (60 g) nonfat dry milk

1 tablespoon (15 ml) water

¾ cup (56 g) graham cracker crumbs

Combine the confectioners' sugar, peanut butter, chocolate chips, dry milk, and water thoroughly in a bowl. Shape teaspoonfuls of the mixture into 1-inch (2.5-cm) balls. You should get about 48 balls. Spread the graham cracker crumbs on a shallow plate. Roll the balls in the graham cracker crumbs until coated.

Yield: 48 servings

Per serving: 68 calories (49% from fat, 11% from protein, 40% from carbohydrate); 2 g protein; 4 g total fat; 1 g saturated fat; 2 g monounsaturated fat; 1 g polyunsaturated fat; 7 g carbohydrate; 1 g fiber; 5 g sugar; 33 mg phosphorus; 18 mg calcium; 16 mg sodium; 67 mg potassium; 23 IU vitamin A; 7 mg ATE vitamin E; 0 mg vitamin C; 1 mg cholesterol

Sweet and Spicy Popcorn

Chili powder and just a little cayenne pepper give this popcorn a bit of a kick. Think of it as kettle corn on steroids.

1 tablespoon (12 g) sugar

1 teaspoon chili powder

½ teaspoon ground cinnamon

Pinch of cayenne pepper

6 cups (48 g) unsalted popcorn

In a large resealable plastic bag, combine the sugar, chili powder, cinnamon, and cayenne pepper. Spray the popcorn with cooking spray. Add the popcorn to the bag, seal the bag, and shake to coat.

Yield: 12 servings

Per serving: 5 calories (6% from fat, 2% from protein, 92% from carbohydrate); 0 g protein; 0 g total fat; 0 g saturated fat; 0 g monounsaturated fat; 0 g polyunsaturated fat; 1 g carbohydrate; 0 g fiber; 1 g sugar; 1 mg phosphorus; 2 mg calcium; 2 mg sodium; 4 mg potassium; 62 IU vitamin A; 0 mg ATE vitamin E; 0 mg vitamin C; 0 mg cholesterol

Fruity Popcorn Balls

Pick your favorite flavor gelatin and combine it with popcorn for a different kind of snack taste. Kids will love this quick and easy snack. But don't be surprised if you catch the adults eating it, too.

3 ounces (85 g) sugar-free gelatin, any flavor

1 cup (200 g) sugar

1 cup (340 g) corn syrup

16 cups (400 g) popcorn

Combine the gelatin, sugar, and corn syrup in a saucepan and bring to a boil over high heat. Pour over popcorn in a large bowl. Quickly shape into balls with buttered hands.

Yield: 32 servings

Per serving: 87 calories (14% from fat, 4% from protein, 82% from carbohydrate); 1 g protein; 2 g total fat; 0 g saturated fat; 0 g monounsaturated fat; 1 g polyunsaturated fat; 20 g carbohydrate; 1 g fiber; 14 g sugar; 48 mg phosphorus; 1 mg calcium; 84 mg sodium; 13 mg potassium; 8 IU vitamin A; 0 mg ATE vitamin E; 0 mg vitamin C; 0 mg cholesterol

5

15-Minute Breakfasts

Breakfast is one of those meals that can take up a sneaky amount of time. You think you'll make something quick and it ends up taking half an hour or more. I find this happens sometimes when I'm trying to get out the door to work. In that case, even 15 minutes is longer than I want to spend on breakfast. So I've developed a number of quick breakfast recipes. Many are the kind of thing you can grab and head out the door with, handy for those of us who work or go to school. But there are also some sit-down meals that let you have a family weekend breakfast without taking half the morning. I've found that having some protein in my breakfast helps keep me from getting hungry in the middle of the morning, so most of these recipes contain some form of protein such as eggs or yogurt. None of them have more than 300 mg of sodium; many of them have less than 100 mg, so you get your low-sodium day off to a good start.

Avocado Omelet for One

I guess you could call this a California omelet, since the avocado, tomato, sprout combination seems to be what we typically think of a California style. If you are looking for a quick and filling breakfast before you rush out the door, you might want to give this omelet a try. You won't be disappointed.

½ cup (125 g) egg substitute, or 2 eggs

1 tablespoon (15 ml) water

1 tablespoon (14 g) unsalted butter

½ avocado, peeled and sliced

¼ cup (45 g) diced tomato

¼ cup (10 g) alfalfa sprouts

2 tablespoons (30 g) plain low-fat yogurt

Beat the eggs and water in a small bowl. Add the butter to an 8-inch (20-cm) omelet pan and heat over medium heat until hot. Pour in the egg mixture, which should set at the edges at once. Carefully push the cooked egg to the center, tilting the pan occasionally so the uncooked egg can flow to the bottom while the top stays moist. Arrange the avocado, tomato, and sprouts on half of the omelet. Fold the omelet over and turn out onto a plate. Top with the yogurt.

Yield: 1 serving

Per serving: 391 calories (66% from fat, 19% from protein, 16% from carbohydrate); 19 g protein; 29 g total fat; 10 g saturated fat; 13 g monounsaturated fat; 4 g polyunsaturated fat; 16 g carbohydrate; 7 g fiber; 8 g sugar; 250 mg phosphorus; 130 mg calcium; 227 mg sodium; 1005 mg potassium; 1269 IU vitamin A; 99 mg ATE vitamin E; 13 mg vitamin C; 33 mg cholesterol

Western Omelet in a Mug

A traditional western omelet can take quite a bit of time to cook. This one cooks in a few minutes in the microwave for a quick breakfast, but one that will satisfy both your hunger and your taste buds.

½ cup (125 g) egg substitute, or 2 eggs, beaten

2 tablespoons (14 g) shredded Swiss cheese

2 tablespoons (20 g) diced onion

1 tablespoon (9 g) diced green bell pepper

Coat a microwave-safe mug with nonstick cooking spray, add all the ingredients, and stir to combine. Microwave, uncovered, on high for 1 minute; stir. Cook for 1 to 1½ minutes longer, or until the eggs are completely set.

Yield: 1 serving

Per serving: 178 calories (45% from fat, 46% from protein, 9% from carbohydrate); 20 g protein; 9 g total fat; 4 g saturated fat; 2 g monounsaturated fat; 2 g polyunsaturated fat; 4 g carbohydrate; 0 g fiber; 2 g sugar; 259 mg phosphorus; 230 mg calcium; 203 mg sodium; 478 mg potassium; 622 IU vitamin A; 35 mg ATE vitamin E; 9 mg vitamin C; 16 mg cholesterol

Tip: I often cook this in a square plastic food storage container and put it between two slices of bread for even better portability.

Devilish Mexican Eggs

This is a quick version of the traditional Mexican huevos ranchero. Depending on how hot or mild your salsa is, these will be more or less devilish. But no matter what, they will be good and easy to fix.

1 cup (260 g) Low-Sodium Salsa (page 232)
2 eggs
¼ teaspoon freshly ground black pepper
¼ cup (28 g) shredded Swiss cheese

Simmer the salsa in a small skillet over medium heat. Crack in the eggs, cover, and cook until the whites set; top with the pepper and cheese.

Yield: 2 servings

Per serving: 184 calories (51% from fat, 29% from protein, 20% from carbohydrate); 14 g protein; 11 g total fat; 5 g saturated fat; 3 g monounsaturated fat; 1 g polyunsaturated fat; 9 g carbohydrate; 2 g fiber; 6 g sugar; 245 mg phosphorus; 229 mg calcium; 212 mg sodium; 375 mg potassium; 1286 IU vitamin A; 115 mg ATE vitamin E; 18 mg vitamin C; 261 mg cholesterol

Eggs with Red Onion and Spinach

Scrambled eggs are enlivened by onion and spinach for a little different take on breakfast. You could put a spoonful of salsa on top to add even more flavor.

1½ tablespoons (21 g) unsalted butter
½ cup (80 g) thinly sliced red onion
2½ cups (625 g) egg substitute, or 10 eggs
2 tablespoons (30 ml) skim milk
¼ teaspoon freshly ground black pepper
5 ounces (140 g) fresh spinach

Heat the butter in a large nonstick skillet over medium heat. Add the onion and sauté until softened, about 5 minutes. Meanwhile, in a large bowl, whisk together the eggs, milk, and pepper. Pour into the pan and cook, stirring occasionally, to desired doneness, 4 to 5 minutes, adding the spinach just before the eggs are set.

Yield: 5 servings

Per serving: 152 calories (46% from fat, 43% from protein, 10% from carbohydrate); 16 g protein; 8 g total fat; 3 g saturated fat; 2 g monounsaturated fat; 2 g polyunsaturated fat; 4 g carbohydrate; 1 g fiber; 2 g sugar; 178 mg phosphorus; 108 mg calcium; 227 mg sodium; 609 mg potassium; 3230 IU vitamin A; 32 mg ATE vitamin E; 9 mg vitamin C; 11 mg cholesterol

Herb Enhanced Eggs

For a fancy breakfast in a hurry, try this broiled egg dish topped with fresh herbs. Vary the flavor by changing the herbs; for example, you can get an Italian access by replacing the thyme with basil and oregano.

¼ teaspoon minced garlic

¼ teaspoon minced fresh thyme

¼ teaspoon minced fresh rosemary

1 tablespoon (4 g) minced fresh parsley

1 tablespoon (5 g) grated Parmesan cheese

4 eggs

2 tablespoons (30 ml) cream

1 tablespoon (14 g) unsalted butter

¼ teaspoon freshly ground black pepper

Preheat the broiler and place the oven rack 6 inches (15 cm) below the heat source. Combine the garlic, thyme, rosemary, parsley, and Parmesan and set aside. Carefully crack 2 eggs into each of 2 small bowls without breaking the yolks. Place 2 individual gratin dishes on a baking sheet. Place 1 tablespoon (15 ml) of cream and ½ tablespoon of butter in each dish and broil for about 3 minutes, until hot and bubbly. Quickly but carefully, pour the eggs into each gratin dish and sprinkle evenly with the herb mixture, then sprinkle with the pepper. Broil for 5 to 6 minutes longer, until the whites of the eggs are almost cooked. The eggs will continue to cook after you take them out of the oven. Allow to set for 60 seconds before serving.

Yield: 2 servings

Per serving: 263 calories (73% from fat, 25% from protein, 3% from carbohydrate); 16 g protein; 21 g total fat; 10 g saturated fat; 7 g monounsaturated fat; 2 g polyunsaturated fat; 2 g carbohydrate; 0 g fiber; 1 g sugar; 253 mg phosphorus; 110 mg calcium; 215 mg sodium; 183 mg potassium; 1031 IU vitamin A; 243 mg ATE vitamin E; 3 mg vitamin C; 519 mg cholesterol

Tip: Serve over toast or English muffins.

Italian Frittata

This Italian-style omelet is delicious with just about any herb combination; I like basil, parsley, and chives, but other combinations would work just as well. If you don't have any ricotta cheese you can substitute no-salt-added cottage cheese.

1 cup (160 g) diced onion

¼ cup (60 ml) water

1 teaspoon oil

½ cup (125 g) egg substitute, or 2 eggs, beaten

2 teaspoons chopped fresh herbs, or ½ teaspoon dried

⅛ teaspoon freshly ground black pepper

2 tablespoons (31 g) ricotta cheese

Bring the onion and water to a boil in a small nonstick skillet over medium-high heat. Cover and cook until the onion is slightly softened, about 2 minutes. Uncover and continue cooking until the water has evaporated, 1 to 2 minutes longer. Drizzle in the oil and stir to coat. Continue cooking, stirring often, until the onion is beginning to brown, 1 to 2 minutes more. Pour in the egg, reduce the heat to medium-low, and continue cooking, stirring constantly, until the egg is starting to set, about 20 seconds. Continue cooking, lifting the edges so the uncooked egg will flow underneath, until mostly set, about 30 seconds more. Reduce the heat to low. Sprinkle the herbs and pepper over the frittata. Spoon the ricotta on top. Lift up an edge of the frittata and drizzle about 1 tablespoon (15 ml) water under it. Cover and cook until the egg is completely set and the cheese is hot, about 2 minutes. Slide the frittata out of the pan using a spatula and serve.

Yield: 2 servings

Per serving: 128 calories (40% from fat, 31% from protein, 29% from carbohydrate); 10 g protein; 6 g total fat; 1 g saturated fat; 1 g monounsaturated fat; 2 g polyunsaturated fat; 9 g carbohydrate; 1 g fiber; 4 g sugar; 126 mg phosphorus; 94 mg calcium; 122 mg sodium; 343 mg potassium; 287 IU vitamin A; 16 mg ATE vitamin E; 5 mg vitamin C; 5 mg cholesterol

Cheesy Hash Brown Skillet Breakfast with Spinach

This dish has everything you need for a tasty, hearty breakfast—potatoes, eggs, cheese, and a bonus of spinach—and it cooks quickly in a covered skillet. In fact, you could even use it for lunch or a light dinner.

1 tablespoon (15 ml) olive oil

1 cup (115 g) frozen hash browns

4 ounces (115 g) frozen spinach, thawed and drained

½ cup (125 g) egg substitute, or 2 eggs

¼ teaspoon freshly ground black pepper

¼ cup (28 g) shredded Swiss cheese

Heat the oil in a small nonstick skillet over medium heat. Layer the hash browns and spinach in the pan. Pour the egg on top and sprinkle with the pepper and cheese. Cover, reduce the heat to medium-low, and cook until the hash browns are starting to brown on the bottom, the egg is set, and the cheese is melted, 4 to 7 minutes.

Yield: 2 servings

Per serving: 363 calories (54% from fat, 18% from protein, 28% from carbohydrate); 17 g protein; 23 g total fat; 8 g saturated fat; 11 g monounsaturated fat; 3 g polyunsaturated fat; 26 g carbohydrate; 4 g fiber; 2 g sugar; 261 mg phosphorus; 292 mg calcium; 184 mg sodium; 740 mg potassium; 7200 IU vitamin A; 35 mg ATE vitamin E; 6 mg vitamin C; 16 mg cholesterol

Open-Faced Mexican Breakfast Sandwich

Here's a quick and flavorful Mexican-inspired breakfast, all in an easy-to-carry form.

¼ cup (63 g) Refried Beans (page 294)

2 Slices Low-Sodium Whole Wheat Bread (page 312), toasted

(continued on page 58)

2 tablespoons (33 g) Low-Sodium Salsa
(page 232)

2 tablespoons (14 g) shredded Swiss cheese

Spread the refried beans on the toast. Top
with the salsa, then the cheese. Microwave on
high until the cheese is melted and the beans
are hot, about 45 seconds.

Yield: 2 servings

Per serving: 158 calories (23% from fat, 19%
from protein, 58% from carbohydrate); 8 g protein;
4 g total fat; 2 g saturated fat; 1 g
monounsaturated fat; 0 g polyunsaturated fat; 24 g
carbohydrate; 4 g fiber; 3 g sugar; 137 mg
phosphorus; 135 mg calcium; 38 mg sodium;
203 mg potassium; 176 IU vitamin A; 17 mg ATE
vitamin E; 4 mg vitamin C; 10 mg cholesterol

Hearty Scrambled Eggs with Cheese and Rice

Adding some rice to your scrambled eggs
makes for a heartier breakfast without adding
to the sodium count or the preparation time.
I like this combination over a piece of whole
wheat toast.

1 cup (165 g) cooked rice

1½ cups (375 g) egg substitute, or 6 eggs,
beaten

¼ cup (28 g) shredded Swiss cheese

¼ teaspoon freshly ground black pepper

Put the rice into a skillet and pour the beaten
eggs over the top. Scramble the egg until set,

about 5 minutes. Sprinkle the cheese and
pepper on top and let melt.

Yield: 3 servings

Per serving: 216 calories (32% from fat, 38%
from protein, 31% from carbohydrate); 20 g protein;
7 g total fat; 3 g saturated fat; 2 g
monounsaturated fat; 2 g polyunsaturated fat; 16 g
carbohydrate; 0 g fiber; 1 g sugar; 241 mg
phosphorus; 178 mg calcium; 202 mg sodium;
447 mg potassium; 542 IU vitamin A; 23 mg ATE
vitamin E; 0 mg vitamin C; 11 mg cholesterol

Tip: You can also add some leftover diced turkey
or chicken.

Ricotta and Spinach Omelet

A simple omelet gets a pickup in flavor and
nutrition from spinach and ricotta cheese. To
make it even better top with a little spaghetti
sauce for an Italian accent or salsa for a
Mexican one.

1 cup (250 g) egg substitute, or 4 eggs

1 tablespoon (15 ml) skim milk

½ teaspoon freshly ground black pepper

3 tablespoons (42 g) unsalted butter, divided

4 ounces (115 g) fresh spinach

⅓ cup (83 g) ricotta cheese

Place the eggs in a small mixing bowl. Add
the milk and pepper. Briskly stir with a fork
until well beaten; set aside. In an 8-inch
(20-cm) nonstick skillet, melt 2 tablespoons

(28 g) of the butter over medium-high heat. Add the spinach and sauté until just wilted. Remove from the pan and set aside. Melt the remaining 1 tablespoon (14 g) butter in the skillet, then slowly pour in the egg mixture, tilting the pan to spread it evenly. Let the eggs firm up a little, allowing some of the remaining liquid to flow to the sides of the pan. Continue to cook for about another minute, then spoon in the ricotta. Spread over half of the omelet and top with the spinach. Fold the other half of the omelet over the filling. Shake the pan gently to slide the omelet to the edge. Holding the pan near the serving plate, tip it so the omelet slides onto the plate.

Yield: 2 servings

Per serving: 332 calories (67% from fat, 26% from protein, 7% from carbohydrate); 22 g protein; 25 g total fat; 14 g saturated fat; 7 g monounsaturated fat; 3 g polyunsaturated fat; 6 g carbohydrate; 1 g fiber; 1 g sugar; 269 mg phosphorus; 253 mg calcium; 299 mg sodium; 808 mg potassium; 6475 IU vitamin A; 191 mg ATE vitamin E; 16 mg vitamin C; 60 mg cholesterol

Tomato-Egg Scramble

Fresh tomatoes and basil add a nice bit of extra flavor to scrambled eggs, giving them an Italian orientation.

1 tablespoon (14 g) unsalted butter

2 cups (500 g) egg substitute, or 8 eggs, beaten

1 cup (180 g) chopped tomatoes

1 teaspoon chopped fresh basil

¼ teaspoon freshly ground black pepper

Melt the butter in a large skillet over medium heat. Pour in the beaten eggs and scramble, stirring with wooden spoon, until the eggs are near the desired doneness. Add the tomatoes and basil and cook, stirring for 1 minute, until the tomatoes are heated through and starting to soften. Season with pepper to taste, and serve immediately.

Yield: 4 servings

Per serving: 139 calories (47% from fat, 45% from protein, 8% from carbohydrate); 15 g protein; 7 g total fat; 3 g saturated fat; 2 g monounsaturated fat; 2 g polyunsaturated fat; 3 g carbohydrate; 0 g fiber; 1 g sugar; 162 mg phosphorus; 70 mg calcium; 204 mg sodium; 499 mg potassium; 773 IU vitamin A; 24 mg ATE vitamin E; 10 mg vitamin C; 9 mg cholesterol

Veggie and Egg Scramble for One

Frozen pepper and onion mix not only adds flavor but also makes this scrambled egg dish even quicker than if fresh ones were used. This quick and easy breakfast for one could easily be expanded to make enough for multiple people.

¼ cup (19 g) sliced mushrooms

½ cup (80 g) frozen pepper and onion mix

¼ cup (63 g) egg substitute, or 1 egg, beaten

¼ cup (28 g) shredded Swiss cheese

(continued on page 60)

In a small skillet coated with nonstick cooking spray, cook the mushrooms and frozen vegetables over medium heat for 2 to 3 minutes, until heated through. Pour the egg into the skillet and stir gently until cooked through, about 5 minutes. Remove from the heat, sprinkle with the cheese, and cover for 2 minutes to melt.

Yield: 1 serving

Per serving: 203 calories (50% from fat, 36% from protein, 14% from carbohydrate); 19 g protein; 11 g total fat; 6 g saturated fat; 3 g monounsaturated fat; 1 g polyunsaturated fat; 7 g carbohydrate; 2 g fiber; 1 g sugar; 310 mg phosphorus; 361 mg calcium; 111 mg sodium; 402 mg potassium; 912 IU vitamin A; 70 mg ATE vitamin E; 67 mg vitamin C; 31 mg cholesterol

Breakfast Pizzas

How about some pizza for breakfast? English muffins provide the base and scrambled eggs are paired with the traditional tomato sauce and cheese for a quick breakfast that will be sure to please.

½ cup (125 g) egg substitute, or 2 eggs, beaten

2 tablespoons (33 g) Low-Sodium Spaghetti Sauce (page 234)

1 English muffin, split and toasted

¼ cup (28 g) shredded Swiss cheese

Preheat the broiler in an oven or a toaster oven and place the oven rack 6 inches

(15 cm) below the heat source. Coat a small skillet with cooking spray and heat over medium-high heat. Add the eggs and cook, stirring often, until set, 1 to 2 minutes. Spread the sauce on the English muffin halves. Top with the scrambled egg and cheese. Broil until the cheese is melted, 1 to 3 minutes.

Yield: 2 servings

Per serving: 198 calories (36% from fat, 30% from protein, 34% from carbohydrate); 15 g protein; 8 g total fat; 4 g saturated fat; 2 g monounsaturated fat; 1 g polyunsaturated fat; 16 g carbohydrate; 1 g fiber; 3 g sugar; 219 mg phosphorus; 245 mg calcium; 238 mg sodium; 323 mg potassium; 457 IU vitamin A; 35 mg ATE vitamin E; 2 mg vitamin C; 16 mg cholesterol

Breakfast Quesadillas

Cheese and eggs fill this breakfast version of the traditional quesadilla. You could also add vegetables such as peppers and onions if you desire. These are easy to make if you have a portable contact grill such as the George Foreman models. If not, you can also grill them in a dry skillet, turning once. Corn tortillas are used because they contain less sodium than flour ones.

1 cup (250 g) egg substitute, or 4 eggs, beaten

¼ cup (65 g) Low-Sodium Salsa (page 232)

¼ cup (30 g) shredded low-fat Cheddar cheese

8 corn tortillas

Coat a skillet with nonstick spray, add the eggs, and scramble over medium heat, stirring in the salsa and cheese when they are almost set, about 4 to 5 minutes. Lightly coat one side of the tortillas with olive oil cooking spray and place 4 of them oil side down on a baking sheet. Divide the egg mixture among the tortillas, spreading to an even thickness. Top with the remaining tortillas, oil side up. Grill the quesadillas until heated through and golden brown, about 3 minutes per side. Cut into quarters to serve.

Yield: 4 servings

Per serving: 152 calories (22% from fat, 31% from protein, 47% from carbohydrate); 12 g protein; 4 g total fat; 1 g saturated fat; 1 g monounsaturated fat; 2 g polyunsaturated fat; 18 g carbohydrate; 3 g fiber; 1 g sugar; 237 mg phosphorus; 102 mg calcium; 2 mg iron; 275 mg sodium; 330 mg potassium; 291 IU vitamin A; 5 mg ATE vitamin E; 0 mg vitamin C; 2 mg cholesterol

Tofu and Egg Stir-Fry

The flavors here aren't a traditional stir-fry, but the wok makes a great tool for quickly cooking this potato, tofu, and egg scramble. Spinach adds flavor and a real nutritional punch.

4 ounces (115 g) firm tofu

2 small red potatoes

2 tablespoons (30 ml) olive oil

½ cup (125 g) egg substitute, or 2 eggs

¼ teaspoon freshly ground black pepper, to taste

1 teaspoon chili powder

2 ounces (55 g) fresh spinach

Slice the tofu lengthwise into slices about ½ inch (1.3 cm) thick and wrap in a paper towel. Put under something heavy, such as a dish. Chop the potatoes into small pieces, place in a microwave-safe bowl, fill with water, and microwave for 5 minutes. Place the olive oil in a wok and heat to very hot over high heat. In a small bowl, beat the eggs, chili powder, and pepper. Chop the spinach into small pieces. Unwrap the tofu and chop into small pieces. Drain the potatoes and add to the hot wok. Stir once to thoroughly coat in oil and then let brown on each side, stirring only occasionally. Add the tofu to the wok. Thoroughly stir the potatoes and tofu together. Reduce the heat to medium. Add the eggs and spinach and stir thoroughly. Let cook for another 3 minutes, until the eggs are set.

Yield: 2 servings

Per serving: 484 calories (33% from fat, 16% from protein, 51% from carbohydrate); 19 g protein; 18 g total fat; 3 g saturated fat; 11 g monounsaturated fat; 3 g polyunsaturated fat; 62 g carbohydrate; 7 g fiber; 5 g sugar; 370 mg phosphorus; 121 mg calcium; 178 mg sodium; 2182 mg potassium; 3282 IU vitamin A; 0 mg ATE vitamin E; 82 mg vitamin C; 1 mg cholesterol

Breakfast-Style Grilled Cheese Sandwich

Some combinations never occur to you until you try them, then they make perfect sense. This is one of them. Adding a layer of egg and some bacon to a grilled cheese sandwich not only makes it more breakfast-like, but it also makes it tastier.

½ cup (125 g) egg substitute, or 2 eggs

2 tablespoons (30 ml) skim milk

¼ teaspoon freshly ground black pepper

3 teaspoons unsalted butter, at room temperature, divided

4 Slices Low-Sodium Whole Wheat Bread (page 312)

2 ounces (55 g) shredded Swiss cheese

4 slices low-sodium bacon, cooked

Beat the eggs, milk, and pepper in a bowl until blended. Heat 1 teaspoon of the butter in a large nonstick skillet over medium heat until hot. Pour in the egg mixture. As the eggs begin to set, spread into a thin layer and cook, pulling, lifting, and folding the eggs, until thickened and no visible liquid egg remains. Remove from the pan and clean the skillet. Spread the remaining 2 teaspoons butter evenly on one side of each slice of bread. Place 2 slices in the skillet, buttered side down. Top evenly with the scrambled eggs, cheese, and bacon. Cover with the remaining 2 slices of bread, buttered side up. Grill the sandwiches over medium heat, turning once, until the bread is toasted and the cheese is melted, 2 to 4 minutes.

Yield: 2 servings

Per serving: 434 calories (51% from fat, 25% from protein, 24% from carbohydrate); 27 g protein; 24 g total fat; 12 g saturated fat; 8 g monounsaturated fat; 3 g polyunsaturated fat; 26 g carbohydrate; 2 g fiber; 4 g sugar; 427 mg phosphorus; 385 mg calcium; 297 mg sodium; 463 mg potassium; 673 IU vitamin A; 119 mg ATE vitamin E; 0 mg vitamin C; 60 mg cholesterol

Tip: Don't spend the money and sodium on the pre-cooked bacon in the grocery store. Instead, fry a big batch when you have time. Cooked bacon will keep for up to a week in the refrigerator or may be frozen for several months.

Breakfast Salmon Patties

Salmon may not be something you think of for breakfast, but besides the fact that it tastes good it has a lot of advantages over most traditional breakfast meats. It's lower in sodium, contains "good fat" rather than "bad fat," and cooks up quickly. I like these patties with fried eggs for a weekend breakfast.

15 ounces (420 g) pink salmon

¼ cup (63 g) egg substitute, or 1 egg, beaten

⅓ cup (55 g) minced onion

½ cup (60 g) all-purpose flour

3 tablespoons (45 ml) olive oil

Drain the salmon. In a bowl, combine the salmon, egg, and onion until sticky. Stir in the flour and form into 4 patties. Add the oil to a large skillet and heat over medium heat. Add the salmon patties and fry until golden brown, about 5 minutes.

Yield: 4 servings

Per serving: 315 calories (49% from fat, 34% from protein, 17% from carbohydrate); 26 g protein; 17 g total fat; 3 g saturated fat; 10 g monounsaturated fat; 3 g polyunsaturated fat; 13 g carbohydrate; 1 g fiber; 1 g sugar; 416 mg phosphorus; 278 mg calcium; 106 mg sodium; 407 mg potassium; 122 IU vitamin A; 19 mg ATE vitamin E; 1 mg vitamin C; 42 mg cholesterol

Shredded Wheat Pancakes

The shredded wheat in these pancakes adds both flavor and texture, not to mention fiber and nutrition. How can you go wrong with that combination?

½ cup (125 g) egg substitute, or 2 eggs

1½ cups (355 ml) skim milk

1½ cups (180 g) Buttermilk Baking Mix (page 27)

3 cups (165 g) shredded wheat, crushed

In a large bowl, beat the eggs and milk until bleaded. Beat in the pancake mix. Stir in the shredded wheat. Let stand for 5 minutes. Pour about ¼ cup (60 ml) per pancake onto a nonstick griddle and cook over medium-high heat until golden brown, about 5 minutes, turning once. You should get 12 pancakes.

Yield: 6 servings

Per serving: 256 calories (11% from fat, 14% from protein, 74% from carbohydrate); 8 g protein; 3 g total fat; 1 g saturated fat; 1 g monounsaturated fat; 0 g polyunsaturated fat; 43 g carbohydrate; 3 g fiber; 9 g sugar; 327 mg phosphorus; 148 mg calcium; 74 mg sodium; 258 mg potassium; 193 IU vitamin A; 57 mg ATE vitamin E; 1 mg vitamin C; 50 mg cholesterol

French Toast

French toast makes a quick and easy breakfast that looks and tastes like you spent a lot of time on it. But because you don't need to mix any batter or bake it it's actually quite a bit faster to fix than pancakes and other breakfast breads. It can also be used for a "breakfast dinner" with the addition of a couple of slices of bacon and some fresh fruit.

1 cup (250 g) egg substitute, or 4 eggs

¾ cup (180 ml) skim milk

1 teaspoon vanilla extract

2 tablespoons (25 g) sugar

1 Loaf Low-Sodium French Bread (page 314), cut into eight ½-inch (1.3-cm)-thick slices

1 teaspoon ground cinnamon

Combine eggs, milk, vanilla, and sugar in a large bowl and mix well. Add the bread and soak well. Lift out the slices and sprinkle with the cinnamon. Cook on a nonstick griddle over medium heat until golden brown on both sides, about 5 to 7 minutes.

Yield: 8 servings

(continued on page 64)

Per serving: 61 calories (19% from fat, 34% from protein, 47% from carbohydrate); 5 g protein; 1 g total fat; 0 g saturated fat; 0 g monounsaturated fat; 1 g polyunsaturated fat; 7 g carbohydrate; 0 g fiber; 3 g sugar; 68 mg phosphorus; 56 mg calcium; 94 mg sodium; 152 mg potassium; 161 IU vitamin A; 14 mg ATE vitamin E; 0 mg vitamin C; 1 mg cholesterol

PB and J French Toast

Everyone likes peanut butter and jelly, so why not for breakfast? This recipe, which coats French toast in chopped peanuts and tops it with jelly, is always popular with children, but you'll find that adults like it too.

½ cup (125 g) egg substitute, or 2 eggs

2 tablespoons (30 ml) skim milk

2 Slices Low-Sodium Whole Wheat Bread (page 312)

½ cup (75 g) unsalted peanuts, finely chopped

¼ cup (80 g) grape jelly

Beat the eggs and milk in a shallow dish until blended. Soak 1 bread slice at a time in the egg mixture, turning once; dip each slice into the peanuts to coat both sides. Coat a large nonstick skillet with cooking spray; heat over medium heat until hot. Place the bread slices in the skillet and cook until golden brown and no visible liquid egg remains, 2 to 3 minutes per side. Adjust the heat as necessary so the peanuts do not burn. Top with the jelly and serve.

Yield: 2 servings

Per serving: 428 calories (40% from fat, 18% from protein, 43% from carbohydrate); 19 g protein; 20 g total fat; 3 g saturated fat; 9 g monounsaturated fat; 6 g polyunsaturated fat; 47 g carbohydrate; 4 g fiber; 23 g sugar; 310 mg phosphorus; 119 mg calcium; 133 mg sodium; 543 mg potassium; 257 IU vitamin A; 9 mg ATE vitamin E; 4 mg vitamin C; 1 mg cholesterol

Tip: If, like me, grape is not your favorite jelly, feel free to substitute.

Apple Oat Bran Cereal

Apple juice and raisins add interest to the otherwise plain taste of oat bran. An added benefit of this easy to fix breakfast is that oat bran is a product that has been shown to reduce cholesterol. Serve with skim milk and honey.

½ cup (40 g) oat bran

½ cup (120 ml) apple juice

¾ cup (180 ml) water

¼ cup (36 g) raisins

½ teaspoon ground cinnamon

Combine all the ingredients in a microwave-safe bowl. Microwave on high for 2½ to 3 minutes.

Yield: 1 serving

Per serving: 182 calories (2% from fat, 3% from protein, 95% from carbohydrate); 1 g protein; 0 g total fat; 0 g saturated fat; 0 g monounsaturated fat; 0 g polyunsaturated fat; 47 g carbohydrate; 2 g fiber; 38 g sugar; 51 mg phosphorus; 45 mg calcium; 17 mg sodium; 465 mg potassium; 3 IU vitamin A; 0 mg ATE vitamin E; 2 mg vitamin C; 0 mg cholesterol

Three Bear's Porridge

There is nothing like a steaming hot bowl of oatmeal on a cold morning. This version adds raisins and honey (and what bear doesn't like raisins and honey) for flavor and wheat germ for extra nutrition.

1¾ cups (411 ml) water

1 tablespoon (7 g) ground cinnamon

¼ cup (36 g) raisins

1⅓ cups (107 g) quick-cooking oats

2 tablespoons (14 g) wheat germ

1 cup (235 ml) skim milk

3 tablespoons (60 g) honey

Bring the water to a boil in a saucepan over high heat, and add the cinnamon and raisins. When the water boils, add the oats and wheat germ. Reduce the heat to low and cook the porridge until all the water is absorbed and the oats are soft, 3 to 5 minutes. Pour the porridge into 3 bowls and cover each with ⅓ cup (80 ml) milk. Dribble 1 tablespoon (20 g) honey over each bowlful.

Yield: 3 servings

Per serving: 301 calories (9% from fat, 14% from protein, 77% from carbohydrate); 11 g protein; 3 g total fat; 1 g saturated fat; 1 g monounsaturated

fat; 1 g polyunsaturated fat; 61 g carbohydrate; 6 g fiber; 26 g sugar; 333 mg phosphorus; 177 mg calcium; 56 mg sodium; 445 mg potassium; 178 IU vitamin A; 50 mg ATE vitamin E; 2 mg vitamin C; 2 mg cholesterol

Tip: Don't wander off or someone may come in and eat it all.

Farina with Apricots and Almonds

A simple cereal such as Cream of Wheat can be made into something special just by adding a topping. In this case we use brown sugar, dried apricots and almonds to transform an otherwise uninteresting bowl of cereal.

2 cups (470 ml) skim milk

⅓ cup farina (40 g), such as Cream of Wheat (not instant)

1 tablespoon (15 g) packed brown sugar

¼ cup (36 g) dried apricots, chopped

2 tablespoons (18 g) roasted unsalted almonds

Bring the milk to a boil in a small saucepan over high heat. Whisk in the farina. Reduce the heat and simmer, whisking occasionally, until thickened, 2 to 3 minutes. Spoon into bowls and top with the sugar, apricots, and almonds, dividing them evenly.

Yield: 2 servings

Per serving: 309 calories (18% from fat, 19% from protein, 63% from carbohydrate); 15 g protein;

(continued on page 66)

6 g total fat; 1 g saturated fat; 4 g monounsaturated fat; 1 g polyunsaturated fat; 49 g carbohydrate; 2 g fiber; 10 g sugar; 355 mg phosphorus; 394 mg calcium; 150 mg sodium; 618 mg potassium; 1015 IU vitamin A; 150 mg ATE vitamin E; 4 mg vitamin C; 5 mg cholesterol

Tip: You can use this same kind of topping on oatmeal or other hot cereals.

New England Oatmeal

Looking for a quick, hot breakfast with a lot of flavor? Try this one. Apples, walnuts, and maple syrup add that North-woods taste to the nutrition of oatmeal. Ready in about 10 minutes, it's perfect for cold mornings.

2 cups (470 ml) water

¼ teaspoon ground cinnamon

1 cup (80 g) quick-cooking oats

⅔ cup (100 g) shredded apple

⅓ cup (50 g) raisins

2 tablespoons (30 ml) maple syrup, divided

2 tablespoons (16 g) chopped walnuts, divided

In a 2-quart (1.8-L) saucepan, combine the water and cinnamon; bring to a boil over medium-high heat. Add the oats and cook for 3 minutes. Stir in the shredded apple, raisins, 1 tablespoon (15 ml) maple syrup, and 1 tablespoon (8 g) walnuts. Cook for 5 minutes longer. Divide the oatmeal between 2 serving bowls. Drizzle the remaining 1 tablespoon (15 ml) maple syrup over top and sprinkle with the 1 tablespoon (8 g) walnuts.

Yield: 2 servings

Per serving: 357 calories (18% from fat, 9% from protein, 73% from carbohydrate); 9 g protein; 8 g total fat; 1 g saturated fat; 1 g monounsaturated fat; 4 g polyunsaturated fat; 68 g carbohydrate; 6 g fiber; 33 g sugar; 250 mg phosphorus; 61 mg calcium; 7 mg sodium; 456 mg potassium; 16 IU vitamin A; 0 mg ATE vitamin E; 2 mg vitamin C; 0 mg cholesterol

Quick Peanut Butter and Banana Breakfast

As a kid I liked peanut butter and banana sandwiches so this just seemed right to me. The whole grain bread adds additional nutritional value, the peanut butter melts into the hot toast and you end up with a treat that is not only good for you but also tastes great. The fact that you can easily grab it on your way out the door is just another added bonus.

2 teaspoons no-salt-added peanut butter

1 Slice Low-Sodium Whole Wheat Bread (page 312), toasted

1 banana, sliced

Spread the peanut butter on the warm toast. Top with the sliced banana.

Yield: 1 serving

Per serving: 262 calories (22% from fat, 9% from protein, 69% from carbohydrate); 6 g protein; 7 g total fat; 1 g saturated fat; 3 g monounsaturated fat; 2 g polyunsaturated fat; 48 g carbohydrate; 6 g fiber; 21 g sugar; 105 mg phosphorus; 38 mg calcium; 12 mg sodium; 668 mg potassium; 96 IU vitamin A; 0 mg ATE vitamin E; 13 mg vitamin C; 0 mg cholesterol

Crunchy Strawberry Yogurt Parfaits

Shredded wheat is one of the only cereals without any sodium. But as a cereal it's probably not very high on many people's lists. However when paired with yogurt and strawberries, it provides that little extra crunch that sends this breakfast over the top. You could also use this for a dessert, but it's the kind of thing that makes breakfast fun, while proving that good nutrition is also tasty.

½ cup (75 g) strawberries

1 cup (55 g) mini shredded wheat cereal, crumbled

2 cups (460 g) low-fat strawberry yogurt

Slice all but 2 of the strawberries. Place a layer of strawberry slices in each of 2 parfait glasses. Sprinkle ¼ cup cereal over the strawberries. Pour about ½ cup (115 g) yogurt over the cereal. Make another layer of strawberries, cereal, and yogurt. Top each with a whole strawberry.

Yield: 2 servings

Per serving: 261 calories (3% from fat, 14% from protein, 83% from carbohydrate); 13 g protein; 1 g total fat; 0 g saturated fat; 0 g monounsaturated fat; 1 g polyunsaturated fat; 75 g carbohydrate; 4 g fiber; 52 g sugar; 377 mg phosphorus; 369 mg

calcium; 143 mg sodium; 636 mg potassium; 52 IU vitamin A; 5 mg ATE vitamin E; 24 mg vitamin C; 5 mg cholesterol

Granola and Yogurt Parfait

This is simple, but it looks impressive and it tastes even better. You can substitute other fruit such as raspberries, blueberries, or peaches depending on what is in season and what flavor you want.

½ cup (85 g) sliced strawberries

¾ cup (195 g) low-fat vanilla yogurt

2 tablespoons (30 g) granola

Into 2 parfait glasses or wine glasses, spoon some berries, vanilla yogurt, and granola. Repeat the layering until all the ingredients are used.

Yield: 2 servings

Per serving: 117 calories (11% from fat, 17% from protein, 72% from carbohydrate); 5 g protein; 1 g total fat; 1 g saturated fat; 0 g monounsaturated fat; 0 g polyunsaturated fat; 22 g carbohydrate; 1 g fiber; 17 g sugar; 145 mg phosphorus; 168 mg calcium; 81 mg sodium; 297 mg potassium; 64 IU vitamin A; 11 mg ATE vitamin E; 23 mg vitamin C; 5 mg cholesterol

Dessert for Breakfast Ambrosia

We usually think of ambrosia as a dessert, but fruit makes a wonderful choice for breakfast, too. I've added apples and melon to the usual recipe. You get a huge 2-cup serving with a creamy orange dressing and it still doesn't quite come to 400 calories.

4 cups (640 g) cubed cantaloupe

4 cups (600 g) orange sections

4 cups (600 g) sliced bananas

4 cups (600 g) peeled and cubed apples

1 cup (110 g) pecans, coarsely chopped

2 ounces (55 g) shredded coconut

¼ cup (60 ml) orange juice

1 cup (225 g) low-fat vanilla yogurt

In a large bowl, arrange layers of cantaloupe, orange sections, bananas, apples, pecans, and coconut. Combine the orange juice and yogurt and pour over. Chill before serving.

Yield: 8 servings

Per serving: 352 calories (31% from fat, 6% from protein, 63% from carbohydrate); 6 g protein; 13 g total fat; 3 g saturated fat; 6 g monounsaturated fat; 3 g polyunsaturated fat; 60 g carbohydrate; 8 g fiber; 39 g sugar; 141 mg phosphorus; 112 mg calcium; 35 mg sodium; 1007 mg potassium; 3314 IU vitamin A; 3 mg ATE vitamin E; 95 mg vitamin C; 1 mg cholesterol

Piña Colada Parfait

Take a trip to the Tropics with this piña colada–inspired parfait. It's full of the traditional flavors of pineapple and coconut as well as the nutrition of yogurt.

⅓ cup (77 g) low-fat vanilla yogurt

½ cup (85 g) crushed pineapple with syrup

1 tablespoon (5 g) shredded coconut, toasted

Top the yogurt with the pineapple and coconut. Serve immediately.

Yield: 1 serving

Per serving: 156 calories (15% from fat, 11% from protein, 74% from carbohydrate); 5 g protein; 3 g total fat; 2 g saturated fat; 0 g monounsaturated fat; 0 g polyunsaturated fat; 30 g carbohydrate; 1 g fiber; 27 g sugar; 124 mg phosphorus; 158 mg calcium; 56 mg sodium; 327 mg potassium; 83 IU vitamin A; 10 mg ATE vitamin E; 10 mg vitamin C; 4 mg cholesterol

Cheddar Breakfast Cookies

These savory breakfast cookies are a favorite grab and go item, either for breakfast or as a mid-morning snack. Along with the distinctive flavor of Cheddar cheese, they contain the fiber and other nutritional benefits of oatmeal and wheat germ.

⅔ cup (150 g) unsalted butter

⅔ cup (132 g) sugar

¼ cup (63 g) egg substitute, or 1 egg

1 teaspoon vanilla extract

¾ cup (90 g) all-purpose flour

½ teaspoon sodium-free baking soda

1½ cups (120 g) quick-cooking oats

4 ounces (115 g) Cheddar cheese, shredded

½ cup (56 g) wheat germ

Preheat the oven to 350°F (180°C, or gas mark 4). Grease a cookie sheet. In a large bowl, beat together the butter, sugar, egg, and vanilla until well blended. In a separate bowl, combine the flour and baking soda; add to the butter mixture and mix well. Stir in the oats, cheese, and wheat germ. Drop by rounded tablespoonfuls onto the prepared cookie sheet. Bake for 12 minutes, or until the edges are golden brown. Transfer to a wire cooling rack. Store in a loosely covered container in the refrigerator or at room temperature.

Yield: 36 cookies, 18 servings

Per serving: 175 calories (50% from fat, 10% from protein, 40% from carbohydrate); 5 g protein; 10 g total fat; 6 g saturated fat; 3 g monounsaturated fat; 1 g polyunsaturated fat; 18 g carbohydrate; 1 g fiber; 8 g sugar; 112 mg phosphorus; 55 mg calcium; 46 mg sodium; 79 mg potassium; 289 IU vitamin A; 73 mg ATE vitamin E; 0 mg vitamin C; 25 mg cholesterol

Peanut Butter and Honey Crispy Squares

A variation of the traditional crispy treats, this version contains peanut butter for added nutrition but retains the grab and go ease.

⅓ cup (87 g) no-salt-added peanut butter

¼ cup (55 g) unsalted butter

¼ cup (80 g) honey

2 tablespoons (30 g) firmly packed brown sugar

3 cups (75 g) crispy rice cereal

Grease an 8-inch (20-cm) square pan. In a saucepan, combine the peanut butter, butter, honey, and brown sugar and bring to a boil over medium-high heat. Reduce the heat to medium and boil for 1 minute, stirring constantly. Pour over the cereal in a large bowl. Press firmly into the prepared pan. Cut into sixteen 2-inch (5-cm) squares. Store in a tightly covered container in the refrigerator.

Yield: 16 servings

Per serving: 100 calories (48% from fat, 6% from protein, 45% from carbohydrate); 2 g protein; 6 g total fat; 2 g saturated fat; 2 g monounsaturated fat; 1 g polyunsaturated fat; 12 g carbohydrate; 0 g fiber; 7 g sugar; 24 mg phosphorus; 6 mg calcium; 41 mg sodium; 55 mg potassium; 320 IU vitamin A; 93 mg ATE vitamin E; 3 mg vitamin C; 8 mg cholesterol

Tip: This is also good with puffed wheat cereal.

Breakfast Banana Shake

This is like having a milkshake for breakfast, but one that is full of nutrition from the yogurt and tofu. Coffee and cinnamon provide additional flavor notes.

1 cup (230 g) low-fat vanilla frozen yogurt

1 cup (235 ml) skim milk

8 ounces (225 g) silken tofu, drained and cut into cubes

2 teaspoons instant coffee granules

2 bananas, sliced and frozen (about 1½ cups [225 g])

Ground cinnamon (optional)

Place the frozen yogurt, milk, tofu, coffee granules, and bananas in a blender; process until smooth and frothy. Sprinkle with the cinnamon, if desired.

Yield: 2 servings

Per serving: 366 calories (19% from fat, 16% from protein, 66% from carbohydrate); 15 g protein; 8 g total fat; 3 g saturated fat; 2 g monounsaturated fat; 2 g polyunsaturated fat; 62 g carbohydrate; 4 g fiber; 37 g sugar; 337 mg phosphorus; 323 mg calcium; 143 mg sodium; 1149 mg potassium; 498 IU vitamin A; 117 mg ATE vitamin E; 15 mg vitamin C; 4 mg cholesterol

Carrot-Pineapple Smoothie

Yes, it may sound like a strange combination, but give it a try. You won't be sorry. It has a vaguely tropical flavor from the fruits, but the carrot give it a unique taste as well as adding nutritional value, especially vitamin A.

¾ cup (124 g) pineapple chunks

½ cup (120 g) ice

⅓ cup (80 ml) orange juice

¼ cup (28 g) grated carrot

½ banana

Place all the ingredients in a blender and process until smooth.

Yield: 1 serving

Per serving: 215 calories (3% from fat, 4% from protein, 93% from carbohydrate); 2 g protein; 1 g total fat; 0 g saturated fat; 0 g monounsaturated fat; 0 g polyunsaturated fat; 54 g carbohydrate; 5 g fiber; 35 g sugar; 50 mg phosphorus; 49 mg calcium; 26 mg sodium; 727 mg potassium; 4036 IU vitamin A; 0 mg ATE vitamin E; 50 mg vitamin C; 0 mg cholesterol

Tip: This makes a good dessert, too.

Mixed Fruit Smoothie

Smoothies make a quick and easy breakfast and they are packed with nutrition. The protein from the yogurt will help keep you from being hungry as the morning goes on. You can substitute other fruits based on your taste; for instance, substitute raspberries for the blueberries and peaches for the bananas to create a peach melba smoothie.

2 cups low-fat peach yogurt

1 cup (145 g) blueberries

2 cups (300 g) sliced bananas

Place all the ingredients in a blender and process until smooth.

Yield: 2 servings

Per serving: 382 calories (3% from fat, 11% from protein, 86% from carbohydrate); 14 g protein; 1 g total fat; 1 g saturated fat; 0 g monounsaturated fat; 0 g polyunsaturated fat; 108 g carbohydrate; 8 g fiber; 81 g sugar; 350 mg phosphorus; 388 mg calcium; 145 mg sodium; 1337 mg potassium; 213 IU vitamin A; 5 mg ATE vitamin E; 28 mg vitamin C; 5 mg cholesterol

Whisk Me Away to the Islands Smoothies

This smoothie *will* whisk you away to the islands, with its flavors of banana, melon, and papaya. The tofu adds protein to keep you from getting hungry in the middle of your morning on the beach.

8 ounces (225 g) silken tofu, drained

2 cups (280 g) peeled and chopped papaya

2 cups (300 g) sliced bananas

1 cup (160 g) cubed cantaloupe

½ cup (120 ml) skim milk

½ cup (120 ml) orange juice

Place all the ingredients in a blender and process until smooth.

Yield: 2 servings

Per serving: 400 calories (9% from fat, 12% from protein, 79% from carbohydrate); 12 g protein; 4 g total fat; 1 g saturated fat; 1 g monounsaturated fat; 2 g polyunsaturated fat; 85 g carbohydrate; 9 g fiber; 44 g sugar; 216 mg phosphorus; 182 mg calcium; 63 mg sodium; 1836 mg potassium; 4842 IU vitamin A; 38 mg ATE vitamin E; 160 mg vitamin C; 1 mg cholesterol

Cappuccino Breakfast Smoothie

Are you the kind of person who only wants (or has time) to grab a quick cup of coffee for breakfast? Take an extra minute and turn it into a protein-rich drink that gives the taste you desire, but will keep you going through the morning.

1 cup (235 ml) skim milk

1 cup (235 ml) coffee

1 cup (230 g) low-fat vanilla yogurt

1 tablespoon (15 g) packed dark brown sugar

¼ teaspoon vanilla extract

⅛ teaspoon ground cinnamon

Place all the ingredients in a blender and process until smooth.

Yield: 2 servings

Per serving: 176 calories (9% from fat, 24% from protein, 67% from carbohydrate); 11 g protein; 2 g total fat; 1 g saturated fat; 0 g monounsaturated fat; 0 g polyunsaturated fat; 29 g carbohydrate; 0 g fiber; 22 g sugar; 292 mg phosphorus; 374 mg calcium; 149 mg sodium; 556 mg potassium; 299 IU vitamin A; 89 mg ATE vitamin E; 2 mg vitamin C; 8 mg cholesterol

6

15-Minute Poultry Dishes

Chicken is one of your best friends when it comes to fixing quick, tasty, low-sodium meals. You'll find that many of these recipes start with boneless skinless chicken breasts. They cook quickly and can be grilled, stir-fried, or sautéed. They are naturally low in fat, and if you find ones that haven't been "enhanced" with a solution to make them juicer, as discussed earlier, they are also naturally low in sodium. And because they become dry if overcooked, they are ideal for fast preparation. Of course, there are recipes that use other chicken and turkey parts and some that take advantage of leftover meat from the roast poultry recipes in chapters 14 and 16.

This chapter also introduces the first of my mock kabobs recipes, typical kabob-flavored dishes that eliminate the time-consuming step of threading the ingredients onto skewers.

Herbed Italian Chicken Breast Tenders

Italian bread crumbs and fresh rosemary and thyme make these chicken tenders different and more flavorful. Once you've tried these, you'll never go back to fast-food chicken tenders. And with the way the lines usually are, you can probably make them in the same amount of time.

½ cup (120 ml) olive oil, for frying

1½ pounds (680 g) boneless skinless chicken breast, cut into strips

¼ teaspoon freshly ground black pepper

1 cup (120 g) all-purpose flour

½ cup (125 g) egg substitute, or 2 eggs

1 tablespoon (15 ml) water

2 cups (220 g) Italian-Style Bread Crumbs (page 33)

¼ cup (20 g) shredded Parmesan cheese

3 tablespoons (5 g) finely chopped fresh rosemary

3 tablespoons (7.5 g) finely chopped fresh thyme

¾ teaspoon finely chopped garlic

Preheat the oven to 350°F (180°C, or gas mark 4). Place a nonstick cookie sheet in the oven. Heat the oil in a large nonstick skillet or frying pan over medium to medium-high heat. Season the chicken tenders with pepper. Place the flour in a shallow dish. Beat the eggs with the water in a second dish alongside the flour. In a third dish, combine the bread crumbs, cheese, rosemary, thyme, and garlic. Coat the chicken in the flour, then in the egg, then in the bread and cheese mixture. Transfer to the skillet and cook until deeply golden on each side, 3 to 4 minutes. Transfer to the cookie sheet in the oven and bake for 5 minutes longer.

Yield: 6 servings

Per serving: 548 calories (38% from fat, 28% from protein, 34% from carbohydrate); 38 g protein; 23 g total fat; 4 g saturated fat; 15 g monounsaturated fat; 3 g polyunsaturated fat; 46 g carbohydrate; 3 g fiber; 0 g sugar; 358 mg phosphorus; 145 mg calcium; 190 mg sodium; 514 mg potassium; 204 IU vitamin A; 13 mg ATE vitamin E; 3 mg vitamin C; 70 mg cholesterol

Honey Mustard Chicken

Tender chicken breasts are cooked in minutes, covered with a tangy, sweet honey mustard glaze. It doesn't get any easier or better than this.

¼ cup (58 g) mayonnaise

2 tablespoons (22 g) mustard

1 tablespoon (20 g) honey

1½ pounds (680 g) boneless skinless chicken breast, cut in half widthwise to make thinner

Combine the mayonnaise, mustard, and honey in a small bowl. Place the chicken in a microwave-safe baking dish. Brush the sauce over the chicken. Microwave, loosely covered with waxed paper, for 6 to 8 minutes, or until the chicken is cooked through.

Yield: 4 servings

Per serving: 242 calories (20% from fat, 68% from protein, 12% from carbohydrate); 40 g protein; 5 g total fat; 1 g saturated fat; 1 g monounsaturated fat; 2 g polyunsaturated fat; 7 g carbohydrate; 0 g fiber; 4 g sugar; 334 mg phosphorus; 24 mg calcium; 126 mg sodium; 452 mg potassium; 40 IU vitamin A; 10 mg ATE vitamin E; 2 mg vitamin C; 102 mg cholesterol

Better than Takeout Chicken Nuggets

The secret to these great tasting nuggets, both is flavor and speed of preparation, is having the Italian-style seasoned bread crumbs already on the shelf or in the freezer. They really don't need anything else to give them the kind of taste that children and adults will both appreciate.

2 boneless chicken breasts

¼ cup (120 g) all-purpose flour

½ cup (220 g) Italian-Style Bread Crumbs (page 33)

½ cup (125 g) egg substitute, or 2 eggs

½ cup canola oil for pan-frying or about 2 cups (570 ml) canola oil for deep frying

Cut the chicken into bite-size pieces. Spread the flour and the bread crumbs on separate plates and beat the egg in a shallow bowl. Dip the chicken pieces into the flour, then the egg, then the bread crumbs. Deep-fry in enough oil to cover for about 5 minutes or until coating is golden brown and chicken is no longer pink

or panfry until golden brown, about 4 minutes per side.

Yield: 4 servings

Per serving: 269 calories (53% from fat, 22% from protein, 25% from carbohydrate); 15 g protein; 163 g total fat; 1 g saturated fat; 9 g monounsaturated fat; 5 g polyunsaturated fat; 17 g carbohydrate; 1 g fiber; 0 g sugar; 136 mg phosphorus; 37 mg calcium; 79 mg sodium; 243 mg potassium; 122 IU vitamin A; 3 mg ATE vitamin E; 0 mg vitamin C; 21 mg cholesterol

Lemon Almond Chicken Breast Fillets

Here's a variation on the lemon chicken typically served in Asian restaurants, but made easier and quicker. The chicken is quickly stir-fried, rather than being breaded and deep-fat fried. Almonds add crunch as well as flavor.

1 tablespoon (15 ml) olive oil, divided

1 clove garlic, minced

1½ pounds (680 g) boneless skinless chicken breast, cut into ¼-inch (6-mm) strips

2 tablespoons (15 g) all-purpose flour

1 cup (235 ml) Low-Sodium Chicken Broth (page 232)

2 tablespoons (30 ml) lemon juice

1 teaspoon sugar

1 teaspoon lemon zest

½ teaspoon dried dillweed

⅓ cup (35 g) sliced unsalted almonds, toasted

2 tablespoons (12 g) sliced scallion

(continued on page 76)

In a large heavy skillet or wok over medium heat, heat 1 teaspoon of the oil. Add the chicken and garlic and cook until chicken is no longer pink, about 5 minutes. Set aside. In the same skillet, add the remaining 2 teaspoons oil. Stir in the flour, then mix in the chicken broth. Bring to a boil, stirring constantly. Remove from the heat; stir in the lemon juice, sugar, lemon zest, and dill. Mix in the chicken and almonds and sprinkle with scallion.

Yield: 4 servings

Per serving: 317 calories (34% from fat, 55% from protein, 10% from carbohydrate); 44 g protein; 12 g total fat; 2 g saturated fat; 7 g monounsaturated fat; 2 g polyunsaturated fat; 8 g carbohydrate; 2 g fiber; 2 g sugar; 414 mg phosphorus; 58 mg calcium; 130 mg sodium; 599 mg potassium; 75 IU vitamin A; 10 mg ATE vitamin E; 7 mg vitamin C; 99 mg cholesterol

Tip: Serve over rice.

Balsamic-Barbecued Chicken

This is really fairly traditional barbecued chicken with one twist. The basic sauce is your typical tomato-based barbecue sauce. But the addition of balsamic vinegar gives this chicken an intense flavor boost while ensuring that the other flavors are absorbed deep into the chicken.

1 cup (235 ml) balsamic vinegar

¾ cup (180 g) no-salt-added ketchup

⅓ cup (75 g) packed brown sugar

¼ teaspoon minced garlic

1 tablespoon (15 ml) Worcestershire sauce

1 tablespoon (11 g) Dijon mustard

½ teaspoon freshly ground black pepper

4 boneless skinless chicken breasts

Combine the vinegar, ketchup, brown sugar, garlic, Worcestershire sauce, mustard, and pepper in a small saucepan and stir until all the ingredients are incorporated and the mixture is smooth. Simmer over medium heat for about 5 minutes. Place a grill pan over medium heat or preheat a gas or charcoal grill. Lightly coat the chicken with some of the sauce. Place the meat on the grill and cook for about 5 minutes per side. Simmer the remaining sauce while the meat cooks until it is reduced by about one-third. Brush the meat with the sauce every few minutes. Remove from the grill and serve with the heated sauce alongside.

Yield: 4 servings

Per serving: 209 calories (5% from fat, 32% from protein, 64% from carbohydrate); 17 g protein; 1 g total fat; 0 g saturated fat; 0 g monounsaturated fat; 0 g polyunsaturated fat; 35 g carbohydrate; 1 g fiber; 32 g sugar; 174 mg phosphorus; 40 mg calcium; 144 mg sodium; 561 mg potassium; 493 IU vitamin A; 4 mg ATE vitamin E; 15 mg vitamin C; 41 mg cholesterol

Weeknight Chicken and Rice Comfort Food

Unlike traditional chicken and rice casseroles that are baked in the oven, this one cooks quickly on the stove. It still has the expected flavors of mushroom soup and broccoli. It still tastes great and gives you that warm feeling both physically and emotionally. But it is quick enough to fix no matter what else you have going on.

1 tablespoon (15 ml) olive oil

4 boneless skinless chicken breasts

1½ cups (355 ml) Condensed Cream of Mushroom Soup (page 31)

1½ cups (355 ml) water

¼ teaspoon paprika, plus more for sprinkling

¼ teaspoon freshly ground black pepper, plus more for sprinkling

2 cups (380 g) instant white rice, uncooked

2 cups (140 g) broccoli florets

Heat the oil in a skillet over medium heat. Add the chicken and cook for 8 to 10 minutes, or until browned. Remove the chicken from the pan. Add the soup, water, paprika, and pepper. Bring to a boil over high heat, then stir in the rice and broccoli. Return the chicken to the pan. Sprinkle additional paprika and pepper over the chicken. Cover and cook on low for 5 minutes, or until the chicken is cooked throughout and the broccoli and rice are tender.

Yield: 4 servings

Per serving: 511 calories (12% from fat, 20% from protein, 68% from carbohydrate); 25 g protein; 7 g total fat; 1 g saturated fat; 3 g monounsaturated fat; 1 g polyunsaturated fat; 85 g carbohydrate; 2 g fiber; 2 g sugar; 337 mg phosphorus; 95 mg calcium; 81 mg sodium; 765 mg potassium; 1163 IU vitamin A; 6 mg ATE vitamin E; 34 mg vitamin C; 44 mg cholesterol

Chicken and Mushrooms Pasta Topping

An easy chicken and mushrooms recipe is a great start to dinner. This one features particularly simple preparation with only 4 ingredients. But, it provides a dinner everyone will like when served over pasta or noodles.

4 boneless skinless chicken breasts

1 pound (454 g) mushrooms, cut in half

2 tablespoons (30 ml) olive oil

3 tablespoons (45 g) Salt-Free Seasoning (page 27)

Preheat the oven to 375°F (190°C, or gas mark 5). Place the chicken breasts and mushrooms in 2 separate bowls. Toss each with 1 tablespoon (15 ml) olive oil and 1½ tablespoons (22 g) seasoning. Place each in separate ovenproof casserole dishes and roast for 6 to 7 minutes, turning each after 4 minutes. Serve the mushrooms over the chicken.

Yield: 4 servings

(continued on page 78)

Per serving: 163 calories (43% from fat, 48% from protein, 9% from carbohydrate); 20 g protein; 8 g total fat; 1 g saturated fat; 5 g monounsaturated fat; 1 g polyunsaturated fat; 4 g carbohydrate; 1 g fiber; 2 g sugar; 236 mg phosphorus; 11 mg calcium; 51 mg sodium; 537 mg potassium; 14 IU vitamin A; 4 mg ATE vitamin E; 4 mg vitamin C; 41 mg cholesterol

Microwaved Chicken Drumsticks

Chicken legs cook quickly in the microwave, flavored by a tomato and herb sauce. Serve with rice or noodles.

1 pound (454 g) chicken drumsticks

1 can (14.5 ounces, or 411 g) no-salt-added stewed tomatoes

¼ teaspoon freshly ground black pepper

¼ teaspoon dried dillweed

¼ teaspoon crumbled sage

Place the chicken in a medium bowl with the large end of the drumstick pointing out, combine the stewed tomatoes, pepper, dill, and sage and pour over the chicken. Microwave for 9 minutes, or until cooked through.

Yield: 4 servings

Per serving: 218 calories (28% from fat, 62% from protein, 10% from carbohydrate); 33 g protein; 7 g total fat; 2 g saturated fat; 2 g monounsaturated fat; 2 g polyunsaturated fat; 5 g carbohydrate; 1 g fiber; 3 g sugar; 232 mg

phosphorus; 52 mg calcium; 120 mg sodium; 556 mg potassium; 232 IU vitamin A; 20 mg ATE vitamin E; 17 mg vitamin C; 105 mg cholesterol

Quick Chicken à la King

This recipe has all the comfort-food taste you could want. Sautéed peppers and onion pair with leftover chicken to provide the great flavor. Using leftovers and make-ahead ingredients make it quick.

1 tablespoon (14 g) unsalted butter

¼ cup (38 g) chopped green bell pepper

¼ cup (40 g) chopped onion

2 cups (470 ml) Condensed Cream of Mushroom Soup (page 31)

½ cup (120 ml) skim milk

1½ cups (210 g) cooked cubed chicken breast

4 cups (660 g) cooked rice

Melt the butter in a saucepan over medium heat. Add the bell pepper and onion and cook until tender, about 5 minutes. Add the soup, milk, and chicken and cook until heated through, about 3 to 4 minutes. Serve over the rice.

Yield: 4 servings

Per serving: 401 calories (17% from fat, 24% from protein, 59% from carbohydrate); 23 g protein; 7 g total fat; 3 g saturated fat; 2 g monounsaturated fat; 1 g polyunsaturated fat; 58 g

carbohydrate; 2 g fiber; 3 g sugar; 291 mg phosphorus; 88 mg calcium; 85 mg sodium; 747 mg potassium; 206 IU vitamin A; 48 mg ATE vitamin E; 8 mg vitamin C; 57 mg cholesterol

Tip: To make an even more complete meal, add some other vegetable, such as peas or carrots.

Crispy Garlic Chicken

You'll love the taste of this chicken, which is just garlicky enough to be noticeable. Panko breadcrumbs provide a nice crunchiness. Slicing the chicken breasts in half widthwise makes them thinner so they cook more quickly without the effort of pounding that many recipes call for. Try this with garlic mashed potatoes for a real treat.

1 pound (454 g) boneless skinless chicken breasts

1 cup (120 g) all-purpose flour

¾ cup (188 g) egg substitute, or 3 eggs, beaten

1 cup (115 g) panko

1 tablespoon (9 g) garlic powder

1 tablespoon (8 g) cornstarch

¼ cup (60 ml) olive oil

3 cloves garlic, crushed

Cut the chicken breasts in half widthwise. Place the flour in a shallow dish and the eggs in a second. In a third shallow dish combine the panko, garlic powder, and cornstarch. Dip the chicken first in the flour, then the egg, then the bread crumbs, pressing so they adhere. Allow the chicken to rest while heating the oil in a large skillet over medium heat. Add the crushed garlic and cook until it begins to brown, about 1 minute. Remove the garlic and fry the chicken in the oil until crisp and golden brown, about 3 minutes per side.

Yield: 4 servings

Per serving: 519 calories (32% from fat, 31% from protein, 37% from carbohydrate); 39 g protein; 18 g total fat; 3 g saturated fat; 11 g monounsaturated fat; 3 g polyunsaturated fat; 47 g carbohydrate; 2 g fiber; 3 g sugar; 367 mg potassium; 93 mg calcium; 159 mg sodium; 554 mg potassium; 192 IU vitamin A; 7 mg ATE vitamin E; 2 mg vitamin C; 66 mg cholesterol

Chicken Breasts Parmesan

I'm sure your Italian grandmother slaved over chicken Parmesan for hours. And this dish has that same classic flavor even though you spend a fraction of time on it. A quick browning followed by microwave cooking will produce a dish that no one will know it took 15 minutes to fix.

½ cup (58 g) Italian-Style Bread Crumbs (page 33)

¼ cup (25 g) grated Parmesan cheese

1½ pounds (680 g) boneless skinless chicken breasts, cut in half widthwise to make thinner

½ cup (125 g) egg substitute, or 2 eggs, beaten

3 tablespoons (45 ml) olive oil

(continued on page 80)

1 can (8 ounces, or 225 g) no-salt-added
   tomato sauce

1 teaspoon Italian seasoning

¼ teaspoon garlic powder

4 ounces (115 g) fresh mozzarella, shredded

On waxed paper, combine the bread crumbs
and Parmesan cheese. Dip the chicken
breasts first in the egg and then in the bread
crumb mixture until coated. Heat the oil in a
large skillet over high heat. Quickly brown the
coated chicken pieces on both sides, about 2
to 3 minutes per side. In a small bowl,
combine the tomato sauce, Italian seasoning,
and garlic powder. Transfer the chicken to a
microwave-safe baking dish. Spoon the
tomato sauce over the chicken. Sprinkle the
mozzarella cheese over the tomato sauce.
Microwave, loosely covered with waxed paper,
for 5 to 6 minutes, or until the sauce is bubbly
and the chicken is tender and cooked
through.

Yield: 4 servings

Per serving: 489 calories (39% from fat, 47%
from protein, 14% from carbohydrate); 56 g protein;
20 g total fat; 6 g saturated fat; 10 g
monounsaturated fat; 2 g polyunsaturated fat; 17 g
carbohydrate; 2 g fiber; 3 g sugar; 607 mg
phosphorus; 340 mg calcium; 274 mg sodium;
855 mg potassium; 562 IU vitamin A; 56 mg ATE
vitamin E; 11 mg vitamin C; 120 mg cholesterol

Crispy Lemon Chicken

Chicken, nicely flavored with lemon juice and
honey mustard, cooks quickly and browns well
under the broiler. Serve with rice or noodles.

¼ cup (55 g) unsalted butter, melted

2 tablespoons (22 g) honey mustard

3 tablespoons (45 ml) lemon juice

1 tablespoon (4 g) dried tarragon

2 boneless skinless chicken breasts, thinly
   sliced

Preheat the broiler and place the oven rack
6 inches (15 cm) below the heat source.
Combine the butter, mustard, lemon juice, and
tarragon in a small bowl. Place the chicken in
an 8-inch (20-cm) square baking dish and
pour the sauce over, turning to coat. Broil the
chicken until cooked through, about 10
minutes, basting occasionally with the sauce.

Yield: 2 servings

Per serving: 300 calories (72% from fat, 23%
from protein, 5% from carbohydrate); 18 g protein;
24 g total fat; 15 g saturated fat; 7 g
monounsaturated fat; 1 g polyunsaturated fat; 4 g
carbohydrate; 1 g fiber; 1 g sugar; 164 mg
phosphorus; 39 mg calcium; 225 mg sodium;
267 mg potassium; 786 IU vitamin A; 195 mg ATE
vitamin E; 12 mg vitamin C; 102 mg cholesterol

Orange Chicken and Mushrooms

The flavor is really only mildly orange, but that is still what sets this dish apart from many others, giving it that subtle citrus tang.

4 boneless skinless chicken breasts

8 ounces (225 g) mushrooms, cut in half

2 tablespoons (30 ml) olive oil

½ teaspoon orange zest

3 tablespoons (45 g) Salt-Free Seasoning (page 27)

Preheat the oven to 375°F (190°C, or gas mark 5). Place the chicken breasts and mushrooms in 2 separate bowls. Toss each with half of the olive oil, orange zest, and seasoning. Place the chicken in a 9-inch (23-cm) square roasting pan. Place the mushrooms in an ovenproof casserole dish. Place both in the oven and cook 6 for 7 minutes, turning each after 4 minutes. Serve the mushrooms over the chicken.

Yield: 4 servings

Per serving: 150 calories (47% from fat, 48% from protein, 5% from carbohydrate); 18 g protein; 8 g total fat; 1 g saturated fat; 5 g monounsaturated fat; 1 g polyunsaturated fat; 2 g carbohydrate; 1 g fiber; 1 g sugar; 187 mg phosphorus; 10 mg calcium; 49 mg sodium; 360 mg potassium; 15 IU vitamin A; 4 mg ATE vitamin E; 3 mg vitamin C; 41 mg cholesterol

Waikiki Beach Chicken

This is a traditional sweet and sour chicken dish, full of all the things you'd expect, and a few you might not, such as snow peas and water chestnuts. The sauce, though, is exactly like the sweet and sour you'd get at an Asian restaurant. The only difference is that it's good for you or quick to fix. It's great with leftover brown rice or thin egg noodles.

⅓ cup (80 g) no-salt-added ketchup

3 tablespoons (45 ml) Low-Sodium Soy Sauce (page 27)

3 tablespoons (38 g) sugar

2 tablespoons (30 ml) rice vinegar

1 tablespoon (8 g) cornstarch

1 tablespoon (15 ml) olive oil

12 ounces (340 g) boneless skinless chicken breasts, cut into ½-inch (1.3-cm) pieces

½ teaspoon ground ginger

½ cup (65 g) sliced carrots

8 ounces (225 g) snow pea pods

8 ounces (225 g) pineapple chunks

1 can (8 ounces, or 225 g) water chestnuts, drained

Combine the ketchup, soy sauce, sugar, vinegar, and cornstarch in a bowl and set aside. Heat the oil in a large skillet over medium heat. Add the chicken, sprinkle with the ginger, and stir-fry until the chicken is cooked through, about 5 minutes. Remove the chicken from the skillet, add the carrots, pea pods, pineapple, and water chestnuts and cook until the carrots are crisp-tender, about

(continued on page 82)

4 minutes. Stir in the chicken and soy sauce mixture and cook until thickened, about 3 to 4 minutes.

Yield: 4 servings

Per serving: 300 calories (14% from fat, 31% from protein, 55% from carbohydrate); 23 g protein; 5 g total fat; 1 g saturated fat; 3 g monounsaturated fat; 1 g polyunsaturated fat; 42 g carbohydrate; 5 g fiber; 25 g sugar; 263 mg phosphorus; 60 mg calcium; 112 mg sodium; 913 mg potassium; 2789 IU vitamin A; 5 mg ATE vitamin E; 46 mg vitamin C; 49 mg cholesterol

Chicken Curry in a Hurry

This is not your usual curry, with a mild sauce made creamy by yogurt and milk. It does, however, have a rich flavor, enhanced by the fresh cilantro garnish. You could add other quick cooking vegetables such as zucchini or broccoli to make it an even more complete meal.

1½ tablespoons (23 ml) olive oil

¾ cup (120 g) thinly sliced onion

2 teaspoons curry powder

½ cup (115 g) low-fat plain yogurt

¾ cup (180 ml) skim milk

¼ teaspoon freshly ground black pepper

1 can (14.5 ounces, or 411 g) no-salt-added tomatoes, drained

3 cups (165 g) cooked rice

3 cups (420 g) sliced or shredded cooked chicken

¼ cup (4 g) fresh cilantro, roughly chopped

Heat the oil in a skillet over medium-low heat. Add the onion and cook, stirring occasionally, for 7 minutes. Sprinkle with the curry powder and cook, stirring, for 1 minute. Add the yogurt and milk and simmer gently for 3 minutes. Stir in the black pepper and tomatoes. Remove from the heat. Divide the rice and chicken among 6 bowls, spoon the sauce over the top, and sprinkle with the cilantro.

Yield: 6 servings

Per serving: 322 calories (26% from fat, 32% from protein, 42% from carbohydrate); 25 g protein; 9 g total fat; 2 g saturated fat; 5 g monounsaturated fat; 2 g polyunsaturated fat; 33 g carbohydrate; 2 g fiber; 7 g sugar; 249 mg phosphorus; 120 mg calcium; 99 mg sodium; 491 mg potassium; 319 IU vitamin A; 32 mg ATE vitamin E; 12 mg vitamin C; 64 mg cholesterol

Have It Your Way Chicken Curry

I'm fond of curries. They fill the house with such a great aroma, not to mention how they taste. This one is moderately spicy from a number of spices that are typical of curry powder. It also contains a nice assortment of vegetables and is really a complete meal in one dish. If you have a favorite curry powder on the shelf, you could substitute a couple of tablespoons of that for the other spices, but I like to experiment, increasing or decreasing the amount of various spices each time I make it just to see if I find a combination I like even better.

4 medium red potatoes, diced

1 cup (150 g) coarsely chopped green bell pepper

1 cup (160 g) coarsely chopped onion

1½ cups (180 g) sliced zucchini

1½ cups (150 g) cauliflower florets

1 pound (454 g) boneless skinless chicken breasts, cubed

1 can (14.5 ounces, or 411 g) no-salt-added tomatoes

1 tablespoon (6 g) coriander

1½ tablespoons (11 g) paprika

1 tablespoon (5.5 g) ground ginger

¼ teaspoon cayenne

½ teaspoon turmeric

¼ teaspoon ground cinnamon

⅛ teaspoon ground cloves

1 cup (235 ml) Low-Sodium Chicken Broth (page 232)

Place all the ingredients in a large saucepan or Dutch oven. Cover and cook until the potatoes are tender and the chicken is cooked through, about 12 minutes.

Yield: 5 servings

Per serving: 382 calories (6% from fat, 31% from protein, 63% from carbohydrate); 30 g protein; 3 g total fat; 1 g saturated fat; 0 g monounsaturated fat; 1 g polyunsaturated fat; 61 g carbohydrate; 9 g fiber; 10 g sugar; 434 mg phosphorus; 94 mg calcium; 115 mg sodium; 2121 mg potassium; 1508 IU vitamin A; 5 mg ATE vitamin E; 97 mg vitamin C; 53 mg cholesterol

Pasta with Rosemary Chicken

Fresh rosemary gives a unique flavor to this quick dish using pasta and shredded leftover chicken. You could also add vegetables if you desire.

12 ounces (340 g) pasta, such as elbows or shells

2 cups (280 g) cooked chicken

2 tablespoons (3 g) chopped fresh rosemary

¼ cup (25 g) grated Parmesan cheese

¼ teaspoon freshly ground black pepper

Cook the pasta according to the package directions until al dente. Reserve 1¼ cups (294 ml) of the cooking water. Drain the pasta and return it to the pot. Meanwhile, shred the chicken, discarding any skin and bones. Toss the pasta with the chicken, rosemary, reserved pasta water, half of the Parmesan, and black pepper. Cook over medium-low heat, stirring, until the sauce has thickened slightly, 2 to 3 minutes. Sprinkle with the remaining half of the Parmesan.

Yield: 4 servings

(continued on page 84)

Per serving: 445 calories (12% from fat, 29% from protein, 59% from carbohydrate); 32 g protein; 6 g total fat; 2 g saturated fat; 1 g monounsaturated fat; 1 g polyunsaturated fat; 64 g carbohydrate; 2 g fiber; 0 g sugar; 321 mg phosphorus; 98 mg calcium; 167 mg sodium; 348 mg potassium; 98 IU vitamin A; 21 mg ATE vitamin E; 2 mg vitamin C; 65 mg cholesterol

Ricotta-Stuffed Chicken Breasts

Stuffed chicken breasts, just oozing with cheese, are bound to be a hit with kids and adults alike.

¾ cup (83 g) shredded Swiss cheese

½ cup (125 g) ricotta cheese

1 tablespoon (2.4 g) chopped fresh thyme

⅛ teaspoon coarsely ground black pepper

6 boneless skinless chicken breasts

2 teaspoons unsalted butter

In a small bowl, fold together the Swiss and ricotta cheeses, thyme, and black pepper. Place a chicken breast on a flat surface. Cut a 2½-inch (6.4-cm) horizontal slit into the side of each chicken breast to form a pocket. Stuff each pocket with 2 tablespoons (30 g) of the cheese mixture. Melt the butter in a skillet over medium-high heat. Add the chicken and cook for 6 minutes. Turn; reduce the heat to medium and cook for 4 to 5 minutes longer, until the chicken is cooked through.

Yield: 6 servings

Per serving: 181 calories (42% from fat, 53% from protein, 4% from carbohydrate); 23 g protein; 8 g total fat; 5 g saturated fat; 2 g monounsaturated fat; 0 g polyunsaturated fat; 2 g carbohydrate; 0 g fiber; 0 g sugar; 278 mg phosphorus; 232 mg calcium; 75 mg sodium; 230 mg potassium; 286 IU vitamin A; 71 mg ATE vitamin E; 1 mg vitamin C; 66 mg cholesterol

Chicken Marsala

Here's another one of those meals that looks and tastes like you spent the hours that a French chef would making it. A classic combination of chicken and mushrooms, subtly flavored with Marsala wine, it is a dish fancy enough for any occasion. Shhhh! Don't tell anyone that it took 15 minutes.

1 tablespoon (15 ml) olive oil

1 pound (454 g) boneless skinless chicken breasts, thinly sliced

½ teaspoon freshly ground black pepper

8 ounces (225 g) mushrooms, sliced

2 teaspoons all-purpose flour

4 cups (940 ml) Marsala wine

¼ cup (60 ml) Low-Sodium Chicken Broth (page 232)

1 teaspoon chopped fresh parsley

Heat the oil in a large skillet over medium heat. Sprinkle the chicken with the black pepper and sauté until cooked through, about 5 minutes. Add the mushrooms and sauté until browned, about 3 minutes. Sprinkle with the flour, add the wine and broth, and bring to a boil. Reduce the heat to medium-low and cook until thickened, about 3 minutes. Stir in the parsley just before serving.

Yield: 4 servings

Per serving: 340 calories (20% from fat, 50% from protein, 30% from carbohydrate); 29 g protein; 5 g total fat; 1 g saturated fat; 3 g monounsaturated fat; 1 g polyunsaturated fat; 17 g carbohydrate; 1 g fiber; 9 g sugar; 286 mg phosphorus; 25 mg calcium; 90 mg sodium; 581 mg potassium; 50 IU vitamin A; 7 mg ATE vitamin E; 3 mg vitamin C; 66 mg cholesterol

Summer Pasta Bolognese

Pasta sauce often calls for long cooking times, but this sauce has plenty of flavor despite taking only minutes to fix. Flavored by fresh basil and with turkey replacing the more common, and less healthy, beef or sausage, it is a sure hit over any kind of pasta.

12 ounces (340 g) spaghetti

2 tablespoons (30 ml) olive oil

1 pound (454 g) ground turkey

½ teaspoon freshly ground black pepper

½ teaspoon chopped garlic

1 can (14.5 ounces, or 411 g) chopped tomatoes

½ cup (120 ml) dry white wine

1 cup (120 g) coarsely grated zucchini

¾ cup (30 g) fresh basil, torn

Cook the pasta according to the package directions until al dente. Meanwhile, heat the oil in a large skillet over medium heat. Add the turkey, season with pepper, and cook, breaking up the turkey with a spoon, for 3 minutes. Add the garlic and cook for 1 minute. Add the tomatoes and wine and simmer, stirring occasionally, until the turkey is cooked through and the sauce has thickened slightly, 4 to 5 minutes. Remove from the heat and fold in the zucchini and basil. Serve over the pasta.

Yield: 4 servings

Per serving: 353 calories (25% from fat, 39% from protein, 36% from carbohydrate); 33 g protein; 10 g total fat; 2 g saturated fat; 5 g monounsaturated fat; 2 g polyunsaturated fat; 31 g carbohydrate; 8 g fiber; 1 g sugar; 373 mg phosphorus; 172 mg calcium; 88 mg sodium; 875 mg potassium; 1120 IU vitamin A; 0 mg ATE vitamin E; 29 mg vitamin C; 68 mg cholesterol

Italian Chicken Stir-Fry

I know that sounds strange, Italian food isn't normally stir-fried. But it seemed like the best description of this Italian-flavored chicken and vegetables combination, which cooks quickly in a wok or skillet and is great over pasta.

2 tablespoons (16 g) all-purpose flour

1 teaspoon garlic powder

¼ teaspoon freshly ground black pepper

1 pound (454 g) boneless skinless chicken breasts, cut into ½-inch (1.3-cm) pieces

(continued on page 86)

1 teaspoon olive oil

1 cup (150 g) sliced red bell pepper

1 cup (160 g) chopped onion

1 cup (120 g) sliced zucchini

8 ounces (225 g) mushrooms, sliced

¼ cup (60 ml) Low-Sodium Chicken Broth
  (page 232)

¼ cup (60 ml) Italian Dressing (page 35)

Add the flour, garlic powder, and pepper to a resealable plastic bag and shake to combine. Add the cubed chicken to the bag and shake until well coated. Heat the oil in a large skillet over medium heat. Add the chicken; cook and stir until the chicken is no longer pink, about 5 minutes. Stir in the bell pepper, onion, zucchini, mushrooms, chicken broth, and Italian dressing. Cover and simmer until the vegetables and meat are tender, about 6 minutes.

Yield: 4 servings

Per serving: 209 calories (17% from fat, 57% from protein, 26% from carbohydrate); 30 g protein; 4 g total fat; 1 g saturated fat; 2 g monounsaturated fat; 1 g polyunsaturated fat; 14 g carbohydrate; 3 g fiber; 6 g sugar; 316 mg phosphorus; 34 mg calcium; 90 mg sodium; 724 mg potassium; 1254 IU vitamin A; 7 mg ATE vitamin E; 81 mg vitamin C; 67 mg cholesterol

Chicken Primavera

This is a simple chicken and veggies dish with only a few ingredients. The flavor is lifted by lemon pepper. Serve with pasta or noodles for a complete meal.

4 boneless skinless chicken breasts

12 ounces (336 g) frozen broccoli, cauliflower, and carrot mix

2 tablespoons (30 ml) olive oil, divided

4 tablespoons (24 g) lemon pepper, divided

Preheat the oven to 375°F (190°C, or gas mark 5). Place the chicken breasts and vegetable medley in 2 separate bowls. Toss each with 1 tablespoon (15 ml) olive oil and 2 tablespoons (12 g) lemon pepper. Place the chicken in a 9-inch (23-cm) square roasting pan. Place the vegetables in an ovenproof casserole dish. Place both in the oven and cook for 6 to 7 minutes, turning each after 4 minutes. Serve the vegetables over the chicken breasts.

Yield: 4 servings

Per serving: 178 calories (41% from fat, 43% from protein, 16% from carbohydrate); 20 g protein; 8 g total fat; 1 g saturated fat; 5 g monounsaturated fat; 1 g polyunsaturated fat; 7 g carbohydrate; 4 g fiber; 1 g sugar; 192 mg phosphorus; 64 mg calcium; 59 mg sodium; 382 mg potassium; 984 IU vitamin A; 4 mg ATE vitamin E; 36 mg vitamin C; 41 mg cholesterol

Ten-Minute Chicken Teriyaki

Even if you didn't make the low-sodium teriyaki sauce on page 30, you can still have chicken teriyaki in a hurry. Mix it up now and still have time to cook this flavorful Asian dish in less than 15 minutes total.

¼ cup (60 ml) Low-Sodium Teriyaki Sauce (page 30)

2 tablespoons (30 g) no-salt-added ketchup

2 tablespoons (18 g) garlic powder

1 tablespoon (12 g) sugar

2 boneless skinless chicken breasts, cut into thin strips

Stir together the teriyaki sauce, ketchup, garlic powder, and sugar in a bowl. Toss the chicken in the sauce to coat, and place on a microwave-safe plate. Cover with plastic wrap and microwave on high for 8 to 10 minutes, until the chicken is no longer pink.

Yield: 2 servings

Per serving: 163 calories (6% from fat, 48% from protein, 47% from carbohydrate); 20 g protein; 1 g total fat; 0 g saturated fat; 0 g monounsaturated fat; 0 g polyunsaturated fat; 19 g carbohydrate; 1 g fiber; 12 g sugar; 215 mg phosphorus; 23 mg calcium; 131 mg sodium; 403 mg potassium; 170 IU vitamin A; 4 mg ATE vitamin E; 5 mg vitamin C; 41 mg cholesterol

Thai-Style Chicken Tenders

I like Thai food because of the mingling of all the different flavors. This quick chicken dish is a good example, balancing the spiciness of ginger and cayenne with peanut butter. Rice

noodles or angel hair pasta would make a good accompaniment.

2 tablespoons (30 ml) sesame oil

1 pound (454 g) boneless skinless chicken breasts, sliced into strips

2 teaspoons minced fresh ginger

¼ cup (60 ml) Low-Sodium Teriyaki Sauce (page 30)

½ cup (130 g) no-salt-added peanut butter

½ teaspoon cayenne pepper

½ cup (50 g) chopped scallion

Heat the oil in a large skillet over medium heat and cook the chicken until it is no longer pink, about 2 to 3 minutes. Reduce the heat to low and add the ginger, teriyaki sauce, peanut butter, and cayenne. Cook, stirring frequently, until the sauce is bubbly and warm, 1 to 2 minutes. Remove from the heat and sprinkle with the scallions. Serve immediately, spooning the sauce over the chicken.

Yield: 5 servings

Per serving: 323 calories (55% from fat, 33% from protein, 12% from carbohydrate); 28 g protein; 20 g total fat; 4 g saturated fat; 9 g monounsaturated fat; 6 g polyunsaturated fat; 10 g carbohydrate; 2 g fiber; 5 g sugar; 268 mg phosphorus; 30 mg calcium; 193 mg sodium; 471 mg potassium; 192 IU vitamin A; 5 mg ATE vitamin E; 3 mg vitamin C; 53 mg cholesterol

Chicken Fried Rice

Fried rice is a favorite of mine because it's so easy to put together a great tasting meal from

(continued on page 88)

things I have already in the refrigerator. This chicken fried rice is a great example. You could add any number of other diced vegetables to liven it up even more, or keep it simple. Either way it's a winner.

¼ cup (63 g) egg substitute, or 1 egg, beaten

1 tablespoon (14 g) unsalted butter

1 tablespoon (15 ml) olive oil

½ cup (80 g chopped onion

1½ cups (250 g) cooked white rice, cold

2 tablespoons (30 ml) Low-Sodium Soy Sauce (page 29)

1 teaspoon freshly ground black pepper

1 cup (140 g) chopped cooked chicken

Melt the butter in a large skillet over medium-low heat. Add the egg and leave flat for 1 to 2 minutes. Remove from the skillet and cut into shreds. Heat the oil in the same skillet; add the onion and sauté until soft, about 5 minutes. Add the rice, soy sauce, black pepper, and chicken. Stir-fry together for about 5 minutes, then stir in the egg. Serve hot.

Yield: 2 servings

Per serving: 420 calories (36% from fat, 26% from protein, 38% from carbohydrate); 27 g protein; 17 g total fat; 6 g saturated fat; 8 g monounsaturated fat; 2 g polyunsaturated fat; 40 g carbohydrate; 1 g fiber; 2 g sugar; 268 mg phosphorus; 57 mg calcium; 159 mg sodium; 441 mg potassium; 339 IU vitamin A; 61 mg ATE vitamin E; 5 mg vitamin C; 75 mg cholesterol

Tip: Substitute leftover pork or shrimp (or some combination) for the chicken.

Apple Chicken Stir-Fry

Stir-frying makes this quick, even though the flavor is not Asian. Apples make an unusual addition to the more usual combination of onion, carrots, and pea pods. Serve over cooked rice.

1 tablespoon (15 ml) vegetable oil

1 pound (454 g) boneless skinless chicken breasts, cubed

½ cup (80 g) sliced onion (sliced through the stem end)

1¾ cups (228 g) thinly sliced carrots

1 teaspoon dried basil

1 cup (80 g) pea pods

1 tablespoon (15 ml) water

1 apple, cored and thinly sliced

Heat the oil in a skillet over medium heat. Add the chicken and stir-fry until lightly browned and cooked through, about 5 minutes. Remove from the skillet. Add the onion, carrots, and basil to the same skillet and stir-fry until the carrots are tender, about 5 minutes. Stir in the pea pods, water, and apple and stir-fry for 2 minutes. Add to the chicken and toss to combine.

Yield: 4 servings

Per serving: 237 calories (30% from fat, 47% from protein, 23% from carbohydrate); 28 g protein; 8 g total fat; 1 g saturated fat; 3 g monounsaturated fat; 3 g polyunsaturated fat; 13 g carbohydrate; 3 g fiber; 8 g sugar; 265 mg phosphorus; 51 mg calcium; 114 mg sodium; 581 mg potassium; 7058 IU vitamin A; 7 mg ATE vitamin E; 22 mg vitamin C; 66 mg cholesterol

Sweet Potato and Chicken Skillet

Sweet potatoes are great not only because they taste so good but also because they cook faster than regular potatoes. For those of you who can't imagine sweet potatoes with a lemon accent, try this and you'll never have that difficulty again.

3 tablespoons (45 ml) olive oil, divided

2 sweet potatoes, cut into 8 wedges each

4 boneless skinless chicken breasts

2 tablespoons (18 g) lemon pepper

Heat 1½ tablespoons (22 ml) of the olive oil in a cast-iron skillet over medium heat. Toss in the sweet potatoes and brown on all sides for 1 minute. Remove to a plate. Add remaining 1½ tablespoons (22 ml) olive oil to the pan; add the chicken, and brown on both sides, about 3 minutes per side. Return the sweet potatoes to the pan and sprinkle all with the lemon pepper. Cook for 3 minutes, or until the chicken is cooked through and the potatoes are tender, then toss and serve.

Yield: 4 servings

Per serving: 323 calories (59% from fat, 22% from protein, 19% from carbohydrate); 18 g protein; 21 g total fat; 3 g saturated fat; 15 g monounsaturated fat; 2 g polyunsaturated fat; 15 g carbohydrate; 3 g fiber; 4 g sugar; 169 mg phosphorus; 42 mg calcium; 69 mg sodium; 395 mg potassium; 11930 IU vitamin A; 4 mg ATE vitamin E; 11 mg vitamin C; 41 mg cholesterol

Chicken Foster

I'll admit this sounds a little strange. It's a main course version of the classic bananas Foster dessert. Don't worry about the amount of alcohol, as long as you follow the instructions to burn it off. It will make quite an impression on your guests. Serve with rice.

½ cup (112 g) unsalted butter

6 tablespoons (90 g) packed brown sugar

1 pound (454 g) boneless skinless chicken breasts, cut into 1-inch (2.5-cm) cubes

¼ teaspoon freshly ground black pepper, to taste

¼ cup (30 g) all-purpose flour

2 small bananas, sliced

¾ cup (180 ml) coconut-flavored rum

Melt the butter in a large skillet over medium heat, and stir in the brown sugar. Season the chicken with pepper, and toss with the flour to coat. Add the chicken and bananas to the skillet, and cook, stirring occasionally, until the chicken is almost cooked through, about 5 minutes. Stir in the rum, and heat through. Remove from the heat, and use a long match or lighter to light the rum. Allow to burn until the alcohol cooks off and the flame goes out.

Yield: 4 servings

Per serving: 598 calories (44% from fat, 22% from protein, 34% from carbohydrate); 28 g protein; 25 g total fat; 15 g saturated fat; 6 g monounsaturated fat; 1 g polyunsaturated fat; 43 g carbohydrate; 2 g fiber; 29 g sugar; 260 mg phosphorus; 42 mg calcium; 86 mg sodium; 647 mg potassium; 780 IU vitamin A; 197 mg ATE vitamin E; 8 mg vitamin C; 127 mg cholesterol

Curried Chicken Mock Kabobs

Chicken gets an unusual flavor treatment here, with curry powder, peanut butter, and lime juice combining. Serve with rice and Curried Fresh Vegetables (page 203).

1½ pounds (680 g) boneless skinless chicken breasts, cut into 1-inch (2.5-cm) cubes

¼ cup (60 ml) coconut milk

2 tablespoons (12 g) curry powder

2 tablespoons (32 g) no-salt-added peanut butter

2 tablespoons (30 ml) lime juice

Preheat the broiler and place the oven rack 6 inches (15 cm) below the heat source. Toss all the ingredients together in a bowl. Spread on a baking sheet and broil until the chicken is cooked through, turning once, 6 to 8 minutes.

Yield: 6 servings

Per serving: 183 calories (32% from fat, 62% from protein, 7% from carbohydrate); 28 g protein; 6 g total fat; 3 g saturated fat; 2 g monounsaturated fat; 1 g polyunsaturated fat; 3 g carbohydrate; 1 g fiber; 1 g sugar; 256 mg phosphorus; 27 mg calcium; 77 mg sodium; 388 mg potassium; 46 IU vitamin A; 7 mg ATE vitamin E; 3 mg vitamin C; 66 mg cholesterol

Fajita Chicken Mock Kabobs

Flavored with garlic, lime, and fresh cilantro, these Mexican chicken cubes can be used for fajitas, taco salad, or just as the meat portion of any Mexican meal.

1 onion, cut into quarters through the stem end

1 green bell pepper, stemmed, seeded, and cut into 1-inch (2.5-cm) cubes

1½ pounds (680 g) boneless skinless chicken breasts

2 tablespoons (30 ml) olive oil

1 teaspoon crushed garlic

1 tablespoon (15 ml) lime juice

¼ cup (4 g) fresh cilantro, minced

Preheat the broiler and place the oven rack 6 inches (15 cm) below the heat source. Toss all the ingredients together in a bowl. Spread on a baking sheet and broil until the vegetables are crisp-tender and the chicken is cooked through, turning once, 6 to 8 minutes.

Yield: 6 servings

Per serving: 183 calories (30% from fat, 60% from protein, 10% from carbohydrate); 27 g protein; 6 g total fat; 1 g saturated fat; 4 g monounsaturated fat; 1 g polyunsaturated fat; 4 g carbohydrate; 1 g fiber; 2 g sugar; 236 mg phosphorus; 23 mg calcium; 77 mg sodium; 386 mg potassium; 234 IU vitamin A; 7 mg ATE vitamin E; 25 mg vitamin C; 66 mg cholesterol

Great Caesar's Chicken Mock Kabobs

Simply flavored with Caesar dressing and Parmesan cheese, this is the perfect topping to make a Caesar's salad a full meal.

1½ pounds (680 g) boneless skinless chicken
    breasts, cut into 1-inch (2.5-cm) cubes
¼ cup Caesar Salad Dressing (page 36)
¼ cup (20 g) shredded Parmesan cheese
2 tablespoons (30 ml) lemon juice

Preheat the broiler and place the oven rack 6 inches (15 cm) below the heat source. Toss all the ingredients together in a bowl. Spread on a baking sheet and broil until the chicken is cooked through, turning once, 6 to 8 minutes.

Yield: 6 servings

Per serving: 144 calories (17% from fat, 81% from protein, 2% from carbohydrate); 28 g protein; 3 g total fat; 1 g saturated fat; 1 g monounsaturated fat; 0 g polyunsaturated fat; 1 g carbohydrate; 0 g fiber; 0 g sugar; 253 mg phosphorus; 59 mg calcium; 137 mg sodium; 301 mg potassium; 42 IU vitamin A; 12 mg ATE vitamin E; 4 mg vitamin C; 69 mg cholesterol

Greek Chicken Mock Kabobs

This dish features Mediterranean-inspired chicken and tomatoes, flavored with garlic and oregano. Other vegetables, such as peppers and zucchini, could also be added.

24 cherry tomatoes
1½ pounds (680 g) boneless skinless chicken
    breasts, cut into 1-inch (2.5-cm) cubes
2 tablespoons (30 ml) olive oil
½ teaspoon crushed garlic
1 teaspoon dried oregano

Preheat the broiler and place the oven rack 6 inches (15 cm) below the heat source. Toss all the ingredients together in a bowl. Spread on a baking sheet and broil until the chicken is cooked through, turning once, 6 to 8 minutes.

Yield: 6 servings

Per serving: 180 calories (31% from fat, 61% from protein, 8% from carbohydrate); 27 g protein; 6 g total fat; 1 g saturated fat; 4 g monounsaturated fat; 1 g polyunsaturated fat; 3 g carbohydrate; 1 g fiber; 0 g sugar; 223 mg phosphorus; 19 mg calcium; 74 mg sodium; 444 mg potassium; 458 IU vitamin A; 7 mg ATE vitamin E; 14 mg vitamin C; 66 mg cholesterol

Indian Chicken Mock Kabobs

This is similar in ingredients and flavor to tandoori chicken, with the yogurt helping to offset the spices. I really like the amount of flavor you get in so little time.

1½ pounds boneless skinless chicken breasts,
    cut into 1-inch (2.5-cm) cubes
¼ cup (60 g) low-fat plain yogurt
2 tablespoons (15 g) garam masala

(continued on page 92)

1 teaspoon crushed garlic

¼ cup (4 g) fresh cilantro, minced

2 tablespoons (30 ml) lime juice

Preheat the broiler and place the oven rack 6 inches (15 cm) below the heat source. Toss all the ingredients together in a bowl. Spread on a baking sheet and broil until the chicken is cooked through, turning once, 6 to 8 minutes.

Yield: 6 servings

Per serving: 134 calories (11% from fat, 84% from protein, 4% from carbohydrate); 27 g protein; 2 g total fat; 0 g saturated fat; 0 g monounsaturated fat; 0 g polyunsaturated fat; 1 g carbohydrate; 0 g fiber; 1 g sugar; 239 mg phosphorus; 34 mg calcium; 82 mg sodium; 330 mg potassium; 148 IU vitamin A; 8 mg ATE vitamin E; 4 mg vitamin C; 66 mg cholesterol

Jerk Chicken Mock Kabobs

This spicy chicken with a taste of the islands is best served over rice.

8 ounces (225 g) pineapple chunks

1½ pounds (680 g) boneless skinless chicken breasts, cut into 1-inch (2.5-cm) cubes

2 tablespoons (30 ml) olive oil

2 tablespoons (30 ml) lime juice

1 tablespoon (9 g) jerk seasoning

Preheat the broiler and place the oven rack 6 inches (15 cm) below the heat source. Toss all

the ingredients together in a bowl. Spread on a baking sheet and broil until the chicken is cooked through, turning once, 6 to 8 minutes.

Yield: 6 servings

Per serving: 178 calories (31% from fat, 61% from protein, 8% from carbohydrate); 26 g protein; 6 g total fat; 1 g saturated fat; 4 g monounsaturated fat; 1 g polyunsaturated fat; 4 g carbohydrate; 0 g fiber; 3 g sugar; 224 mg phosphorus; 19 mg calcium; 74 mg sodium; 343 mg potassium; 40 IU vitamin A; 7 mg ATE vitamin E; 6 mg vitamin C; 66 mg cholesterol

Smoky Chicken Mock Kabobs

Simple barbecued chicken in minutes, smoky and delicious. Serve with a quick salad for a great meal.

1½ pounds (680 g) boneless skinless chicken breasts, cut into 1-inch (2.5-cm) cubes

¼ cup (60 ml) Barbecue Sauce (page 30)

1 teaspoon liquid smoke

Preheat the broiler and place the oven rack 6 inches (15 cm) below the heat source. Toss all the ingredients together in a bowl. Spread on a baking sheet and broil until the chicken is cooked through, turning once, 6 to 8 minutes.

Yield: 6 servings

Per serving: 146 calories (9% from fat, 76% from protein, 15% from carbohydrate); 26 g protein; 1 g total fat; 0 g saturated fat; 0 g monounsaturated fat; 0 g polyunsaturated fat; 5 g carbohydrate; 0 g fiber; 4 g sugar; 222 mg phosphorus; 12 mg calcium; 77 mg sodium; 289 mg potassium; 23 IU vitamin A; 7 mg ATE vitamin E; 1 mg vitamin C; 66 mg cholesterol

Teriyaki Chicken Mock Kabobs

Sweet Asian-flavored chicken chunks. Serve with stir-fried veggies and rice.

1½ pounds (680 g) boneless skinless chicken breasts, cut into 1-inch (2.5-cm) cubes

¼ cup (60 ml) Low-Sodium Teriyaki Sauce (page 30)

2 tablespoons (30 ml) sesame oil

Preheat the broiler and place the oven rack 6 inches (15 cm) below the heat source. Toss all the ingredients together in a bowl. Spread on a baking sheet and broil until the chicken is cooked through, turning once, 6 to 8 minutes.

Yield: 6 servings

Per serving: 179 calories (33% from fat, 61% from protein, 6% from carbohydrate); 26 g protein; 6 g total fat; 1 g saturated fat; 2 g monounsaturated fat; 2 g polyunsaturated fat; 2 g carbohydrate; 0 g fiber; 2 g sugar; 225 mg phosphorus; 13 mg calcium; 180 mg sodium; 295 mg potassium; 23 IU vitamin A; 7 mg ATE vitamin E; 1 mg vitamin C; 66 mg cholesterol

Turkey Meatballs Mock Kabobs

Relive the taste of Thanksgiving in these quick cranberry sauce–flavored turkey meatballs.

1½ pounds (680 g) ground turkey

½ cup (160 g) cranberry sauce

1½ tablespoons (23 ml) Barbecue Sauce (page 30)

1½ tablespoons (23 ml) cider vinegar

Preheat the broiler and place the oven rack 6 inches (15 cm) below the heat source. Combine all the ingredients in a bowl and mix well. Form into 1-inch (2.5-cm) balls. You should get about 36 balls. Place on a baking sheet and broil until the turkey is cooked through, turning once, 6 to 8 minutes.

Yield: 6 servings

Per serving: 174 calories (10% from fat, 64% from protein, 26% from carbohydrate); 27 g protein; 2 g total fat; 1 g saturated fat; 0 g monounsaturated fat; 0 g polyunsaturated fat; 11 g carbohydrate; 0 g fiber; 10 g sugar; 233 mg phosphorus; 15 mg calcium; 79 mg sodium; 356 mg potassium; 10 IU vitamin A; 0 mg ATE vitamin E; 0 mg vitamin C; 68 mg cholesterol

Chicken Liver Mock Kabobs

Liver and onions, one of my favorite meals. If you feel the same way, this is for you.

(continued on page 94)

Traditional tastes of liver, onion, and bacon, but in a fraction of the time it usually takes.

1 onion, cut into quarters through the stem end

1½ pounds (680 g) chicken livers

6 slices low-sodium bacon, cut into 1-inch (2.5-cm) pieces

2 tablespoons (30 ml) olive oil

½ teaspoon freshly ground black pepper

Preheat the broiler and place the oven rack 6 inches (15 cm) below the heat source. Toss all the ingredients together in a bowl. Spread on a baking sheet and broil until the liver is cooked through, turning once, 6 to 8 minutes.

Yield: 6 servings

Per serving: 290 calories (48% from fat, 46% from protein, 6% from carbohydrate); 32 g protein; 15 g total fat; 4 g saturated fat; 6 g monounsaturated fat; 2 g polyunsaturated fat; 4 g carbohydrate; 0 g fiber; 1 g sugar; 551 mg phosphorus; 19 mg calcium; 188 mg sodium; 443 mg potassium; 16309 IU vitamin A; 4869 mg ATE vitamin E; 5 mg vitamin C; 648 mg cholesterol

Pennsylvania Dutch Chicken Corn Soup

When I was growing up along the Maryland/ Pennsylvania border, chicken corn soup was always one of the highlights at volunteer fire company carnivals and suppers. This soup has a similar flavor, rich with vegetables and chicken.

4 cups (940 ml) Low-Sodium Chicken Broth (page 232)

2 cups (280 g) chopped cooked chicken

½ cup (50 g) chopped celery

½ cup (65 g) sliced carrots

½ cup (80 g) chopped onion

12 ounces (336 g) frozen corn

1 tablespoon (4 g) chopped fresh parsley

¼ teaspoon garlic powder

2 cups (470 ml) water

12 ounces (340 g) egg noodles

Place all the ingredients in a large kettle and simmer over medium heat until the noodles and vegetables are tender, about 12 minutes.

Yield: 8 servings

Per serving: 185 calories (19% from fat, 32% from protein, 45% from carbohydrate); 15 g protein; 4 g total fat; 1 g saturated fat; 1 g monounsaturated fat; 1 g polyunsaturated fat; 23 g carbohydrate; 4 g fiber; 2 g sugar; 182 mg phosphorus; 21 mg calcium; 86 mg sodium; 379 mg potassium; 1167 IU vitamin A; 6 mg ATE vitamin E; 5 mg vitamin C; 31 mg cholesterol

Ready in a Jiffy Chicken Vegetable Soup

Maybe this isn't quite like Mom used to make, but it's pretty close. It's the kind of comfort food that can't help but make people feel better, full of chicken, noodles, and vegetables in a rich broth. And being able to get it on the table in 15 minutes will make you feel even better.

1 tablespoon (15 ml) olive oil

½ cup (50 g) sliced celery

½ cup (65 g) sliced carrots

¼ cup (40 g) chopped onion

6 cups (1.4 L) Low-Sodium Chicken Broth (page 232)

4 ounces (112 g) egg noodles

8 ounces (225 g) boneless skinless chicken breasts, thinly sliced

1 teaspoon chopped fresh parsley

¼ teaspoon white pepper

Heat the oil in a Dutch oven over medium heat and sauté the celery, carrots, and onion until soft, about 3 minutes. Stir in the chicken broth. Bring to a boil over high heat and add the noodles, chicken, parsley, and pepper. Reduce the heat to a simmer and cook until the chicken is cooked through and the noodles and vegetables are tender, about 10 to 12 minutes.

Yield: 4 servings

Per serving: 271 calories (24% from fat, 36% from protein, 40% from carbohydrate); 25 g protein; 8 g total fat; 2 g saturated fat; 4 g monounsaturated fat; 1 g polyunsaturated fat; 28 g carbohydrate; 2 g fiber; 2 g sugar; 292 mg phosphorus; 44 mg calcium; 174 mg sodium; 627 mg potassium; 2049 IU vitamin A; 8 mg ATE vitamin E; 3 mg vitamin C; 60 mg cholesterol

Shotgun Wedding Soup

Italian wedding soup is a favorite around our house. This hurry-up version has the traditional flavors, but not the usual long cooking. Pull some of the meatballs you made ahead of time from the freezer and have the whole thing on the table in 15 minutes.

1 tablespoon (15 ml) olive oil

¼ cup (40 g) chopped onion

1 pound (454 g) Basic Turkey Meatballs (page 244)

6 cups (1.4 L) Low-Sodium Chicken Broth (page 232)

8 ounces (225 g) orzo or other small pasta

10 ounces (280 g) frozen spinach, chopped

¼ teaspoon freshly ground black pepper

Heat the oil in a heavy saucepan over medium heat and sauté the onion until soft, about 5 minutes. Add the meatballs, broth, pasta, spinach, and pepper and cook until the pasta is tender, about 10 minutes.

Yield: 4 servings

Per serving: 474 calories (36% from fat, 28% from protein, 36% from carbohydrate); 40 g protein; 23 g total fat; 9 g saturated fat; 10 g monounsaturated fat; 2 g polyunsaturated fat; 52 g carbohydrate; 3 g fiber; 1 g sugar; 453 mg phosphorus; 156 mg calcium; 256 mg sodium; 984 mg potassium; 8549 IU vitamin A; 0 mg ATE vitamin E; 2 mg vitamin C; 78 mg cholesterol

Tip: Don't have any meatballs? Use 1 pound (454 g) ground beef and brown it along with the onion.

White Chili

Chili is usually a long cooking project, but it doesn't have to be. This chicken and white bean chili goes together quickly, but it tastes like you toiled for hours. Serve with a dollop of sour cream.

2 tablespoons (30 ml) olive oil

12 ounces (340 g) boneless skinless chicken breasts, chopped into ½-inch (1.3-cm) pieces

¾ cup (120 g) chopped onion

1 teaspoon minced garlic

1 teaspoon dried oregano

1 tablespoon (7 g) ground cumin

¼ teaspoon freshly ground black pepper

1 jalapeño pepper, seeded and chopped

¼ teaspoon hot pepper sauce

2 cups (470 ml) Low-Sodium Chicken Broth (page 232)

4 cups (728 g) no-salt-added navy beans

Heat the oil in a Dutch oven over medium heat. Add the chicken, onion, garlic, oregano, cumin, black pepper, and jalapeño. Sauté until the chicken is cooked through, about 5 minutes. Add the hot pepper sauce, broth, and beans, bring to a boil, reduce the heat to medium-low, and simmer for 5 minutes, until heated through.

Yield: 4 servings

Per serving: 452 calories (20% from fat, 34% from protein, 47% from carbohydrate); 39 g protein; 10 g total fat; 2 g saturated fat; 6 g monounsaturated fat; 2 g polyunsaturated fat; 54 g carbohydrate; 12 g fiber; 1 g sugar; 507 mg phosphorus; 168 mg calcium; 99 mg sodium; 1077 mg potassium; 91 IU vitamin A; 5 mg ATE vitamin E; 7 mg vitamin C; 49 mg cholesterol

Moroccan Chicken Salad

This different kind of chicken salad contains flavorful chicken seasoned with cumin then paired with the sweetness of carrots, raisins, spinach, and a generous amount of fresh cilantro in a moderately spicy dressing.

5 tablespoons (75 ml) olive oil, divided

1½ pounds (680 g) boneless skinless chicken breasts, cut into strips

1 teaspoon ground cumin

¼ teaspoon freshly ground black pepper

3 tablespoons (45 ml) lime juice

¼ teaspoon red pepper flakes

5 ounces (140 g) fresh spinach

2 cups (32 g) chopped fresh cilantro

1 to 2 carrots, peeled into strips (1 cup [110 g])

½ cup (75 g) raisins

Heat 2 tablespoons (30 ml) of the oil in a large skillet over medium-high heat. Season the chicken with the cumin and pepper. Cook the chicken until golden brown and cooked through, about 2 minutes per side. In a small bowl, whisk together the lime juice, red pepper flakes, and remaining 3 tablespoons

(45 ml) oil. In a large bowl, combine the cooked chicken, spinach, cilantro, carrots, and raisins, pour over the dressing, and toss to combine.

Yield: 4 servings

Per serving: 430 calories (40% from fat, 38% from protein, 21% from carbohydrate); 42 g protein; 20 g total fat; 3 g saturated fat; 13 g monounsaturated fat; 2 g polyunsaturated fat; 23 g carbohydrate; 3 g fiber; 14 g sugar; 399 mg phosphorus; 97 mg calcium; 177 mg sodium; 1029 mg potassium; 8637 IU vitamin A; 11 mg ATE vitamin E; 26 mg vitamin C; 99 mg cholesterol

Creamy Chicken Salad

The dressing of this chicken salad starts like a traditional mayonnaise-based dressing, then is made extra creamy by the addition of cream cheese. The addition of sunflower seeds and sprouts gives it a delicious, nutty crunch. This is great simply served over lettuce or as a sandwich filling stuffed into pita pockets.

2 cups (280 g) cooked diced chicken breast

1 cup (120 g) finely diced celery

1 tablespoon (4 g) finely chopped fresh parsley

½ teaspoon lemon juice

2 teaspoons skim milk

1 tablespoon (14 g) cream cheese

2 tablespoons (28 g) mayonnaise

½ cup (70 g) unsalted sunflower seeds

½ cup (20 g) alfalfa sprouts

Combine the chicken, celery, parsley, and lemon juice in a large bowl. In a small bowl, combine the milk, cream cheese, and mayonnaise. Spoon over the chicken mixture, toss to coat evenly, and chill in the refrigerator for at least a half hour. Just before serving, add the sunflower seeds and top with the alfalfa sprouts.

Yield: 6 servings

Per serving: 163 calories (48% from fat, 42% from protein, 10% from carbohydrate); 17 g protein; 9 g total fat; 2 g saturated fat; 2 g monounsaturated fat; 4 g polyunsaturated fat; 4 g carbohydrate; 2 g fiber; 1 g sugar; 241 mg phosphorus; 29 mg calcium; 65 mg sodium; 275 mg potassium; 195 IU vitamin A; 13 mg ATE vitamin E; 2 mg vitamin C; 43 mg cholesterol

California Chicken Wrap

You almost know if the name says "California" that you're going to find avocado. And you'd be right in this case where it's paired with leftover chicken (or turkey breast) and red onion in these tasty wraps.

4 tablespoons (56 g) mayonnaise

4 whole wheat tortillas

1 cup (70 g) shredded lettuce

1 tomato, thinly sliced

1 red onion, thinly sliced

1 avocado, peeled, pitted, and sliced lengthwise

6 ounces (168 g) chicken breast, cooked, cooled, and thinly sliced

(continued on page 98)

Spread 1 tablespoon (14 g) of mayonnaise on each tortilla. Place some lettuce in the center of each wrap and top with the tomato, onion, avocado, and sliced chicken. Fold in the left and right sides of the wrap toward the center, and roll the bottom edge of the tortilla into a burrito shape. Cut the wrap in half to serve.

Yield: 4 servings

Per serving: 304 calories (39% from fat, 23% from protein, 38% from carbohydrate); 18 g protein; 13 g total fat; 2 g saturated fat; 7 g monounsaturated fat; 3 g polyunsaturated fat; 30 g carbohydrate; 5 g fiber; 3 g sugar; 183 mg phosphorus; 40 mg calcium; 208 mg sodium; 538 mg potassium; 427 IU vitamin A; 3 mg ATE vitamin E; 12 mg vitamin C; 40 mg cholesterol

Chicken Soft Tacos

Leftover chicken makes quick and easy work of these simple tacos. The flavor is not typically Mexican, with only chicken, veggies, and cheese, but with the flavor of the guacamole and fresh tomatoes you won't miss the seasonings. If you prefer more Mexican flavor, add a dollop of salsa or sprinkle with Mexican seasoning.

¼ cup (65 g) guacamole

8 corn tortillas, warmed

1 cup (140 g) shredded cooked chicken, warmed

1 cup (70 g) shredded iceberg lettuce

¼ cup (45 g) finely chopped Roma tomatoes

½ cup (60 g) grated Cheddar cheese

Spread ½ tablespoon (8 g) of the guacamole down the center of each warmed tortilla. Top with 2 tablespoons (18 g) of the warmed chicken and the lettuce, tomato, and cheese. Fold into a taco and serve.

Yield: 8 tacos, 4 servings

Per serving: 233 calories (40% from fat, 28% from protein, 32% from carbohydrate); 17 g protein; 10 g total fat; 5 g saturated fat; 4 g monounsaturated fat; 1 g polyunsaturated fat; 19 g carbohydrate; 3 g fiber; 1 g sugar; 279 mg phosphorus; 194 mg calcium; 195 mg sodium; 247 mg potassium; 320 IU vitamin A; 48 mg ATE vitamin E; 3 mg vitamin C; 48 mg cholesterol

Quick Chick Burritos

There are no fancy seasonings here, just simple food that goes together well. Leftover rice and chicken make these burritos especially quick to fix. Or microwave a bag of "Instant" Rice (page 228).

1⅓ cups (95 g) broccoli florets

2 cups (280 g) sliced cooked chicken breast

1⅓ cups (215 g) cooked brown rice

4 flour tortillas

2 cups (220 g) shredded Swiss cheese

Place the broccoli in a microwave-safe bowl, cover loosely with waxed paper, and steam in the microwave until tender, 3 minutes. Heat the chicken and rice in the microwave. Warm the tortillas in the microwave for 10 seconds. Place ½ cup (70 g) of chicken on the bottom third of each tortilla, followed by ⅓ cup (55 g) of brown rice, then ⅓ cup (24 g) of broccoli. Evenly sprinkle ½ cup (55 g) of cheese over the broccoli. Roll each tortilla into a burrito. Cut each burrito in half, on the diagonal, and serve hot.

Yield: 4 servings

Per serving: 602 calories (37% from fat, 32% from protein, 31% from carbohydrate); 48 g protein; 24 g total fat; 13 g saturated fat; 8 g monounsaturated fat; 2 g polyunsaturated fat; 46 g carbohydrate; 5 g fiber; 2 g sugar; 696 mg phosphorus; 729 mg calcium; 286 mg sodium; 451 mg potassium; 1240 IU vitamin A; 143 mg ATE vitamin E; 25 mg vitamin C; 120 mg cholesterol

Leftover Turkey Casserole

This makes a great use for leftover Thanksgiving turkey when you are tired of "another Thanksgiving dinner that couldn't be beat" (as Arlo Guthrie put it). Since I also make a batch of condensed cream of mushroom soup for a Thanksgiving green bean casserole, I make extra for a dinner like this one.

2 cups (280 g) chopped cooked turkey

2 cups (330 g) cooked rice

1 cup (235 ml) Condensed Cream of Mushroom Soup (page 31)

12 ounces (336 g) frozen mixed vegetables

½ cup (55 g) shredded Swiss cheese

Combine the turkey, rice, soup, and vegetables in a skillet. Simmer over medium heat until the vegetables are cooked through, about 10 minutes. Sprinkle the cheese over the top and serve.

Yield: 3 servings

Per serving: 465 calories (21% from fat, 36% from protein, 44% from carbohydrate); 40 g protein; 10 g total fat; 5 g saturated fat; 3 g monounsaturated fat; 2 g polyunsaturated fat; 50 g carbohydrate; 5 g fiber; 5 g sugar; 462 mg phosphorus; 275 mg calcium; 116 mg sodium; 779 mg potassium; 4228 IU vitamin A; 48 mg ATE vitamin E; 3 mg vitamin C; 114 mg cholesterol

Easter Monday Turkey Casserole

Here's a little different take on leftover turkey than the last one. I used to make a similar dish with leftover ham and hard-cooked eggs after Easter, but now we usually have turkey to keep the sodium level lower, so I've converted to this recipe. It is good over noodles or potatoes.

1 cup (140 g) chopped cooked turkey

2 hard-boiled eggs, chopped

1 cup (235 ml) Condensed Cream of Mushroom Soup (page 31)

1 cup (100 g) chopped celery

½ cup (225 g) mayonnaise

1 teaspoon onion flakes

(continued on page 100)

Combine all the ingredients in a large saucepan. Simmer over medium heat until warmed through, about 10 minutes.

Yield: 2 servings

Per serving: 416 calories (48% from fat, 30% from protein, 22% from carbohydrate); 31 g protein; 22 g total fat; 5 g saturated fat; 6 g monounsaturated fat; 8 g polyunsaturated fat; 22 g carbohydrate; 2 g fiber; 4 g sugar; 343 mg phosphorus; 90 mg calcium; 266 mg sodium; 914 mg potassium; 678 IU vitamin A; 117 mg ATE vitamin E; 2 mg vitamin C; 374 mg cholesterol

Tip: This is also an excellent casserole to use with leftover chicken.

Thanksgiving Friday Turkey Sandwich

It seems like most of my turkey recipes are uses for the remainder of holiday birds. But what a great way to use leftover turkey. The guacamole really sets off the turkey flavor and makes it different from the traditional turkey dinner, so you don't get tired of the same old thing.

1 tablespoon (14 g) mayonnaise

2 Slices Low-Sodium Whole Wheat Bread (page 312), toasted if desired

1 teaspoon Dijon mustard

2 ounces (56 g) turkey breast, sliced

2 tablespoons (28 g) guacamole

½ cup (26 g) salad greens

2 ounces (56 g) Swiss cheese, sliced

2 slices tomato

Spread the mayonnaise on one slice of toast, then spread mustard on the other. Arrange the sliced turkey on one side. Spread guacamole over the turkey. Pile on the salad greens and top with the cheese and tomato slices, then place the remaining slice of toast on top.

Yield: 1 serving

Per serving: 518 calories (42% from fat, 28% from protein, 31% from carbohydrate); 36 g protein; 24 g total fat; 12 g saturated fat; 8 g monounsaturated fat; 3 g polyunsaturated fat; 40 g carbohydrate; 6 g fiber; 11 g sugar; 584 mg phosphorus; 622 mg calcium; 140 mg sodium; 752 mg potassium; 1348 IU vitamin A; 120 mg ATE vitamin E; 15 mg vitamin C; 90 mg cholesterol

Turkey Almond Pitas

With just enough added flavor from celery and scallions, this is a great use for leftover turkey. The almonds add a little extra flavor to what might otherwise be considered boring turkey salad.

2 cups (280 g) diced cooked turkey

½ cup (50 g) sliced celery

¼ cup (25 g) sliced scallion

¼ teaspoon freshly ground black pepper

¼ cup (27 g) sliced unsalted almonds

½ cup (112 g) mayonnaise

6 lettuce leaves

3 pita breads, cut in half

Combine the turkey, celery, scallion, pepper, almonds, and mayonnaise in a medium bowl, mixing well. Cover and refrigerate for several hours to allow the flavors to blend. When ready to serve, place a lettuce leaf in each pita pocket and then stuff with the filling.

Yield: 6 servings

Per serving: 233 calories (32% from fat, 31% from protein, 37% from carbohydrate); 18 g protein; 8 g total fat; 1 g saturated fat; 3 g monounsaturated fat; 3 g polyunsaturated fat; 22 g carbohydrate; 2 g fiber; 1 g sugar; 159 mg phosphorus; 55 mg calcium; 223 mg sodium; 240 mg potassium; 91 IU vitamin A; 0 mg ATE vitamin E; 1 mg vitamin C; 50 mg cholesterol

Tip: This filling may also be served heated.

Turkey Salad with Tomato and Avocado

This is a particularly easy salad, full of flavorful ingredients such as turkey, avocado, and red onion, with a simple balsamic vinaigrette dressing.

6 cups (330 g) lettuce, torn into pieces

8 ounces (225 g) cooked turkey, thinly sliced

2 tomatoes, cut into wedges

1 avocado, seeded, peeled, and cut into bite-size pieces

½ cup (80 g) thinly sliced red onion

½ cup (50 g) grated Parmesan cheese

¼ cup (60 ml) olive oil

2 tablespoons (30 ml) balsamic vinegar

¼ teaspoon freshly ground black pepper

Divide the lettuce, turkey, tomatoes, avocado, onion, and Parmesan among 4 bowls. In a small bowl, whisk together the oil, vinegar, and pepper. Drizzle over the salad and toss.

Yield: 4 servings

Per serving: 364 calories (62% from fat, 26% from protein, 13% from carbohydrate); 24 g protein; 26 g total fat; 5 g saturated fat; 16 g monounsaturated fat; 3 g polyunsaturated fat; 12 g carbohydrate; 5 g fiber; 3 g sugar; 274 mg phosphorus; 181 mg calcium; 248 mg sodium; 713 mg potassium; 849 IU vitamin A; 15 mg ATE vitamin E; 28 mg vitamin C; 67 mg cholesterol

7

15-Minute Beef Dishes

You may think that beef is not a good choice for quick meals, but that is not necessarily the case. You just need to be careful about the cut of beef and preparation method you choose. You probably don't want to start with something such as chuck, which benefits from long, slow cooking to make it tender, but ground beef cooks quickly and is used in a number of these recipes. And then there's steak. It can easily be cooked in less than 15 minutes (especially if you are like me and prefer it medium-rare). I also make use of the microwave to speed cooking times for things such as meatloaf that usually require a long time in the conventional oven. And there are more mock kabobs, which provide a number of international flavor options and cook quickly under the broiler.

15-Minute Meatloaf

Yes, you can fix a meatloaf in 15 minutes, as this recipe demonstrates. And the best part about it is that it still tastes just like you expect meatloaf to taste, which is to say great!

2 pounds (908 g) extra-lean ground beef

¼ cup (62 g) egg substitute, or 1 egg

¼ cup (60 g) no-salt-added ketchup

¾ cup (60 g) quick-cooking oats

½ teaspoon freshly ground black pepper

2 tablespoons (18 g) Onion Soup Mix (page 34)

Combine all the ingredients in a large bowl and mix well. Form a ring with the meat mixture in a round microwave-safe pan, leaving a hole in the middle at least 2 inches (5 cm) wide. Microwave on high for 12 to 15 minutes, until the meatloaf is firm and no longer pink in the center.

Yield: 6 servings

Per serving: 315 calories (60% from fat, 31% from protein, 10% from carbohydrate); 31 g protein; 27 g total fat; 10 g saturated fat; 12 g monounsaturated fat; 1 g polyunsaturated fat; 10 g carbohydrate; 1 g fiber; 3 g sugar; 278 mg phosphorus; 24 mg calcium; 119 mg sodium; 550 mg potassium; 142 IU vitamin A; 0 mg ATE vitamin E; 2 mg vitamin C; 104 mg cholesterol

Meatloaf in a Mug

Ever have that feeling that you really wish you had a nice slice of leftover meatloaf for lunch? If there isn't one in the refrigerator, try this quick solution. It is a little more subtly flavored than most oven-baked meatloaf, with its Worcestershire sauce and scallions instead of the more traditional tomato and egg, but it is most definitely a real meatloaf.

1 Slice Low-Sodium Bread (page 312), torn into pieces

2 tablespoons (30 ml) skim milk

½ teaspoon Worcestershire sauce

4 ounces (115 g) extra-lean ground beef

2 tablespoons (12 g) thinly sliced scallion

⅛ teaspoon freshly ground black pepper

Place the torn bread into a small bowl and pour in the milk and Worcestershire sauce; set aside for a few minutes for the bread to absorb the liquid. Add the ground beef, scallion, and pepper to the bread; mix well and place in a 10-ounce (280-g) microwave-safe mug. Cook in the microwave at 70 percent power until the meatloaf is firm and no longer pink in the center, 4 to 5½ minutes depending on the microwave. Remove the meatloaf from the microwave, and allow to stand for 2 minutes before serving.

Yield: 1 serving

Per serving: 276 calories (54% from fat, 29% from protein, 17% from carbohydrate); 25 g protein; 20 g total fat; 8 g saturated fat; 9 g monounsaturated fat; 1 g polyunsaturated fat; 15 g

(continued on page 104)

carbohydrate; 1 g fiber; 2 g sugar; 240 mg phosphorus; 88 mg calcium; 128 mg sodium; 486 mg potassium; 191 IU vitamin A; 19 mg ATE vitamin E; 7 mg vitamin C; 79 mg cholesterol

Beef Cutlets in Mushroom Sauce

Quick and easy beef patties simmer in a creamy mushroom sauce so they come out loaded with flavor. The sauce is perfect over mashed potatoes or noodles for a real comfort food meal.

1 pound (454 g) extra-lean ground beef

½ cup (120 ml) skim milk, divided

¼ teaspoon freshly ground black pepper

1½ teaspoons Worcestershire sauce

1 tablespoon (8 g) all-purpose flour

1 tablespoon (15 ml) olive oil

1 cup (235 ml) Condensed Cream of Mushroom Soup (page 31)

Combine the beef, ¼ cup (60 ml) of the milk, the pepper, and the Worcestershire sauce in a bowl, mixing well. Shape into 4 oblong patties ½-inch (1.3-cm) thick. Dip into the flour. Heat the oil in a skillet over medium heat, add the patties, and brown on both sides, about a minute per side. Drain off the fat. Dilute the soup with remaining ¼ cup (60 ml) milk and pour over the patties. Cover and simmer over medium heat for 10 minutes, or until desired doneness.

Yield: 4 servings

Per serving: 276 calories (63% from fat, 27% from protein, 10% from carbohydrate); 23 g protein; 24 g total fat; 9 g saturated fat; 11 g monounsaturated fat; 2 g polyunsaturated fat; 9 g carbohydrate; 0 g fiber; 1 g sugar; 230 mg phosphorus; 60 mg calcium; 124 mg sodium; 630 mg potassium; 76 IU vitamin A; 20 mg ATE vitamin E; 4 mg vitamin C; 81 mg cholesterol

Microwave Shepherd's Pie

Everyone knows what to expect when you say "shepherd's pie," layers of beef, vegetables, and potatoes topped with cheese. That's exactly what this classic comfort food is. The only difference from most shepherd's pie is that this one cooks quickly in the microwave.

1 can (8 ounces, or 225 g) no-salt-added tomato sauce

1 pound (454 g) extra-lean ground beef

2 cups (140 g) broccoli florets

2 cups (450 g) mashed potatoes, leftover or instant

1 cup (110 g) shredded Swiss cheese

In a medium bowl, combine the tomato sauce and ground beef, mixing well. Spread into a high-sided 9-inch (23-cm) square microwave-safe dish. Spread the broccoli on top. Spread the mashed potatoes over the broccoli, then sprinkle with the cheese. Microwave on high for 10 minutes, or until the beef is no longer pink in the middle.

Yield: 4 servings

Per serving: 471 calories (57% from fat, 25% from protein, 18% from carbohydrate); 35 g protein; 35 g total fat; 15 g saturated fat; 13 g monounsaturated fat; 3 g polyunsaturated fat; 24 g carbohydrate; 4 g fiber; 4 g sugar; 466 mg phosphorus; 405 mg calcium; 138 mg sodium; 953 mg potassium; 988 IU vitamin A; 114 mg ATE vitamin E; 57 mg vitamin C; 113 mg cholesterol

Open-Faced Flavor Burgers

This recipe had me stumped for a title. I can describe these burgers, with their complex sauce, featuring things such as horseradish, Worcestershire, mustard, and onion. They're classy, classic, rich, and any number of other adjectives. But they really are hard to define in any term that tells you what to expect. So you may just have to try them and see what you'd call them.

1 pound (454 g) extra-lean ground beef

1½ teaspoons Worcestershire sauce

1½ teaspoons prepared horseradish

1 teaspoon freshly ground black pepper

⅓ cup (75 g) Chili Sauce (page 233)

1½ teaspoons mustard

1 teaspoon minced onion

2 hamburger buns

Preheat the broiler and place the oven rack 6 inches (15 cm) below the heat source. In a large bowl, combine the beef, Worcestershire sauce, horseradish, pepper, chili sauce, mustard, and onion, mixing well. Cut the buns

in half and spread with the meat mixture. Place on a baking sheet and broil until cooked through, about 8 to 10 minutes.

Yield: 4 servings

Per serving: 263 calories (57% from fat, 29% from protein, 15% from carbohydrate); 24 g protein; 21 g total fat; 8 g saturated fat; 9 g monounsaturated fat; 1 g polyunsaturated fat; 12 g carbohydrate; 1 g fiber; 3 g sugar; 190 mg phosphorus; 38 mg calcium; 225 mg sodium; 387 mg potassium; 340 IU vitamin A; 0 mg ATE vitamin E; 8 mg vitamin C; 78 mg cholesterol

Tip: If you have homemade low-sodium buns, you can save about half the sodium.

Smoky Hamburgers

Liquid smoke and Worcestershire sauce set off the flavor of these burgers, giving them a taste that's not quite classic barbecue, but is really good.

1 pound (454 g) extra-lean ground beef

1 tablespoon (15 ml) Worcestershire sauce

1 tablespoon (15 ml) liquid smoke

1 teaspoon garlic powder

1 tablespoon (15 ml) olive oil

Prepare a grill for high heat. In a medium bowl, lightly mix together the ground beef, Worcestershire sauce, liquid smoke, and garlic powder. Form into 3 patties, handling as little as possible. Brush both sides of each patty with some oil. Place the patties on the grill

(continued on page 106)

grate, and cook for about 5 minutes per side, until desired doneness.

Yield: 3 servings

Per serving: 303 calories (69% from fat, 29% from protein, 2% from carbohydrate); 29 g protein; 30 g total fat; 11 g saturated fat; 15 g monounsaturated fat; 2 g polyunsaturated fat; 2 g carbohydrate; 0 g fiber; 0 g sugar; 222 mg phosphorus; 11 mg calcium; 149 mg sodium; 480 mg potassium; 5 IU vitamin A; 0 mg ATE vitamin E; 9 mg vitamin C; 104 mg cholesterol

Asian Burgers

There used to be a mix to make Asian-style hamburgers. I don't believe it exists anymore, and even if it did, it would be loaded with sodium. But these burgers, flavored with soy sauce, ginger, and typical Asian vegetables, recreate that taste. They make great sandwiches or the meat portion of a more complete meal with rice and stir-fried vegetables.

1 tablespoon (15 ml) sesame oil

1 tablespoon (15 ml) Low-Sodium Soy Sauce (page 29)

½ teaspoon garlic powder

½ teaspoon ground ginger

½ teaspoon onion powder

½ teaspoon freshly ground black pepper

1 pound (454 g) extra-lean ground beef

¼ cup (25 g) chopped scallion

½ can (4 ounces, or 115 g) water chestnuts, drained and diced

1 tablespoon (15 ml) olive oil

In a medium bowl, knead together the sesame oil, soy sauce, garlic powder, ginger, onion powder, pepper, ground beef, scallion, and water chestnuts until evenly combined; form into 4 patties. Heat the oil in a skillet over medium-high heat. Cook the burgers to the desired doneness, about 5 minutes per side for well done.

Yield: 4 servings

Per serving: 294 calories (65% from fat, 24% from protein, 11% from carbohydrate); 22 g protein; 26 g total fat; 9 g saturated fat; 12 g monounsaturated fat; 3 g polyunsaturated fat; 10 g carbohydrate; 1 g fiber; 2 g sugar; 192 mg phosphorus; 20 mg calcium; 91 mg sodium; 566 mg potassium; 63 IU vitamin A; 0 mg ATE vitamin E; 3 mg vitamin C; 78 mg cholesterol

Open-Faced Mexican Hamburgers

Great-tasting Mexican-spiced beef atop toasted buns. And all in 15 minutes or less. To set it off even more, top with a slice of Swiss cheese and a dollop of salsa.

2 hamburger buns, split in half

1 pound (454 g) extra-lean ground beef

¼ cup (62 g) egg substitute, or 1 egg

2 tablespoons (16 g) all-purpose flour

1 tablespoon (8 g) chili powder

1 teaspoon ground cumin

Place the oven rack about 5 inches (12.7 cm) from the heat source. Place the buns on a baking sheet and broil on one side until toasted, about 1 minute. Combine the beef, egg, flour, chili powder, and cumin in a bowl, mixing well, and spread the meat to the edge of each bun. Return to the oven and broil for 10 minutes, or to the desired doneness.

Yield: 4 servings

Per serving: 284 calories (55% from fat, 29% from protein, 16% from carbohydrate); 26 g protein; 22 g total fat; 8 g saturated fat; 9 g monounsaturated fat; 1 g polyunsaturated fat; 14 g carbohydrate; 2 g fiber; 2 g sugar; 217 mg phosphorus; 47 mg calcium; 218 mg sodium; 457 mg potassium; 619 IU vitamin A; 0 mg ATE vitamin E; 1 mg vitamin C; 78 mg cholesterol

Parmesan Beef Patties

These are almost like mini Italian meatloaves. They are tasty beef patties in a creamy Italian accented onion sauce and are great over egg noodles or just about anything.

1 cup (160 g) sliced onion

1 tablespoon (14 g) unsalted butter

¼ cup (60 g) sour cream

¼ teaspoon Italian seasoning

1 pound (454 g) extra-lean ground beef

¼ cup (30 g) Italian-Style Bread Crumbs (page 33)

¼ cup (25 g) grated Parmesan cheese

⅓ cup (80 ml) skim milk

⅛ teaspoon freshly ground black pepper

Combine the onion and butter in a small microwave-safe dish. Microwave on high, uncovered, for 4 to 5 minutes, or until the onion is tender, stirring once. Add the sour cream and seasoning; set aside. Combine the beef, bread crumbs, cheese, milk, and pepper in a medium bowl; mix well. Shape into 4 patties. Place on a meat rack or glass dish and cover with waxed paper. Microwave on high for 6 to 7 minutes, or until desired doneness. Top each with some of the onion mixture.

Yield: 4 servings

Per serving: 318 calories (61% from fat, 27% from protein, 12% from carbohydrate); 26 g protein; 26 g total fat; 12 g saturated fat; 10 g monounsaturated fat; 1 g polyunsaturated fat; 11 g carbohydrate; 1 g fiber; 2 g sugar; 265 mg phosphorus; 140 mg calcium; 193 mg sodium; 467 mg potassium; 223 IU vitamin A; 59 mg ATE vitamin E; 3 mg vitamin C; 98 mg cholesterol

Quick and Sloppy Joes

Well, if you're quick, you are often sloppy. But in this case, these sandwiches are just sloppy enough to be a hit. And the taste is exactly what you'd expect with their lightly seasoned tomato sauce. It's meal I have found that kids just love.

1 pound (454 g) extra-lean ground beef

1 can (8 ounces, or 225 g) no-salt-added tomato sauce

1 tablespoon (11 g) mustard

(continued on page 108)

1 tablespoon (10 g) minced onion

6 hamburger buns

Cook the beef in a skillet over medium heat until browned, about 5 minutes. Pour off the fat. Add the tomato sauce, mustard, and onion, stir to combine, and cook until heated through, 1 to 2 minutes. Serve on the hamburger buns.

Yield: 6 servings

Per serving: 258 calories (46% from fat, 25% from protein, 29% from carbohydrate); 19 g protein; 16 g total fat; 6 g saturated fat; 7 g monounsaturated fat; 1 g polyunsaturated fat; 22 g carbohydrate; 2 g fiber; 4 g sugar; 172 mg phosphorus; 53 mg calcium; 251 mg sodium; 431 mg potassium; 133 IU vitamin A; 0 mg ATE vitamin E; 5 mg vitamin C; 52 mg cholesterol

Barbecue Sloppy Joes

This is a classic family meal and so easy you can have it any night you want. Starting with prepared barbecue sauce means that you can get a lot of flavor with few ingredients and little fuss.

2 tablespoons (30 ml) olive oil

1 cup (160 g) diced onion

1 pound (454 g) extra-lean ground beef

2 cups (500 g) Barbecue Sauce (page 30)

4 hamburger buns

Heat the oil in a skillet and sauté the onion over low heat until lightly browned, 5 minutes. Add the ground beef and cook until browned,

about 5 minutes. Add the barbecue sauce and cook, stirring, until heated through, 1 to 2 minutes. Serve on the hamburger buns.

Yield: 4 servings

Per serving: 467 calories (44% from fat, 17% from protein, 39% from carbohydrate); 23 g protein; 26 g total fat; 9 g saturated fat; 13 g monounsaturated fat; 2 g polyunsaturated fat; 52 g carbohydrate; 1 g fiber; 38 g sugar; 171 mg phosphorus; 17 mg calcium; 108 mg sodium; 380 mg potassium; 1 IU vitamin A; 0 mg ATE vitamin E; 3 mg vitamin C; 78 mg cholesterol

Tip: Top with a slice of Swiss cheese for extra flavor.

Hamburger Hash

This variation on hash contains ground meat and rice, rather than the more common roast beef and potatoes. This is the kind of thing I love to make for lunch on the weekend, something quick, filling, and tasty that doesn't keep me in the kitchen for long.

1 pound (454 g) extra-lean ground beef

1 cup (160 g) chopped onion

1 cup (150 g) chopped green bell pepper

1 garlic clove, minced

1 teaspoon freshly ground black pepper

1 tablespoon (8 g) chili powder

1 can (14.5 ounces, or 411 g) no-salt-added tomatoes

¾ cup (124 g) cooked rice

In a large heavy pan, brown the meat over medium heat, stirring continuously to break up any large pieces, about 5 minutes. Drain off all but 1 tablespoon (15 ml) of fat. Stir in the onion, bell pepper, and garlic. Cook, stirring, until the onion is tender, about 5 minutes. Season with black pepper and chili powder, then add the tomatoes and rice and cook until heated through, 2 to 3 minutes.

Yield: 4 servings

Per serving: 280 calories (51% from fat, 27% from protein, 22% trom carbohydrate); 24 g protein; 20 g total fat; 8 g saturated fat; 9 g monounsaturated fat; 1 g polyunsaturated fat; 19 g carbohydrate; 3 g fiber; 6 g sugar; 215 mg phosphorus; 58 mg calcium; 106 mg sodium; 716 mg potassium; 825 IU vitamin A; 0 mg ATE vitamin E; 48 mg vitamin C; 78 mg cholesterol

Bourbon-Sauced Steak

Not many sauces are good enough that I want to put them on a rib-eye steak, but this one is. Longer marinating would give it even more flavor, but I like the subtle flavor that is imparted in minutes. The use of ingredients such as lemon juice, Worcestershire sauce, and bourbon ensures that the flavor will be absorbed quickly.

1 cup (235 ml) water

⅔ cup (160 ml) bourbon

2 tablespoons (30 ml) Low-Sodium Soy Sauce (page 29)

¼ cup (60 g) packed brown sugar

3 tablespoons (45 ml) Worcestershire sauce

2 tablespoons (30 ml) lemon juice

1½ pounds (680 g) beef rib-eye steak

Whisk together the water, bourbon, soy sauce, brown sugar, Worcestershire sauce, and lemon juice in a bowl, and pour into a resealable bag large enough to hold the steak. Add the steak, turn to coat with the marinade, squeeze out the excess air, and seal the bag. Let marinate for 5 minutes.

While the steak marinates, prepare a grill for high heat, and lightly oil the grate. Remove the steak from the marinade, letting the extra drip back into the bag. Grill the steak over high heat, 1 to 2 minutes per side, to sear the meat. Move the steak to a cooler part of the grill and cook for an additional 2 to 3 minutes per side for medium-rare, or until the desired doneness. Brush with the marinade during grilling.

Yield: 4 servings

Per serving: 433 calories (38% from fat, 42% from protein, 20% from carbohydrate); 35 g protein; 14 g total fat; 5 g saturated fat; 6 g monounsaturated fat; 0 g polyunsaturated fat; 17 g carbohydrate; 0 g fiber; 14 g sugar; 359 mg phosphorus; 32 mg calcium; 244 mg sodium; 797 mg potassium; 13 IU vitamin A; 0 mg ATE vitamin E; 24 mg vitamin C; 100 mg cholesterol

Even Better Steak

Usually I say that there is nothing better than plain grilled steak, but this recipe just might

(continued on page 110)

be the one to change my mind. Flank steak is a great choice for quick recipes because it is most tender when cooked quickly and thinly sliced.

1½ cups (90 g) fresh parsley leaves

¼ cup (25 g) coarsely chopped scallion

2 tablespoons (30 ml) lemon juice

½ teaspoon minced garlic

½ teaspoon Dijon mustard

⅓ cup (80 ml) olive oil

1½ pounds (680 g) flank steak

Pulse the parsley, scallion, lemon juice, garlic, mustard, and olive oil in a food processor until slightly chunky. Prepare a grill for high heat or place a grill pan over high heat. Grill the steak until the desired doneness, 4 to 5 minutes per side for medium-rare, turning once. Transfer to a cutting board and thinly slice the steak against the grain. Serve with the sauce.

Yield: 5 servings

Per serving: 402 calories (59% from fat, 39% from protein, 2% from carbohydrate); 39 g protein; 26 g total fat; 7 g saturated fat; 15 g monounsaturated fat; 2 g polyunsaturated fat; 2 g carbohydrate; 1 g fiber; 0 g sugar; 301 mg phosphorus; 50 mg calcium; 93 mg sodium; 583 mg potassium; 1568 IU vitamin A; 0 mg ATE vitamin E; 28 mg vitamin C; 75 mg cholesterol

Montreal Steak

This dish is a classic steakhouse steak. The seasoning blend is similar in flavor to the commercial Montreal steak seasoning, but without all the sodium.

2 teaspoons paprika

1½ teaspoons freshly ground black pepper

¾ teaspoon onion powder

¾ teaspoon garlic powder

¼ teaspoon cayenne pepper

¾ teaspoon coriander

¾ teaspoon turmeric

1½ pounds (680 g) beef rib-eye steak, at room temperature

Prepare a grill for high heat and lightly oil the grate. Stir the spices together in a small bowl. Rub the steak on both sides with the seasoning mixture. Grill until the desired doneness, 3 to 3½ minutes per side for medium-rare, turning once.

Yield: 4 servings

Per serving: 285 calories (47% from fat, 50% from protein, 3% from carbohydrate); 35 g protein; 14 g total fat; 6 g saturated fat; 6 g monounsaturated fat; 1 g polyunsaturated fat; 2 g carbohydrate; 1 g fiber; 0 g sugar; 344 mg phosphorus; 27 mg calcium; 109 mg sodium; 699 mg potassium; 661 IU vitamin A; 0 mg ATE vitamin E; 2 mg vitamin C; 100 mg cholesterol

Garlic Beer Steak

Garlic and beer provide all the subtle flavor boosts that this steak needs. When you start with great steak you don't need very much.

12 ounces (355 ml) beer

1 teaspoon minced garlic

1 teaspoon freshly ground black pepper

2 tablespoons (30 ml) lemon juice

1½ pounds (680 g) beef rib-eye steak

Prepare a grill for high heat and lightly oil the grate. In a shallow glass dish, combine the beer, garlic, pepper, and lemon juice. Mix well. Place the steak in the marinade, turning to coat. Allow to sit for 5 minutes. Remove the steak from the marinade, and discard the marinade. Grill the steak for about 5 minutes on each side, or to the desired doneness.

Yield: 4 servings

Per serving: 321 calories (46% from fat, 50% from protein, 3% from carbohydrate); 35 g protein; 14 g total fat; 6 g saturated fat; 6 g monounsaturated fat; 0 g polyunsaturated fat; 2 g carbohydrate; 0 g fiber; 0 g sugar; 346 mg phosphorus; 25 mg calcium; 110 mg sodium; 669 mg potassium; 3 IU vitamin A; 0 mg ATE vitamin E; 4 mg vitamin C; 100 mg cholesterol

Country-Fried Steak

You might know country-fried steak as chicken-fried steak, depending on where you live. It is another classic Southern comfort food with lightly breaded cube steak fried and served with a cream gravy. Serve it the classic way with mashed potatoes to soak up the gravy.

3 tablespoons skim milk

2 egg whites

8 tablespoons (60 g) all-purpose flour, divided

½ teaspoon onion powder

¼ teaspoon garlic powder

¼ teaspoon freshly ground black pepper

1 pound (454 g) beef cube steaks

2 teaspoons olive oil

8 ounces (225 g) mushrooms, quartered

2 cups (470 ml) Low-Sodium Beef Broth (page 231)

Combine the milk and egg whites in a shallow dish, stirring with a whisk. Combine 5 tablespoons (38 g) of the flour, onion powder, garlic powder, and pepper in a shallow dish. Working with 1 steak at a time, dip into the egg mixture, then dredge in the flour mixture. Repeat with the remaining steaks. Heat the oil in a large nonstick skillet over medium-high heat. Add the steaks; cook for 3 minutes on each side, or until browned. Remove the steaks from the pan and keep warm. Add the mushrooms to the pan and sauté for 3 minutes. In a small bowl, combine the remaining 3 tablespoons (22 g) flour and the broth, stirring with a whisk. Add the broth mixture to the pan, bring to a boil over high heat, and cook for 1 minute, stirring constantly. Spoon over the steaks.

Yield: 4 servings

Per serving: 259 calories (24% from fat, 52% from protein, 24% from carbohydrate); 33 g protein; 7 g total fat; 2 g saturated fat; 3 g monounsaturated fat; 1 g polyunsaturated fat; 15 g

(continued on page 112)

carbohydrate; 1 g fiber; 1 g sugar; 352 mg phosphorus; 56 mg calcium; 180 mg sodium; 737 mg potassium; 24 IU vitamin A; 7 mg ATE vitamin E; 2 mg vitamin C; 52 mg cholesterol

Beef with Snow Peas

This dish is just like you would get from a Chinese takeout place, and is just as fast. It's made with a traditional, slightly sweet soy and ginger sauce and typical ingredients, but it has a lot less sodium and is a lot less expensive. Serve over rice for a complete meal.

3 tablespoons (45 ml) Low-Sodium Soy Sauce (page 29)

2 tablespoons (30 ml) rice wine

1 tablespoon (15 g) packed brown sugar

½ teaspoon cornstarch

1 tablespoon (15 ml) olive oil

1 tablespoon (6 g) minced fresh ginger

1 tablespoon (10 g) minced garlic

1 pound (454 g) beef round steak, cut into thin strips

8 ounces (225 g) snow pea pods

In a small bowl, combine the soy sauce, rice wine, brown sugar, and cornstarch. Set aside. Heat the oil in a wok or skillet over medium-high heat. Stir-fry the ginger and garlic for 30 seconds. Add the steak and stir-fry for 2 minutes, or until evenly browned. Add the snow peas and stir-fry for an additional 3 minutes. Add the soy sauce mixture and bring to a boil, stirring constantly. Lower the

heat to medium and simmer until the sauce is thick and smooth, 3 to 4 minutes. Serve immediately.

Yield: 4 servings

Per serving: 240 calories (29% from fat, 50% from protein, 20% from carbohydrate); 29 g protein; 7 g total fat; 2 g saturated fat; 4 g monounsaturated fat; 1 g polyunsaturated fat; 11 g carbohydrate; 2 g fiber; 6 g sugar; 304 mg phosphorus; 60 mg calcium; 108 mg sodium; 603 mg potassium; 618 IU vitamin A; 0 mg ATE vitamin E; 35 mg vitamin C; 52 mg cholesterol

Quick Beef and Pasta Skillet Meal

This goes Hamburger Helper one better, both in time to prepare and in the healthiness of the ingredients, while producing a meal that kids and adults will both like. In fact you may just find that you like the flavor better.

1 pound (454 g) extra-lean ground beef

1 cup (160 g) chopped onion

10¾ ounces (300 g) condensed low-sodium tomato soup

¼ cup (60 ml) water

1 tablespoon (15 ml) Worcestershire sauce

½ cup (55 g) shredded Swiss cheese

2 cups (280 g) cooked pasta, such as elbows or spirals

Cook the beef and onion in a skillet over medium heat until browned, about 5 minutes. Pour off the fat. Add the soup, water,

Worcestershire, cheese, and pasta and heat through, 2 to 3 minutes.

Yield: 4 servings

Per serving: 495 calories (41% from fat, 24% from protein, 36% from carbohydrate); 34 g protein; 25 g total fat; 11 g saturated fat; 10 g monounsaturated fat; 2 g polyunsaturated fat; 50 g carbohydrate; 2 g fiber; 6 g sugar; 364 mg phosphorus; 189 mg calcium; 134 mg sodium; 595 mg potassium; 340 IU vitamin A; 40 mg ATE vitamin E; 30 mg vitamin C; 93 mg cholesterol

Steak Stroganoff

Stroganoff is another of those classic dishes that looks and tastes like it took a long while to prepare. But it doesn't have to. This stroganoff is a perfect example, classic in ingredients and taste, yet ready in minutes.

3 tablespoons (45 ml) olive oil, divided

1 cup (160 g) sliced onion

4 ounces (112 g) mushrooms, sliced

1 pound (454 g) round steak, thinly sliced

¼ cup (30 g) all-purpose flour

½ teaspoon freshly ground black pepper

8 ounces (225 g) sour cream

In skillet, heat 1 tablespoon (15 ml) of the oil and sauté the onion and mushrooms over medium heat until softened, about 5 minutes; remove from the heat and set aside. Dredge the steak in the flour. In the same skillet, heat the remaining 2 tablespoons (30 ml) oil and cook the steak over medium heat until desired

doneness, 6 to 8 minutes. Season with the pepper. Transfer to a platter and drain the fat from the skillet. Return the onion and mushrooms with their liquid to the skillet and add the sour cream. Cook over medium heat, stirring occasionally, until heated through. Serve the sauce over the steak.

Yield: 4 servings

Per serving: 402 calories (50% from fat, 37% from protein, 14% from carbohydrate); 36 g protein; 22 g total fat; 7 g saturated fat; 12 g monounsaturated fat; 2 g polyunsaturated fat; 14 g carbohydrate; 1 g fiber; 2 g sugar; 304 mg phosphorus; 78 mg calcium; 69 mg sodium; 499 mg potassium; 213 IU vitamin A; 57 mg ATE vitamin E; 4 mg vitamin C; 88 mg cholesterol

Tip: Serve with noodles.

Mama's Nacho Dinner

Or at least it might be if your mama is from Mexico. Put this Mexican dinner together in minutes. It's super quick, but healthy, with a traditional taco taste that's sure to please.

1 pound (454 g) extra-lean ground beef

1 tablespoon (9 g) Salt-Free Taco Seasoning (page 28)

1 can (8 ounces, or 225 g) no-salt-added tomato sauce

1½ cups (355 ml) water

1½ cups (285 g) instant white rice, uncooked

¼ cup (65 g) Low-Sodium Salsa (page 232)

(continued on page 114)

¼ cup (30 g) shredded Cheddar cheese

½ cup (27 g) shredded lettuce

Cook the beef and taco seasoning in a skillet over medium heat until browned, about 5 minutes. Pour off any fat. Add the tomato sauce, water, and rice and bring to a boil. Cover and cook over low heat for 5 minutes, or until the rice is tender. Top with the salsa, cheese, and lettuce.

Yield: 4 servings

Per serving: 505 calories (36% from fat, 21% from protein, 43% from carbohydrate); 29 g protein; 23 g total fat; 10 g saturated fat; 9 g monounsaturated fat; 1 g polyunsaturated fat; 61 g carbohydrate; 2 g fiber; 3 g sugar; 306 mg phosphorus; 103 mg calcium; 154 mg sodium; 665 mg potassium; 410 IU vitamin A; 21 mg ATE vitamin E; 10 mg vitamin C; 87 mg cholesterol

Mexican Roll-Ups

Take some of your leftover roast beef from the recipe on page 254 and turn it into these tasty roll-ups. Full of great tasting fresh veggies and with just a hint of Southwestern spice, they are great for a quick lunch on the run.

6 whole wheat tortillas

6 leaves romaine lettuce

1¼ pounds (568 g) roast beef, sliced

1 cup (180 g) chopped tomatoes

1 cup (150 g) chopped red bell pepper

1 cup (150 g) chopped yellow bell pepper

2 tablespoons (30 ml) olive oil

3 tablespoons (45 ml) red wine vinegar

2 tablespoons (14 g) ground cumin

For each roll-up place a tortilla on a piece of waxed paper or foil. Place a romaine lettuce leaf on the bottom third of the tortilla. Add about 3 ounces (84 g) beef on top of the lettuce. Divide the tomatoes, red and yellow bell peppers, oil, vinegar, and cumin among the tortillas. Fold the bottom over the filling, fold the sides in, and roll the tortilla closed.

Yield: 6 servings

Per serving: 349 calories (38% from fat, 34% from protein, 27% from carbohydrate); 30 g protein; 15 g total fat; 4 g saturated fat; 8 g monounsaturated fat; 1 g polyunsaturated fat; 24 g carbohydrate; 2 g fiber; 2 g sugar; 232 mg phosphorus; 45 mg calcium; 194 mg sodium; 459 mg potassium; 1020 IU vitamin A; 0 mg ATE vitamin E; 111 mg vitamin C; 81 mg cholesterol

Beef Satay with Peanut Sauce

Flavorful beef strips with a peanut-based dipping sauce flavored with onion and garlic are a treat for everyone and proof that kids do like foods from other cultures.

½ cup (130 g) no-salt-added peanut butter

2 teaspoons Low-Sodium Soy Sauce (page 29)

2 teaspoons balsamic vinegar

1 tablespoon (15 ml) lemon juice

2 tablespoons (18 g) Onion Soup Mix (page 34), divided

2 teaspoons garlic powder, divided

¾ cup (180 ml) water

1 pound (454 g) beef round steak, sliced into strips

1 tablespoon (15 ml) sesame oil

Preheat the broiler and place the oven rack 6 inches (15 cm) below the heat source. In a small bowl, stir together the peanut butter, soy sauce, vinegar, lemon juice, 1 tablespoon (9 g) of the soup mix, 1 teaspoon of the garlic powder, and the water and set aside. Gently pound the beef strips with a rolling pin to flatten. In a bowl, combine the beef, oil, remaining 1 tablespoon (9 g) soup mix, and remaining 1 teaspoon garlic powder and toss to coat each strip of beef well. Spread on a baking sheet and broil for 2 to 3 minutes per side. Serve hot with the sauce on the side for dipping.

Yield: 4 servings

Per serving: 374 calories (55% from fat, 36% from protein, 9% from carbohydrate); 34 g protein; 23 g total fat; 5 g saturated fat; 11 g monounsaturated fat; 6 g polyunsaturated fat; 9 g carbohydrate; 2 g fiber; 3 g sugar; 365 mg phosphorus; 41 mg calcium; 86 mg sodium; 691 mg potassium; 1 IU vitamin A; 0 mg ATE vitamin E; 2 mg vitamin C; 52 mg cholesterol

Traditional Beef Kabobs

These beef bites follow the classic formula for kabobs, marinating for a short while in a well-spiced vinaigrette. They go together quickly, especially if you use my mock kabob technique and don't even bother with the skewers.

½ teaspoon minced garlic

2 teaspoons smoked paprika

½ teaspoon turmeric

1 teaspoon ground cumin

½ teaspoon freshly ground black pepper

⅓ cup (80 ml) red wine vinegar

½ cup (120 ml) olive oil

1½ pounds (680 g) beef round steak, cut into 1½-inch (3.8-cm) cubes

Prepare a grill for medium-high heat. In the bowl of a food processor, combine the garlic, paprika, turmeric, cumin, pepper, and red wine vinegar. With the motor running, drizzle in the olive oil until emulsified. Pour the marinade over the meat in a large bowl and toss to coat. Thread the meat onto skewers, leaving about ½ inch (1.3 cm) between pieces of meat. Place on the grill and cook, with the lid closed, for 2 to 3 minutes per side, 8 to 12 minutes in all.

Yield: 4 servings

Per serving: 468 calories (64% from fat, 34% from protein, 2% from carbohydrate); 40 g protein; 33 g total fat; 6 g saturated fat; 22 g monounsaturated fat; 3 g polyunsaturated fat; 3 g carbohydrate; 1 g fiber; 1 g sugar; 391 mg phosphorus; 48 mg calcium; 111 mg sodium; 703 mg potassium; 614 IU vitamin A; 0 mg ATE vitamin E; 1 mg vitamin C; 78 mg cholesterol

Bacon Beef Mock Kabobs

This is good eating, Southern-style. Bacon, steak, and vegetables are cooked quickly with a barbecue sauce glaze for a tasty treat.

4 slices low-sodium bacon

1 cup (160 g) quartered onion

1 cup (150 g) 1-inch (2.5-cm) pieces green bell pepper

24 cherry tomatoes

1½ pounds (680 g) beef round steak, cut into 1-inch (2.5-cm) cubes

2 tablespoons (30 ml) olive oil

2 tablespoons (30 ml) Barbecue Sauce (page 30)

1 teaspoon freshly ground black pepper

Preheat the broiler and place the oven rack 6 inches (15 cm) below the heat source. Broil the bacon strips until partially cooked, 3 to 4 minutes, then cut into pieces. Combine all the ingredients in a large bowl. Spread on a baking sheet and broil until the vegetables are crisp-tender and the steak is the desired doneness, turning once, 6 to 8 minutes.

Yield: 6 servings

Per serving: 257 calories (38% from fat, 46% from protein, 15% from carbohydrate); 29 g protein; 11 g total fat; 3 g saturated fat; 6 g monounsaturated fat; 1 g polyunsaturated fat; 10 g carbohydrate; 2 g fiber; 4 g sugar; 295 mg phosphorus; 39 mg calcium; 131 mg sodium; 691 mg potassium; 519 IU vitamin A; 1 mg ATE vitamin E; 35 mg vitamin C; 58 mg cholesterol

Tip: Serve with rice.

Chili Beef Mock Kabobs

Spicy Southwestern steak bites make a great meal, or they can also be served as an appetizer. Cut them a little smaller and this also makes a great start to a really flavorful pot of chili.

1½ pounds (680 g) beef round steak, cut into 1-inch (2.5-cm) cubes

1 tablespoon (15 ml) cider vinegar

2 tablespoons (16 g) chili powder

2 tablespoons (30 g) packed brown sugar

½ teaspoon freshly ground black pepper

½ teaspoon dried thyme

Preheat the broiler and place the oven rack 6 inches (15 cm) below the heat source. Combine all the ingredients in a bowl. Spread on a baking sheet and broil until the steak is the desired doneness, turning once, 6 to 8 minutes.

Yield: 6 servings

Per serving: 172 calories (23% from fat, 63% from protein, 15% from carbohydrate); 27 g protein; 4 g total fat; 1 g saturated fat; 2 g monounsaturated fat; 0 g polyunsaturated fat; 6 g carbohydrate; 1 g fiber; 5 g sugar; 263 mg phosphorus; 38 mg calcium; 100 mg sodium; 492 mg potassium; 745 IU vitamin A; 0 mg ATE vitamin E; 2 mg vitamin C; 52 mg cholesterol

Hungarian Mock Kabobs

This is the kabob version of beef paprikash, with steak, onions, and peppers seasoned with paprika and garlic, and is great over rice or noodles.

1 cup (160 g) quartered onion

1 cup (150 g) 1-inch (2.5-cm) pieces green bell pepper

1½ pounds (680 g) beef round steak, cut into 1-inch (2.5-cm) cubes

2 tablespoons (30 ml) olive oil

1½ teaspoons minced garlic

1 teaspoon paprika

1 teaspoon caraway seed

Preheat the broiler and place the oven rack 6 inches (15 cm) below the heat source. Combine all the ingredients in a bowl. Spread on a baking sheet and broil until the vegetables are crisp-tender and the steak is the desired doneness, turning once, 6 to 8 minutes.

Yield: 6 servings

Per serving: 206 calories (38% from fat, 53% from protein, 9% from carbohydrate); 27 g protein; 8 g total fat; 2 g saturated fat; 5 g monounsaturated fat; 1 g polyunsaturated fat; 4 g carbohydrate; 1 g fiber; 2 g sugar; 271 mg phosphorus; 38 mg calcium; 75 mg sodium; 522 mg potassium; 296 IU vitamin A; 0 mg ATE vitamin E; 22 mg vitamin C; 52 mg cholesterol

Indonesian Beef Mock Kabobs

With the flavor of beef satay, these steak bites are spicy, but with the edge taken off by the lime juice. They go well with curried vegetables and rice.

1½ pounds (680 g) beef round steak, thinly sliced

2 tablespoons (30 ml) lime juice

2 tablespoons (30 ml) Low-Sodium Soy Sauce (page 29)

1 tablespoon (15 g) Chili Sauce (page 233)

¼ teaspoon hot pepper sauce

1 tablespoon (4 g) chopped fresh cilantro

Preheat the broiler and place the oven rack 6 inches (15 cm) below the heat source. Combine all the ingredients in a bowl. Spread on a baking sheet and broil until the steak is the desired doneness, turning once, 6 to 8 minutes.

Yield: 6 servings

Per serving: 152 calories (24% from fat, 73% from protein, 3% from carbohydrate); 27 g protein; 4 g total fat; 1 g saturated fat; 2 g monounsaturated fat; 0 g polyunsaturated fat; 1 g carbohydrate; 0 g fiber; 0 g sugar; 261 mg phosphorus; 27 mg calcium; 91 mg sodium; 441 mg potassium; 77 IU vitamin A; 0 mg ATE vitamin E; 2 mg vitamin C; 52 mg cholesterol

Korean Beef Mock Kabobs

Similar in flavor to the traditional Korean *bulgogi*, with lots of garlic flavor, this is a real hit around our house.

½ cup (50 g) 2-inch (5-cm) pieces scallion

8 ounces (225 g) mushrooms

1 ½ pounds (680 g) beef round steak, thinly sliced

2 tablespoons (25 g) sugar

2 tablespoons (30 ml) dry white wine

2 tablespoons (30 ml) sesame oil

½ teaspoon crushed garlic

2 tablespoons (30 ml) Low-Sodium Soy Sauce (page 29)

Preheat the broiler and place the oven rack 6 inches (15 cm) below the heat source. Combine all the ingredients in a bowl. Spread on a baking sheet and broil until the vegetables are crisp-tender and the steak is the desired doneness, turning once, 6 to 8 minutes.

Yield: 6 servings

Per serving: 220 calories (36% from fat, 52% from protein, 12% from carbohydrate); 28 g protein; 9 g total fat; 2 g saturated fat; 3 g monounsaturated fat; 2 g polyunsaturated fat; 7 g carbohydrate; 1 g fiber; 5 g sugar; 296 mg phosphorus; 34 mg calcium; 89 mg sodium; 579 mg potassium; 83 IU vitamin A; 0 mg ATE vitamin E; 3 mg vitamin C; 52 mg cholesterol

Middle Eastern Beef Mock Kabobs

These meatballs are flavored with typical Middle Eastern spices throughout, making them a real taste treat. They are also very popular as an appetizer.

1 ½ pounds (680 g) extra-lean ground beef

2 tablespoons (12.5 g) minced scallion

¾ teaspoon minced garlic

¼ cup (15 g) minced fresh parsley

2 teaspoons ground cumin

1 teaspoon dried mint

1 teaspoon paprika

1 tablespoon (6 g) coriander

½ teaspoon ground cinnamon

Preheat the broiler and place the oven rack 6 inches (15 cm) below the heat source. Combine all the ingredients in a bowl, mixing well. Form into 1-inch (2.5-cm) balls. You should get 36 balls. Spread on a baking sheet and broil until the meatballs are cooked through, turning occasionally, 6 to 8 minutes.

Yield: 6 servings

Per serving: 199 calories (66% from fat, 32% from protein, 2% from carbohydrate); 22 g protein; 20 g total fat; 8 g saturated fat; 9 g monounsaturated fat; 1 g polyunsaturated fat; 1 g carbohydrate; 1 g fiber; 0 g sugar; 169 mg phosphorus; 27 mg calcium; 79 mg sodium; 379 mg potassium; 473 IU vitamin A; 0 mg ATE vitamin E; 6 mg vitamin C; 78 mg cholesterol

Steakhouse Mock Kabobs

If you like the traditional steakhouse taste of steak with sautéed mushrooms and onions then this recipe is for you. These tender morsels of steak and vegetables cook quickly but pack a lot of flavor.

1 cup (160 g) quartered onion

8 ounces (225 g) mushrooms

1½ pounds (680 g) beef round steak, cut into 1-inch (2.5-cm) cubes

1 tablespoon (15 ml) olive oil

1 tablespoon (15 ml) Worcestershire sauce

1 teaspoon chopped parsley

1 teaspoon dried thyme

Preheat the broiler and place the oven rack 6 inches (15 cm) below the heat source. Combine all the ingredients in a bowl. Spread on a baking sheet and broil until the vegetables are crisp-tender and the steak is the desired doneness, turning once, 6 to 8 minutes.

Yield: 6 servings

Per serving: 188 calories (30% from fat, 60% from protein, 10% from carbohydrate); 28 g protein; 6 g total fat; 2 g saturated fat; 3 g monounsaturated fat; 0 g polyunsaturated fat; 4 g carbohydrate; 1 g fiber; 2 g sugar; 296 mg phosphorus; 35 mg calcium; 100 mg sodium; 603 mg potassium; 27 IU vitamin A; 0 mg ATE vitamin E; 7 mg vitamin C; 52 mg cholesterol

Tip: Serve with rice.

No-Fuss Beef Stew

This is another one of those classic dishes that typically takes a large portion of the day to cook. I've kept the classic beef, potato, carrot, and onion combination and the traditional flavor, but speeded up the preparation so you can have it any night that you want.

¼ cup (30 g) all-purpose flour

2 tablespoons (18 g) Onion Soup Mix (page 34)

¼ cup (60 ml) water

3 cups (705 ml) Low-Sodium Beef Broth (page 231)

1 cup (130 g) sliced carrots

1 large red potato, diced

12 ounces (336 g) frozen green beans

1 pound (454 g) cooked beef, round roast or steak, cut into 1 inch cubes

Combine the flour, soup mix, and water in a small bowl and set aside. Bring the broth to a boil in a large skillet or heavy saucepan over high heat. Stir in the vegetables and beef. Cover; reduce the heat to low, and cook for about 10 minutes, or until the vegetables are tender. Stir in the flour mixture and cook until slightly thickened, 1 to 2 minutes.

Yield: 4 servings

Per serving: 440 calories (39% from fat, 34% from protein, 27% from carbohydrate); 37 g protein; 19 g total fat; 7 g saturated fat; 8 g monounsaturated fat; 1 g polyunsaturated fat; 29 g carbohydrate; 5 g fiber; 2 g sugar; 358 mg phosphorus; 67 mg calcium; 208 mg sodium; 1106 mg potassium; 4250 IU vitamin A; 0 mg ATE vitamin E; 21 mg vitamin C; 98 mg cholesterol

Zesty Vegetable Soup

My mom used to make hamburger vegetable soup all the time, but never this quickly. This soup has a lot of the same kind of flavor, which is definitely a good thing. Oregano adds a slightly Mediterranean taste and goes nicely with the stewed tomatoes to provide a depth of flavor.

1 pound (454 g) extra-lean ground beef

½ cup (80 g) chopped onion

2 cans (14.5 ounces, or 411 g each) no-salt-added stewed tomatoes

4 cups (940 ml) Low-Sodium Beef Broth (page 231)

10 ounces (280 g) mixed vegetables

½ cup (50 g) egg noodles, uncooked

½ teaspoon dried oregano

In a large pot over medium-high heat, brown the beef with the onion until the beef is no longer pink and the onion is tender, about 5 minutes. Drain off the fat. Stir in the tomatoes, broth, vegetables, noodles, and oregano. Bring to a boil over high heat, reduce the heat to a simmer, cover, and simmer until the noodles and vegetables are tender, about 10 minutes.

Yield: 8 servings

Per serving: 164 calories (46% from fat, 29% from protein, 25% from carbohydrate); 15 g protein; 10 g total fat; 4 g saturated fat; 4 g monounsaturated fat; 1 g polyunsaturated fat; 13 g carbohydrate; 3 g fiber; 5 g sugar; 144 mg phosphorus; 60 mg calcium; 133 mg sodium; 579 mg potassium; 1679 IU vitamin A; 1 mg ATE vitamin E; 19 mg vitamin C; 41 mg cholesterol

Calf Liver with Lemon Thyme

Liver is usually a big production, with flour coating, lots of oil to cook it in, and bacon and onion to accompany it. This liver is quickly and simply prepared, so you can have it any night, but the classic flavors are all still there. If you can't find lemon thyme, regular thyme will work.

8 ounces (225 g) calf liver

1 tablespoon (15 ml) olive oil

¼ cup (10 g) chopped fresh lemon thyme

½ teaspoon freshly ground black pepper

Rinse the liver and pat dry. Heat the oil in a large nonstick skillet over medium heat. Place the fresh thyme in a layer on the bottom of the pan, then place the liver on top. Cook for about 4 to 5 minutes on each side. Calf liver may be eaten slightly pink, but be careful not to overcook it. Remove from the bed of thyme, season with pepper, and serve.

Yield: 2 servings

Per serving: 580 calories (34% from fat, 56% from protein, 10% from carbohydrate); 79 g protein; 21 g total fat; 6 g saturated fat; 7 g monounsaturated fat; 2 g polyunsaturated fat; 14 g carbohydrate; 0 g fiber; 0 g sugar; 1352 mg phosphorus; 19 mg calcium; 215 mg sodium; 963 mg potassium; 86188 IU vitamin A; 25622 mg ATE vitamin E; 5 mg vitamin C; 876 mg cholesterol

8

15-Minute Pork and Lamb Dishes

As with beef, some pork recipes need longer cooking. You probably don't want to try to cook ribs in 15 minutes, but there are a lot of pork recipes that can be cooked in that time. Most of these recipes start with a whole boneless pork loin. This is available in my area at most large grocery stores and is usually even cheaper at the membership clubs. I buy one, then cut most of it up into boneless loin chops that can be frozen and quickly thawed when needed. Some of the end pieces that don't make good chops I cut into cubes or strips or grind into ground pork that is cheaper and a lot lower in fat than the ground pork you'll find in the meat case. Most of these recipes use either those chops, strips, or ground pork. There are also more mock kabobs, some using lamb, which lends itself well to quick cubing and broiling.

Breaded Pork Chops

Simply prepared, crispy delicious pork chops with a minimum of fuss. For variety use the Italian Bread Crumbs on page 33 instead of the Southern-style ones.

¼ cup (62 g) egg substitute, or 1 egg, beaten

½ cup (120 ml) skim milk

1½ cups (173 g) Southern-Style Bread Crumbs (page 32)

6 boneless pork loin chops

¼ cup (60 ml) olive oil

In a shallow bowl, combine the egg and milk. Place the bread crumbs in another shallow bowl. Dip each pork chop in the egg mixture, then dredge in the crumbs, patting them on to make a thick coating. Heat the oil in a large skillet over medium heat and cook the chops for 4 to 5 minutes on each side, or until a meat thermometer registers 160°F (71°C) when inserted into the center of a chop.

Yield: 6 servings

Per serving: 336 calories (39% from fat, 33% from protein, 27% from carbohydrate); 28 g protein; 14 g total fat; 3 g saturated fat; 9 g monounsaturated fat; 2 g polyunsaturated fat; 22 g carbohydrate; 1 g fiber; 0 g sugar; 296 mg phosphorus; 78 mg calcium; 93 mg sodium; 527 mg potassium; 90 IU vitamin A; 16 mg ATE vitamin E; 1 mg vitamin C; 64 mg cholesterol

Beer-Braised Pork Chops

Kind of sweet and sour flavored, with the added kick of beer, these chops are a sure winner.

4 boneless pork loin chops

½ teaspoon freshly ground black pepper

1 tablespoon (15 ml) canola oil

¾ cup (180 ml) beer or nonalcoholic beer

3 tablespoons (45 g) no-salt-added ketchup

2 tablespoons (30 g) packed brown sugar

Sprinkle both sides of the pork chops with pepper. Heat the oil in a large skillet over medium heat and brown the pork on both sides, about 3 minutes per side. Combine the beer, ketchup, and brown sugar in a small bowl; pour over the pork. Bring to a boil over high heat. Reduce the heat to a simmer and cook, uncovered, for 10 to 12 minutes, or until a meat thermometer registers 160°F (71°C) when inserted into the center of a chop.

Yield: 4 servings

Per serving: 220 calories (35% from fat, 44% from protein, 21% from carbohydrate); 22 g protein; 8 g total fat; 2 g saturated fat; 4 g monounsaturated fat; 1 g polyunsaturated fat; 10 g carbohydrate; 0 g fiber; 9 g sugar; 231 mg phosphorus; 23 mg calcium; 58 mg sodium; 460 mg potassium; 136 IU vitamin A; 2 mg ATE vitamin E; 3 mg vitamin C; 64 mg cholesterol

Tip: Serve over rice.

Cajun Pork Chops

These are great with the Cajun Rice on page 209.

1 teaspoon paprika

½ teaspoon ground cumin

½ teaspoon freshly ground black pepper

½ teaspoon cayenne pepper

½ teaspoon crumbled sage

½ teaspoon garlic powder

4 boneless pork loin chops

1½ teaspoons olive oil

Mix the paprika, cumin, black pepper, cayenne pepper, sage, and garlic powder on a plate. Liberally coat each pork chop with the spice mixture. Heat the olive oil in a large skillet over high heat. Place the pork chops in the skillet and reduce the heat to medium. Cook until the pork is no longer pink in the center, 8 to 10 minutes, or until a meat thermometer registers 160°F (71°C) when inserted into the center of a chop.

Yield: 4 servings

Per serving: 150 calories (38% from fat, 59% from protein, 3% from carbohydrate); 22 g protein; 6 g total fat; 2 g saturated fat; 3 g monounsaturated fat; 1 g polyunsaturated fat; 1 g carbohydrate; 0 g fiber; 0 g sugar; 226 mg phosphorus; 20 mg calcium; 52 mg sodium; 404 mg potassium; 411 IU vitamin A; 2 mg ATE vitamin E; 2 mg vitamin C; 64 mg cholesterol

Tip: If these are too spicy for your liking, reduce or eliminate the cayenne.

Asian Pork Chops

Mushrooms and onions cook around these Asian-flavored chops. You can combine these with either rice or in a more American-type setting with pasta or potatoes.

1 tablespoon (15 ml) oil

4 boneless loin pork chops

1 cup (160 g) sliced onion

8 ounces (225 g) mushrooms, sliced

¼ teaspoon freshly ground black pepper

1 teaspoon ground ginger

¼ cup (60 ml) orange juice

Heat the oil in a large skillet over medium-high heat and brown the chops on each side for 3 minutes. Add the onion and mushrooms around the chops, sprinkle with the pepper and ginger, and pour the orange juice over. Cover and cook until a meat thermometer registers 160°F (71°C) when inserted into the center of a chop, 10 to 15 minutes.

Yield: 4 servings

Per serving: 197 calories (36% from fat, 48% from protein, 16% from carbohydrate); 24 g protein; 8 g total fat; 2 g saturated fat; 3 g monounsaturated fat; 3 g polyunsaturated fat; 8 g carbohydrate; 1 g fiber; 3 g sugar; 282 mg phosphorus; 26 mg calcium; 55 mg sodium; 647 mg potassium; 21 IU vitamin A; 2 mg ATE vitamin E; 10 mg vitamin C; 64 mg cholesterol

Sweet and Spicy Glazed Pork Chops

A slightly sweet, slightly spicy glaze coats these grilled pork chops. The addition of mayonnaise gives it all a creamy goodness that is different from most glazes, which are usually sugar-based.

2 tablespoons (30 g) packed dark brown sugar

½ cup (120 g) no-salt-added ketchup

½ cup (115 g) mayonnaise

2 tablespoons (22 g) mustard

2 tablespoons (30 ml) Worcestershire sauce

6 boneless pork loin chops

Prepare a grill for medium-high heat, and lightly oil the grate. Place the sugar, ketchup, mayonnaise, mustard, and Worcestershire sauce in a bowl, and stir until blended. Place the pork chops on the preheated grill, and cook the chops until the surface is seared but the meat is just barely pink in the middle, about 5 minutes. Brush the chops with the glaze mixture, and flip to cook the glaze onto the meat. When the glazed side shows good grill marks, flip again, brush the glaze onto the other side, flip, and grill until the second side shows nice brown grill marks, about 5 minutes, or until a meat thermometer registers 160°F (71°C) when inserted into the center of a chop.

Yield: 6 servings

Per serving: 218 calories (34% from fat, 41% from protein, 25% from carbohydrate); 22 g protein; 8 g total fat; 2 g saturated fat; 3 g monounsaturated fat; 2 g polyunsaturated fat; 14 g carbohydrate; 0 g fiber; 9 g sugar; 233 mg phosphorus; 20 mg calcium; 125 mg sodium; 521 mg potassium; 224 IU vitamin A; 2 mg ATE vitamin E; 13 mg vitamin C; 68 mg cholesterol

Creole Pork Chops

Cooked in a spicy tomato sauce containing the Cajun holy trinity of celery, onion, and green pepper, these chops are a New Orleans–style treat.

¼ cup (60 g) all-purpose flour

4 boneless pork loin chops

5 tablespoons (75 ml) olive oil

1 cup (160 g) thinly sliced onion

½ cup (75 g) thinly sliced green bell pepper

¼ cup (30 g) finely chopped celery

½ teaspoon minced garlic

1 can (14.5 ounces, or 411 g) no-salt-added stewed tomatoes

½ teaspoon sugar

1 tablespoon (2.7 g) minced fresh thyme

¼ teaspoon freshly ground black pepper

¼ teaspoon hot pepper sauce

¼ cup (15 g) chopped fresh parsley

Place the flour in a large resealable plastic bag. Add the pork chops, one at a time, and shake to coat. Heat the oil in a large skillet over medium-high heat and cook the pork chops for about 4 minutes per side. Remove the chops from the skillet and keep warm. In the drippings, sauté the onion, green pepper, celery, and garlic until tender, 5 minutes. Stir in the tomatoes, sugar, thyme, pepper, and hot pepper sauce. Return the pork chops to the pan, reduce the heat to a simmer, cover, and cook for 4 to 5 minutes, or until a meat thermometer registers 160°F (71°C) when inserted into the center of a chop. Spoon the sauce over the top, sprinkle with the parsley, and serve.

Yield: 4 servings

Per serving: 354 calories (54% from fat, 27% from protein, 19% from carbohydrate); 24 g protein; 22 g total fat; 4 g saturated fat; 14 g monounsaturated fat; 2 g polyunsaturated fat; 17 g carbohydrate; 3 g fiber; 6 g sugar; 268 mg phosphorus; 79 mg calcium; 74 mg sodium; 748 mg potassium; 590 IU vitamin A; 2 mg ATE vitamin E; 38 mg vitamin C; 64 mg cholesterol

Honey Mustard Pork Chops

Tasty honey mustard chops cook quickly and get a flavor and nutrition boost from orange juice. They are good with just about anything, but I especially like them with the Broccoli with Orange Sauce on page 194 to carry out the flavor theme.

4 boneless pork loin chops

1 teaspoon lemon pepper

2 teaspoons olive oil

½ cup (120 ml) orange juice

1 tablespoon (11 g) Dijon mustard

1 tablespoon (20 g) honey

Sprinkle the pork chops with the lemon pepper. Heat the oil in a large nonstick skillet over medium heat, add the chops, and cook for 2 to 3 minutes per side, or until lightly browned. In a small bowl, combine the orange juice, mustard, and honey; pour over the pork. Bring to a boil, reduce the heat to a simmer, cover, and cook for 5 to 8 minutes, or until a meat thermometer registers 160°F (71°C) when inserted into the center of a chop. Serve the sauce over the chops.

Yield: 4 servings

Per serving: 183 calories (34% from fat, 48% from protein, 18% from carbohydrate); 22 g protein; 7 g total fat; 2 g saturated fat; 4 g monounsaturated fat; 1 g polyunsaturated fat; 8 g carbohydrate; 0 g fiber; 4 g sugar; 228 mg phosphorus; 22 mg calcium; 96 mg sodium; 448 mg potassium; 38 IU vitamin A; 2 mg ATE vitamin E; 11 mg vitamin C; 64 mg cholesterol

Instant Sweet-and-Sour Pork Chops

This is like traditional sweet-and-sour pork in flavor, with the aspects of tomato, honey, and soy sauce. But as chops, they are more versatile in the number of things that they go well with.

(continued on page 126)

3 tablespoons (45 g) Chili Sauce (page 233)

3 tablespoons (60 g) honey

2 tablespoons (30 ml) Low-Sodium Soy Sauce (page 29)

4 boneless pork loin chops

Preheat the broiler and place the oven rack 4 to 6 inches (10 to 15 cm) from the heat source. In a small bowl, combine the chili sauce, honey, and soy sauce. Brush on both sides of the pork, place on a baking sheet, and broil for 3 to 4 minutes per side, or until a meat thermometer registers 160°F (71°C) when inserted into the center of a chop.

Yield: 4 servings

Per serving: 187 calories (21% from fat, 47% from protein, 32% from carbohydrate); 22 g protein; 4 g total fat; 1 g saturated fat; 2 g monounsaturated fat; 0 g polyunsaturated fat; 15 g carbohydrate; 0 g fiber; 14 g sugar; 230 mg phosphorus; 18 mg calcium; 87 mg sodium; 396 mg potassium; 195 IU vitamin A; 2 mg ATE vitamin E; 3 mg vitamin C; 64 mg cholesterol

Pork Chops Mole

In a style similar to traditional mole recipes, these Mexican chops get a flavor boost from cocoa and cinnamon, imparting a slightly sweet and surprisingly delicious taste.

1 teaspoon ground cumin

1 teaspoon chili powder

4 boneless pork loin chops

1 tablespoon (15 ml) olive oil

1¼ cups (325 g) Low-Sodium Salsa (page 232)

1 teaspoon cocoa powder

⅛ teaspoon ground cinnamon

2 tablespoons (2 g) minced fresh cilantro

2 tablespoons (12 g) chopped scallion

Combine the cumin and chili powder in a small bowl; rub over both sides of the pork. Heat the oil in a large skillet over medium heat, add the chops, and cook for 2 to 3 minutes per side, or until lightly browned. In a small bowl, combine the salsa, cocoa, and cinnamon; pour over the pork. Bring the sauce to a boil, reduce the heat to a simmer, and cook, uncovered, for 3 to 4 minutes per side, or until a meat thermometer registers 160°F (71°C) when inserted into the center of a chop, stirring sauce occasionally. Sprinkle with the cilantro and scallion and serve.

Yield: 4 servings

Per serving: 188 calories (39% from fat, 48% from protein, 13% from carbohydrate); 23 g protein; 8 g total fat; 2 g saturated fat; 5 g monounsaturated fat; 1 g polyunsaturated fat; 6 g carbohydrate; 2 g fiber; 3 g sugar; 251 mg phosphorus; 48 mg calcium; 140 mg sodium; 590 mg potassium; 860 IU vitamin A; 2 mg ATE vitamin E; 14 mg vitamin C; 64 mg cholesterol

Pork Chops with Apple Mustard Sauce

Pork chops are cooked in apple juice to a tender, moist perfection, and then mustard is added to take the sauce to the next level.

4 boneless pork loin chops

1/8 teaspoon freshly ground black pepper

2 tablespoons (28 g) unsalted butter

1/3 cup (80 ml) apple juice

1 tablespoon (6 g) dried minced onion

1 tablespoon (11 g) Dijon mustard

Sprinkle the pork chops with the pepper. Heat the butter in a large skillet over medium-high heat, add the pork chops, and cook for 2 to 3 minutes per side, or until lightly browned. Stir in the apple juice and reduce the heat to medium. Cover and cook for 5 to 6 minutes per side, or until a meat thermometer registers 160°F (71°C) when inserted into the center of a chop. Transfer to a serving platter and keep warm. Add the onion and mustard to the skillet. Cook, uncovered, over low heat until heated through, 1 minute. Spoon over the chops and serve.

Yield: 4 servings

Per serving: 198 calories (47% from fat, 45% from protein, 8% from carbohydrate); 22 g protein; 10 g total fat; 5 g saturated fat; 4 g monounsaturated fat; 1 g polyunsaturated fat; 4 g carbohydrate; 0 g fiber; 3 g sugar; 233 mg phosphorus; 25 mg calcium; 98 mg sodium; 423 mg potassium; 193 IU vitamin A; 50 mg ATE vitamin E; 2 mg vitamin C; 79 mg cholesterol

Tip: Serve with rice or noodles and garnish with apple slices if desired.

Pork Chops with Sautéed Vegetables

Call it an American stir-fry if you want. Simple seasonings and fresh vegetables highlight the flavor of the pork.

2 boneless pork loin chops

1/4 teaspoon olive oil

1 cup (160 g) chopped onion

1/2 cup (75 g) chopped red bell pepper

1 cup (70 g) shredded cabbage

1/2 cup (90 g) chopped tomato

1/3 cup (80 ml) Low-Sodium Chicken Broth (page 232)

1/4 teaspoon freshly ground black pepper

1/8 teaspoon paprika

In a large nonstick skillet coated with cooking spray, cook the pork chops for 2 to 3 minutes per side, or until lightly browned. Transfer to a plate and keep warm. In the same skillet, add the oil, onion, and red pepper. Cook for 3 to 5 minutes, or until the vegetables are tender. Stir in the cabbage, tomato, broth, pepper, and paprika. Return the chops to the pan, reduce the heat to a simmer, cover, and cook for 6 to 8 minutes, or until a meat thermometer registers 160°F (71°C) when inserted into the center of a chop and the vegetables are tender.

Yield: 2 servings

Per serving: 202 calories (24% from fat, 47% from protein, 29% from carbohydrate); 24 g protein; 5 g total fat; 2 g saturated fat; 3 g

(continued on page 128)

monounsaturated fat; 1 g polyunsaturated fat; 15 g carbohydrate; 3 g fiber; 8 g sugar; 284 mg phosphorus; 61 mg calcium; 77 mg sodium; 806 mg potassium; 1638 IU vitamin A; 2 mg ATE vitamin E; 96 mg vitamin C; 64 mg cholesterol

Cranberry Orange Pork

Dried cranberries, Dijon mustard and orange juice transform these chops from ordinary to something really special. This dish is good enough for guests or a holiday dinner, but quick enough for even the busiest weeknight.

4 boneless pork loin chops

1 tablespoon (15 ml) olive oil

½ cup (120 ml) Low-Sodium Beef Broth (page 231), divided

2 tablespoons (18 g) dried cranberries

1½ teaspoons Dijon mustard

1 tablespoon (15 g) orange juice concentrate

1 teaspoon cornstarch

Place the chops on a cutting board and pound with a meat mallet or rolling pin to ¼ inch (6 mm) thick. Heat the oil in a large skillet over medium heat, add the pork chops, and cook for 2 to 3 minutes per side, or until lightly browned. Add ¼ cup (60 ml) of the beef broth, reduce the heat to a simmer, cover, and cook for 5 to 8 minutes, or until a meat thermometer registers 160°F (71°C) when inserted into the center of a chop. Transfer the meat to a serving dish and keep warm. In the same skillet, add the cranberries, mustard, and remaining ¼ cup (60 ml) broth.

Combine the orange juice concentrate and cornstarch in a small bowl until smooth; gradually add to the broth mixture. Bring to a boil; cook and stir for 1 to 2 minutes, or until thickened. Pour over the pork and serve.

Yield: 4 servings

Per serving: 174 calories (41% from fat, 52% from protein, 7% from carbohydrate); 22 g protein; 8 g total fat; 2 g saturated fat; 4 g monounsaturated fat; 1 g polyunsaturated fat; 3 g carbohydrate; 0 g fiber; 2 g sugar; 229 mg phosphorus; 18 mg calcium; 91 mg sodium; 426 mg potassium; 29 IU vitamin A; 2 mg ATE vitamin E; 8 mg vitamin C; 64 mg cholesterol

Hawaiian Pork Stir-Fry

Here's a variation on sweet-and-sour pork, with traditional taste, lots of fruit and vegetables for nutrition, and a fast preparation for busy people. Serve over rice for a complete meal.

8 ounces (225 g) pineapple chunks with juice

1 tablespoon (15 g) packed brown sugar

2 teaspoons cornstarch

¼ cup (60 ml) Low-Sodium Chicken Broth (page 232)

2 tablespoons (30 ml) lemon juice

1 teaspoon lemon zest

1 tablespoon (15 ml) Low-Sodium Soy Sauce (page 29)

1 pound (454 g) pork loin roast, cut into thin strips

1½ teaspoons olive oil

1 cup (150 g) sliced red bell pepper

½ cup (80 g) quartered and thinly sliced onion

½ teaspoon minced garlic

1 orange, peeled, sectioned, and sections cut in half

Drain the pineapple, reserving the juice; set the juice and pineapple aside. In a bowl, combine the brown sugar and cornstarch. Stir in the broth, lemon juice, lemon zest, soy sauce, and reserved pineapple juice until blended; set aside. In a nonstick skillet coated with cooking spray, stir-fry the pork over high heat for 3 to 4 minutes, or until the meat is no longer pink; transfer to a plate and keep warm. Heat the oil in the same skillet and stir-fry the bell pepper, onion, and garlic for 3 to
4 minutes, or until crisp-tender. Stir the broth mixture and add to the vegetables. Bring to a boil and cook, stirring, for 2 minutes, until thickened. Return the pork to the pan, add the orange pieces and pineapple, and cook until heated through, 1 to 2 minutes.

Yield: 4 servings

Per serving: 243 calories (25% from fat, 42% from protein, 33% from carbohydrate); 26 g protein; 7 g total fat; 2 g saturated fat; 3 g monounsaturated fat; 1 g polyunsaturated fat; 20 g carbohydrate; 3 g fiber; 15 g sugar; 282 mg phosphorus; 55 mg calcium; 76 mg sodium; 726 mg potassium; 1301 IU vitamin A; 2 mg ATE vitamin E; 106 mg vitamin C; 71 mg cholesterol

Pork and Apple Stir-Fry

This sweet and spicy stir-fry is excellent over plain rice. It starts off with the usual vegetables you would find in a stir-fry, but the addition of apple pie filling takes the flavor to a much higher level.

½ teaspoon cornstarch

½ cup (120 ml) apple cider

2 tablespoons (30 ml) Low-Sodium Soy Sauce (page 29)

2 teaspoons canola oil

8 ounces (225 g) boneless pork loin chops, cut into strips

½ cup (50 g) sliced celery

⅓ cup (43 g) sliced carrot

⅓ cup (53 g) sliced onion

⅓ cup (50 g) sliced red bell pepper

⅓ cup (41 g) sliced water chestnuts

¼ teaspoon ground ginger

1 cup (250 g) apple pie filling

In a small bowl, combine the cornstarch, cider, and soy sauce and whisk until smooth; set aside. Heat the oil in a large skillet or wok over medium heat and stir-fry the pork for 5 to 7 minutes, or until no longer pink. Add the celery, carrot, onion, red pepper, water chestnuts, and ginger; stir-fry until the vegetables are tender, about 5 minutes. Add the pie filling, and then stir the cornstarch mixture and add to the pan. Bring to a boil over high heat and cook, stirring, for 1 to 2 minutes, or until thickened.

(continued on page 130)

Yield: 3 servings

Per serving: 230 calories (26% from fat, 30% from protein, 44% from carbohydrate); 17 g protein; 7 g total fat; 1 g saturated fat; 3 g monounsaturated fat; 1 g polyunsaturated fat; 26 g carbohydrate; 3 g fiber; 18 g sugar; 211 mg phosphorus; 37 mg calcium; 97 mg sodium; 635 mg potassium; 2361 IU vitamin A; 2 mg ATE vitamin E; 36 mg vitamin C; 48 mg cholesterol

Pork and Pasta Skillet

Here's a quick, one-skillet Asian-flavored meal. The flavor and composition is similar to traditional lo mein recipes, but the angel hair pasta and the choice of vegetables makes it something more.

3 ounces (84 g) angel hair pasta

4 boneless pork loin chops, cut into thin strips

¼ teaspoon freshly ground black pepper

1 teaspoon canola oil, divided

10 ounces (280 g) fresh or frozen green beans

½ cup (75 g) sliced celery

¼ cup (40 g) chopped onion

3 tablespoons (45 ml) water

4 teaspoons (20 ml) Low-Sodium Soy Sauce (page 29)

Cook the pasta according to package directions until al dente. Meanwhile, sprinkle the pork with the pepper. Heat ½ teaspoon of the oil in a large nonstick skillet or wok coated with cooking spray, and stir-fry the pork over high heat until no longer pink, 3 to

4 minutes. Remove from the pan and keep warm. In the same pan, heat the remaining ½ teaspoon oil and stir-fry the beans, celery, and onion until crisp-tender, about 5 minutes. Add the water, soy sauce, and reserved pork; heat through. Drain the pasta, add to the pork mixture, and toss to coat.

Yield: 2 servings

Per serving: 394 calories (26% from fat, 48% from protein, 26% from carbohydrate); 47 g protein; 11 g total fat; 3 g saturated fat; 5 g monounsaturated fat; 2 g polyunsaturated fat; 26 g carbohydrate; 8 g fiber; 4 g sugar; 551 mg phosphorus; 98 mg calcium; 163 mg sodium; 1184 mg potassium; 1164 IU vitamin A; 4 mg ATE vitamin E; 28 mg vitamin C; 127 mg cholesterol

Hot Pork and Pasta Salad

A mustard and vinaigrette dressing highlight this salad of pork, spaghetti, and vegetables, including the bonus of asparagus. You could use any other pasta in place of the spaghetti.

8 ounces (225 g) spaghetti

1 cup (150 g) sliced red bell pepper

8 ounces (225 g) asparagus, trimmed and cut into 1-inch (2.5-cm) pieces

6 tablespoons (90 ml) olive oil, divided

12 ounces (340 g) pork loin roast, cut into ½-inch (1.3-cm) slices

4 teaspoons (15 g) Dijon mustard

1 tablespoon (15 ml) cider vinegar

½ teaspoon minced garlic

½ teaspoon dried thyme

¼ teaspoon freshly ground black pepper

Cook the spaghetti according to the package directions until al dente, stirring in the red pepper during the last 6 minutes and the asparagus during the last 3 minutes. Meanwhile, heat 2 tablespoons (30 ml) of the oil in a large skillet over high heat and cook the pork for 3 to 4 minutes, or until no longer pink in the center. In a small bowl, combine the remaining oil, mustard, vinegar, garlic, thyme, and black pepper. Drain the spaghetti mixture and add to the skillet. Add the dressing, toss to coat, and cook until heated through, 1 to 2 minutes.

Yield: 4 servings

Per serving: 384 calories (56% from fat, 23% from protein, 21% from carbohydrate); 23 g protein; 25 g total fat; 4 g saturated fat; 17 g monounsaturated fat; 3 g polyunsaturated fat; 20 g carbohydrate; 5 g fiber; 3 g sugar; 281 mg phosphorus; 44 mg calcium; 106 mg sodium; 549 mg potassium; 1615 IU vitamin A; 2 mg ATE vitamin E; 75 mg vitamin C; 54 mg cholesterol

Pork and Pineapple

If you cook a large pork roast, this is an excellent way to use the leftovers. It has a delicate sweet-and-sour flavor from the simple combination of ingredients. Serve over rice or noodles.

2 pounds (908 g) cooked pork loin roast, thinly sliced

10 ounces (280 g) crushed pineapple with juice

1 teaspoon packed brown sugar

¼ teaspoon nutmeg

Combine all the ingredients in a saucepan. Bring to a boil, reduce the heat to a simmer, and cook until the mixture is heated through, 4 to 6 minutes.

Yield: 6 servings

Per serving: 199 calories (30% from fat, 67% from protein, 3% from carbohydrate); 32 g protein; 6 g total fat; 2 g saturated fat; 3 g monounsaturated fat; 1 g polyunsaturated fat; 1 g carbohydrate; 0 g fiber; 1 g sugar; 330 mg phosphorus; 21 mg calcium; 77 mg sodium; 567 mg potassium; 12 IU vitamin A; 3 mg ATE vitamin E; 2 mg vitamin C; 95 mg cholesterol

Tip: Add some sliced red and green bell peppers and chopped onion for a complete sweet-and-sour meal.

Mexican-Flavored Pork

If you've been missing the boxed skillet meal mixes, this is the recipe for you. This one-skillet Mexican meal goes together in minutes, much faster than the mixes, yet has great flavor and nutrition. This makes enough for a large family or leftovers for lunch.

2 tablespoons (16 g) all-purpose flour

1 teaspoon chili powder

(continued on page 132)

¾ teaspoon freshly ground black pepper

1 pound (454 g) boneless pork loin chops, cut into strips

1 tablespoon (15 ml) canola oil

1 tablespoon (14 g) unsalted butter

2 cups (140 g) sliced mushrooms

1 cup (160 g) chopped onion

1 cup (150 g) chopped red bell pepper

1 teaspoon dried oregano

1 teaspoon minced garlic

3 cups (705 ml) skim milk

2 cans (8 ounces, or 225 g, each) no-salt-added tomato sauce

1 pound (454 g) elbow macaroni, uncooked

12 ounces (336 g) frozen corn

In a large resealable plastic bag, combine the flour, chili powder, and black pepper. Add the pork, a few pieces at a time, and shake to coat. Heat the oil and butter in a large skillet over medium heat, add the pork, mushrooms, onion, red bell pepper, and oregano, and cook for 4 to 6 minutes, or until the pork is browned. Add the garlic; cook 1 minute longer. Add the milk, tomato sauce, pasta, and corn. Bring to a boil over high heat, reduce the heat to a simmer, and cook, uncovered, until the pasta is tender, about 8 minutes.

Yield: 8 servings

Per serving: 429 calories (16% from fat, 24% from protein, 60% from carbohydrate); 26 g protein; 7 g total fat; 2 g saturated fat; 3 g monounsaturated fat; 2 g polyunsaturated fat; 65 g carbohydrate; 4 g fiber; 7 g sugar; 394 mg phosphorus; 169 mg calcium; 104 mg sodium; 920 mg potassium; 1206 IU vitamin A; 69 mg ATE vitamin E; 50 mg vitamin C; 41 mg cholesterol

Pork Lo Mein

This is exactly the kind of lo mein you get at Chinese restaurants. Lo mien is the kind of meal that looks like it takes a long time to prepare, but it doesn't have to. In the time it takes to cook the spaghetti (yes, even in the 6 minutes that angel hair takes), you can have the rest of the ingredients ready to stir into the noodles.

1 pound (454 g) spaghetti

2 pounds (908 g) ground pork

½ teaspoon minced garlic

2 teaspoons minced fresh ginger

¼ teaspoon red pepper flakes

2 tablespoons (16 g) cornstarch

2 cups (470 ml) water

½ cup (120 ml) Low-Sodium Soy Sauce (page 29)

¼ cup (60 ml) Low-Sodium Chicken Broth (page 232)

1 cup (100 g) sliced scallion

Cook the spaghetti according to the package directions until al dente. Meanwhile, in a skillet, cook the pork, garlic, ginger, and pepper flakes over medium heat until the meat is no longer pink, about 6 to 8 minutes; drain off the fat. In a bowl, combine the cornstarch, water, soy sauce, and broth and whisk until smooth. Add to the pork mixture along with the scallion. Bring to a boil over high heat and cook, stirring, for 1 minute, or until thickened. Drain the spaghetti and place in a large serving bowl. Add the pork mixture and toss to coat.

Yield: 6 servings

Per serving: 522 calories (56% from fat, 24% from protein, 20% from carbohydrate); 31 g protein; 33 g total fat; 12 g saturated fat; 14 g monounsaturated fat; 3 g polyunsaturated fat; 26 g carbohydrate; 4 g fiber; 1 g sugar; 366 mg phosphorus; 51 mg calcium; 148 mg sodium; 571 mg potassium; 211 IU vitamin A; 3 mg ATE vitamin E; 4 mg vitamin C; 109 mg cholesterol

Pork Skillet Supper

This tasty one-skillet meal goes together so fast that you could microwave the potato if you don't have any leftovers and still finish in less than 15 minutes. The creamy sauce has lots of flavor and the combination gives you a complete meal in one dish. For a real country meal, serve with cornbread or biscuits.

1 tablespoon (15 ml) olive oil

¾ cup (120 g) chopped onion

1½ cups (355 ml) Condensed Cream of Mushroom Soup (page 31)

½ cup (120 ml) skim milk

1 teaspoon Worcestershire sauce

⅛ teaspoon freshly ground black pepper

1 cup (140 g) cooked pork loin

1 large cooked potato, diced

1 cup (130 g) no-salt-added frozen peas

Heat the oil in a large skillet over medium heat and sauté the onion until tender, 5 minutes. Stir in the soup, milk, Worcestershire, and pepper; mix well. Add the pork, potato, and peas and cook until heated through, 2 to 3 minutes.

Yield: 3 servings

Per serving: 278 calories (22% from fat, 13% from protein, 65% from carbohydrate); 9 g protein; 7 g total fat; 1 g saturated fat; 4 g monounsaturated fat; 1 g polyunsaturated fat; 46 g carbohydrate; 7 g fiber; 6 g sugar; 234 mg phosphorus; 115 mg calcium; 113 mg sodium; 1222 mg potassium; 1230 IU vitamin A; 28 mg ATE vitamin E; 24 mg vitamin C; 5 mg cholesterol

Quick Schnitzel

This is not quite traditional breaded schnitzel, but with the delicious honey lemon sauce, I'd be willing to bet you don't get any complaints.

4 boneless pork loin chops

2 tablespoons (16 g) all-purpose flour

½ teaspoon freshly ground black pepper

2 tablespoons (28 g) unsalted butter

¼ cup (60 ml) lemon juice

¼ cup (80 g) honey

With a meat mallet or rolling pin, pound the chops to ¼ inch (6 mm) thick. In a large resealable plastic bag, combine the flour and pepper. Add the pork, 2 pieces at a time, and shake to coat. Heat the butter in a large skillet over medium heat and cook the pork

(continued on page 134)

for 3 to 4 minutes per side, or until no longer pink in the center. Remove from the heat and keep warm. Add the lemon juice and honey to the skillet; cook and stir for 3 minutes, or until thickened. Return the pork to the pan and cook for 2 to 3 minutes longer, or until heated through.

Yield: 4 servings

Per serving: 263 calories (34% from fat, 33% from protein, 33% from carbohydrate); 22 g protein; 10 g total fat; 5 g saturated fat; 3 g monounsaturated fat; 1 g polyunsaturated fat; 22 g carbohydrate; 0 g fiber; 18 g sugar; 228 mg phosphorus; 19 mg calcium; 53 mg sodium; 413 mg potassium; 188 IU vitamin A; 50 mg ATE vitamin E; 8 mg vitamin C; 79 mg cholesterol

Stir-Fried Pork and Cabbage

This is as quick and easy a stir-fry as you'll find. The fresh ginger provides an extra spark.

1 tablespoon (15 ml) olive oil, divided

6 cups (540 g) 1-inch (2.5-cm) pieces cabbage

1 cup (130 g) julienned carrot

1 pound (454 g) pork loin roast, cut into
    ¾-inch (2-cm) pieces

2 tablespoons (12 g) minced fresh ginger

1 cup (235 ml) Low-Sodium Chicken Broth
    (page 232), divided

¼ cup (60 ml) Low-Sodium Soy Sauce
    (page 29)

4 teaspoons (11 g) cornstarch

Heat 1 teaspoon of the oil in a large nonstick skillet or wok over high heat and stir-fry the cabbage for 1 to 2 minutes, or until crisp-tender. Add the carrots and stir-fry for 2 to 3 minutes longer, or until the carrots are crisp-tender. Remove from the skillet and keep warm. In the same pan, heat the remaining 2 teaspoons oil and stir-fry the pork for 2 minutes. Add the ginger and stir-fry for 2 minutes longer, or until the pork is lightly browned. Stir in ¾ cup (180 ml) of the broth and the soy sauce. Bring to a boil over high heat, reduce the heat to a simmer, cover, and cook for 3 minutes, or until the pork is no longer pink in the center. Combine the cornstarch and remaining ¼ cup (55 ml) broth in a small bowl and whisk until smooth. Gradually stir into the pan. Return the cabbage mixture to the pan, bring to a boil, and cook, stirring, for 2 to 3 minutes, or until thickened.

Yield: 4 servings

Per serving: 258 calories (31% from fat, 43% from protein, 26% from carbohydrate); 28 g protein; 9 g total fat; 2 g saturated fat; 5 g monounsaturated fat; 1 g polyunsaturated fat; 17 g carbohydrate; 5 g fiber; 7 g sugar; 329 mg phosphorus; 96 mg calcium; 163 mg sodium; 967 mg potassium; 4092 IU vitamin A; 2 mg ATE vitamin E; 46 mg vitamin C; 71 mg cholesterol

Island in the Sun Pork Burgers

These may be the tastiest burgers you've ever had, with a sweet-and-sour flavor cooked right in, highlighted by a grilled pineapple slice.

3 tablespoons (45 ml) vinegar

2 tablespoons (30 g) packed brown sugar

½ cup (80 g) chopped onion

2 tablespoons (30 ml) Low-Sodium Soy Sauce (page 29)

1 teaspoon garlic powder

1 pound (454 g) ground pork

10 ounces (280 g) pineapple slices, drained

5 hamburger buns, split

Preheat the broiler and place the oven rack 6 inches (15 cm) below the heat source or prepare a grill for medium-high heat. Combine the vinegar, sugar, onion, soy sauce, and garlic powder in a large bowl. Crumble the pork over the mixture and mix well. Shape into 5 patties. Broil or grill the pork and the pineapple slices for 4 to 5 minutes on each side, or until a meat thermometer registers 160°F (71°C) when inserted into the center of a burger. Serve on the buns.

Yield: 5 servings

Per serving: 430 calories (45% from fat, 19% from protein, 36% from carbohydrate); 20 g protein; 22 g total fat; 8 g saturated fat; 10 g monounsaturated fat; 2 g polyunsaturated fat; 39 g carbohydrate; 2 g fiber; 19 g sugar; 231 mg phosphorus; 72 mg calcium; 267 mg sodium; 457 mg potassium; 15 IU vitamin A; 2 mg ATE vitamin E; 6 mg vitamin C; 65 mg cholesterol

Pork and Slaw Wraps

Quick to fix, but nutritious and flavorful, these wraps get a head start by using prepared coleslaw mix. You could save a little money at the cost of a few extra minutes by shredding your own. The dressing is a typical creamy coleslaw dressing.

⅔ cup (46 g) coleslaw mix

4 teaspoons (12.5 g) finely chopped onion

1 tablespoon (14 g) mayonnaise

2 teaspoons sugar

½ teaspoon rice vinegar

½ teaspoon lemon juice

Pinch of celery seed

Pinch of freshly ground black pepper

1 teaspoon olive oil

6 ounces (168 g) boneless pork loin, cut into strips

2 flour tortillas, warmed

In a large bowl, combine the coleslaw, onion, mayonnaise, sugar, vinegar, lemon juice, celery seed, and pepper; set aside. Heat the oil in a small skillet over medium heat and cook the pork until it is no longer pink in the center, 6 to 8 minutes. Spoon the coleslaw mixture and pork down the center of each tortilla and roll up.

Yield: 2 servings

Per serving: 378 calories (42% from fat, 23% from protein, 35% from carbohydrate); 21 g protein; 18 g total fat; 5 g saturated fat; 8 g monounsaturated fat; 3 g polyunsaturated fat; 33 g

(continued on page 136)

carbohydrate; 2 g fiber; 5 g sugar; 231 mg phosphorus; 85 mg calcium; 273 mg sodium; 433 mg potassium; 36 IU vitamin A; 2 mg ATE vitamin E; 11 mg vitamin C; 55 mg cholesterol

Pork Burritos

Quick and tasty, these pork wraps with avocado and chiles turn a burrito into a full meal with the addition of vegetables.

1 tablespoon (15 ml) olive oil

12 ounces (340 g) boneless pork loin chops

¼ teaspoon freshly ground black pepper

4 flour tortillas

1 avocado, pitted, peeled, and thinly sliced

⅓ cup (53 g) thinly sliced red onion

4 ounces (112 g) diced green chiles

4 cups (220 g) salad greens

Heat the oil in a medium skillet over medium-high heat. Sprinkle the pork chops with the pepper, add to the skillet, and cook until browned and a meat thermometer registers 155°F (68°C) when inserted into the center of a chop, about 3 minutes per side. Cut the chops into ¼-inch (6-mm) slices. Microwave the tortillas on high until slightly warm and softened, about 20 seconds. Place the pork, avocado, onion, chiles, and salad greens on the bottom third of each tortilla, fold the bottom edge up and over the filling, tuck the filling in tightly, fold the sides in, then roll the tortilla up, securing with a toothpick if necessary.

Yield: 4 servings

Per serving: 426 calories (36% from fat, 22% from protein, 42% from carbohydrate); 24 g protein; 17 g total fat; 3 g saturated fat; 10 g monounsaturated fat; 2 g polyunsaturated fat; 45 g carbohydrate; 7 g fiber; 12 g sugar; 305 mg phosphorus; 86 mg calcium; 266 mg sodium; 892 mg potassium; 528 IU vitamin A; 2 mg ATE vitamin E; 13 mg vitamin C; 54 mg cholesterol

Pork Fajitas

Easy-to-make fajitas are always popular at our house. This version uses pork, rather than the more common chicken or beef, but the other ingredients and spices are just what you'd expect

1 tablespoon (15 ml) olive oil

1 pound (454 g) boneless pork loin, cut into ¼-inch (6-mm) slices

½ cup (75 g) sliced red bell pepper

½ cup (75 g) sliced green bell pepper

1 cup (160 g) sliced onion

½ cup (130 g) Low-Sodium Salsa (page 232)

4 flour tortillas, warmed

½ cup (58 g) shredded Cheddar cheese

¼ cup (60 g) sour cream

Heat the oil in a large skillet over medium heat, add the pork, bell peppers, and onion, and cook until the pork is no longer pink and the vegetables are tender, 6 to 8 minutes. Stir in the salsa and cook until heated through, 1 to 2 minutes. Place about ¾ cup (180 g) filling down the center of each tortilla; top with the shredded cheese and sour cream. Fold in the sides of the tortilla and roll up.

Yield: 4 servings

Per serving: 457 calories (45% from fat, 25% from protein, 30% from carbohydrate); 28 g protein; 23 g total fat; 7 g saturated fat; 11 g monounsaturated fat; 3 g polyunsaturated fat; 34 g carbohydrate; 3 g fiber; 4 g sugar; 322 mg phosphorus; 115 mg calcium; 315 mg sodium; 681 mg potassium; 934 IU vitamin A; 17 mg ATE vitamin E; 58 mg vitamin C; 77 mg cholesterol

Pork Pockets

Like a gyro, only a whole lot faster and easier to make, these pockets make a great lunch or the start of a simple dinner accompanied by a big salad.

1 pound (454 g) pork loin, sliced

½ cup (120 ml) Caesar Salad Dressing (page 91)

1 teaspoon olive oil

2 pita breads, cut in half

½ cup (60 g) chopped cucumber

½ cup (80 g) sliced red onion, separated into rings

¼ cup (60 ml) Ranch Dressing (page 34)

Place the pork in a large resealable plastic bag, add the Caesar dressing, seal the bag, and turn to coat. Heat the oil in a large nonstick skillet over medium heat and cook the pork for 7 to 8 minutes, or until the meat is no longer pink. Fill each pita half with pork, cucumber, and onion, and then drizzle with the ranch dressing.

Yield: 4 servings

Per serving: 305 calories (34% from fat, 36% from protein, 30% from carbohydrate); 27 g protein; 11 g total fat; 3 g saturated fat; 4 g monounsaturated fat; 3 g polyunsaturated fat; 23 g carbohydrate; 1 g fiber; 2 g sugar; 289 mg phosphorus; 49 mg calcium; 227 mg sodium; 505 mg potassium; 54 IU vitamin A; 4 mg ATE vitamin E; 3 mg vitamin C; 75 mg cholesterol

Asian Ground Pork Mock Kabobs

These tasty little Chinese-style meatballs are another example of quick-cooking meat recipes that can be added to other dishes such as soups and stir-fries.

1½ pounds (680 g) ground pork

¼ cup (25 g) minced scallion

2 teaspoons Low-Sodium Soy Sauce (page 29)

1 teaspoon sesame oil

1 teaspoon ground ginger

1 teaspoon crushed garlic

1 teaspoon paprika

1 tablespoon (6 g) coriander

½ teaspoon ground cinnamon

Preheat the broiler and place the oven rack 6 inches (15 cm) below the heat source. Combine all the ingredients in a bowl, mixing well. Form into 1-inch (2.5-cm) balls. You should get about 36 balls. Spread on a baking sheet and broil until the meatballs are cooked through, turning occasionally, 6 to 8 minutes.

(continued on page 138)

Yield: 6 servings

Per serving: 311 calories (73% from fat, 25% from protein, 2% from carbohydrate); 19 g protein; 25 g total fat; 9 g saturated fat; 11 g monounsaturated fat; 3 g polyunsaturated fat; 1 g carbohydrate; 0 g fiber; 0 g sugar; 206 mg phosphorus; 27 mg calcium; 70 mg sodium; 369 mg potassium; 270 IU vitamin A; 2 mg ATE vitamin E; 4 mg vitamin C; 82 mg cholesterol

Cajun Pork Mock Kabobs

A spicy little number, just the way Cajun food should be. Perfect with rice.

1½ pounds (680 g) pork loin roast, cut into
    1-inch (2.5-cm) cubes

2 tablespoons (30 ml) cider vinegar

1 tablespoon (8 g) Salt-Free Cajun Seasoning
    (page 29)

2 tablespoons (30 g) packed brown sugar

Preheat the broiler and place the oven rack 6 inches (15 cm) below the heat source. Combine all the ingredients in a bowl, mixing well. Spread on a baking sheet and broil until the pork is cooked through, turning once, 6 to 8 minutes.

Yield: 6 servings

Per serving: 163 calories (27% from fat, 61% from protein, 12% from carbohydrate); 24 g protein; 5 g total fat; 2 g saturated fat; 2 g monounsaturated fat; 1 g polyunsaturated fat; 5 g carbohydrate; 0 g fiber; 5 g sugar; 249 mg

phosphorus; 19 mg calcium; 60 mg sodium; 440 mg potassium; 8 IU vitamin A; 2 mg ATE vitamin E; 1 mg vitamin C; 71 mg cholesterol

Curried Pork Mock Kabobs

These are simple, curry-flavored pork cubes. You can add veggies to this if you want. Zucchini, bell peppers, and cherry tomatoes would all be good choices.

1½ pounds (680 g) pork loin roast, cut into
    1-inch (2.5-cm) cubes

¼ cup (60 ml) coconut milk

2 tablespoons (16 g) curry powder

2 tablespoons (32 g) no-salt-added peanut
    butter

2 tablespoons (30 ml) lime juice

Preheat the broiler and place the oven rack 6 inches (15 cm) below the heat source. Combine all the ingredients in a bowl, mixing well. Spread on a baking sheet and broil until the pork is cooked through, turning once, 6 to 8 minutes.

Yield: 6 servings

Per serving: 204 calories (43% from fat, 51% from protein, 6% from carbohydrate); 26 g protein; 10 g total fat; 4 g saturated fat; 4 g monounsaturated fat; 1 g polyunsaturated fat; 3 g carbohydrate; 1 g fiber; 1 g sugar; 281 mg phosphorus; 29 mg calcium; 61 mg sodium; 518 mg potassium; 31 IU vitamin A; 2 mg ATE vitamin E; 3 mg vitamin C; 71 mg cholesterol

Barbecued Pork Mock Kabobs

This dish contains the traditional flavors of long-cooked pulled pork, even though it is cooked quickly. It is great served with potatoes or noodles. Or cut the pieces a little smaller and make into a sandwich.

1 cup (160 g) quartered onion

1½ pounds (680 g) pork loin roast, cut into 1-inch (2.5-cm) cubes

¼ cup (60 ml) Barbecue Sauce (page 30)

Preheat the broiler and place the oven rack 6 inches (15 cm) below the heat source. Combine all the ingredients in a bowl, mixing well. Spread on a baking sheet and broil until the pork is cooked through, turning once, 6 to 8 minutes.

Yield: 6 servings

Per serving: 177 calories (25% from fat, 57% from protein, 18% from carbohydrate); 24 g protein; 5 g total fat; 2 g saturated fat; 2 g monounsaturated fat; 1 g polyunsaturated fat; 8 g carbohydrate; 0 g fiber; 5 g sugar; 254 mg phosphorus; 21 mg calcium; 62 mg sodium; 458 mg potassium; 8 IU vitamin A; 2 mg ATE vitamin E; 3 mg vitamin C; 71 mg cholesterol

Squash and Pork Mock Kabobs

This New England–style pork, flavored with maple syrup and pared with butternut squash, is a real fall or winter treat.

2 cups (300 g) 2-inch (5-cm) chunks butternut squash

1½ pounds (680 g) pork loin roast, cut into 1-inch (2.5-cm) cubes

2 tablespoons (30 ml) red wine vinegar

2 tablespoons (30 ml) maple syrup

1 teaspoon chili powder

Preheat the broiler and place the oven rack 6 inches (15 cm) below the heat source. Combine all the ingredients in a bowl, mixing well. Spread on a baking sheet and broil until the pork is cooked through and the squash is tender, turning once, 6 to 8 minutes.

Yield: 6 servings

Per serving: 186 calories (24% from fat, 53% from protein, 23% from carbohydrate); 24 g protein; 5 g total fat; 2 g saturated fat; 2 g monounsaturated fat; 1 g polyunsaturated fat; 10 g carbohydrate; 1 g fiber; 5 g sugar; 264 mg phosphorus; 43 mg calcium; 65 mg sodium; 611 mg potassium; 5092 IU vitamin A; 2 mg ATE vitamin E; 11 mg vitamin C; 71 mg cholesterol

Thai Pork Mock Kabobs

The flavors of Southeast Asia are mixed into these quick-cooking balls of ground pork. They are great as the main part of a meal, and are also really good in soups and other dishes.

1½ pounds (680 g) ground pork

3 tablespoons (18 g) minced fresh mint

3 tablespoons (3 g) minced fresh cilantro

(continued on page 140)

3 tablespoons (7.5 g) minced fresh basil

2 tablespoons (30 ml) Low-Sodium Soy Sauce (page 29)

1 teaspoon lime juice

1 teaspoon paprika

1 tablespoon (6 g) coriander

½ teaspoon ground cinnamon

Preheat the broiler and place the oven rack 6 inches (15 cm) below the heat source. Combine all the ingredients in a bowl, mixing well. Form into 1-inch (2.5-cm) balls. You should get 36 balls. Spread on a baking sheet and broil until the meatballs are cooked through, turning occasionally, 6 to 8 minutes.

Yield: 6 servings

Per serving: 308 calories (71% from fat, 26% from protein, 3% from carbohydrate); 20 g protein; 24 g total fat; 9 g saturated fat; 11 g monounsaturated fat; 2 g polyunsaturated fat; 2 g carbohydrate; 1 g fiber; 0 g sugar; 215 mg phosphorus; 52 mg calcium; 80 mg sodium; 416 mg potassium; 531 IU vitamin A; 2 mg ATE vitamin E; 5 mg vitamin C; 82 mg cholesterol

Ground Lamb Mock Kabobs

These lamb meatballs feature Middle Eastern spices, including cumin, mint, and coriander.

1½ pounds (680 g) ground lamb

2 tablespoons (12 g) minced scallion

½ teaspoon minced garlic

¼ cup (16 g) minced fresh parsley

2 teaspoons ground cumin

1 teaspoon minced fresh mint

1 teaspoon paprika

1 tablespoon (6 g) coriander

½ teaspoon ground cinnamon

Preheat the broiler and place the oven rack 6 inches (15 cm) below the heat source. Combine all the ingredients in a bowl, mixing well. Form into 1-inch (2.5-cm) balls. You should get about 36 balls. Spread on a baking sheet and broil until the meatballs are cooked through, turning occasionally, 6 to 8 minutes.

Yield: 6 servings

Per serving: 328 calories (63% from fat, 35% from protein, 2% from carbohydrate); 28 g protein; 23 g total fat; 9 g saturated fat; 10 g monounsaturated fat; 2 g polyunsaturated fat; 1 g carbohydrate; 1 g fiber; 0 g sugar; 237 mg phosphorus; 44 mg calcium; 96 mg sodium; 442 mg potassium; 473 IU vitamin A; 0 mg ATE vitamin E; 6 mg vitamin C; 110 mg cholesterol

Indian Lamb Mock Kabobs

Indian spices and yogurt add flavor and moistness to these lamb chunks.

1½ pounds (680 g) leg of lamb, cut into 1-inch (2.5-cm) cubes

¼ cup (60 g) low-fat plain yogurt

2 tablespoons (20 g) finely chopped onion

¼ cup (4 g) minced fresh cilantro

2 teaspoons garam masala

Preheat the broiler and place the oven rack 6 inches (15 cm) below the heat source. Combine all the ingredients in a bowl, mixing well. Spread on a baking sheet and broil until the lamb is cooked through, turning once, 6 to 8 minutes.

Yield: 6 servings

Per serving: 283 calories (54% from fat, 44% from protein, 2% from carbohydrate); 30 g protein; 17 g total fat; 7 g saturated fat; 7 g monounsaturated fat; 1 g polyunsaturated fat; 1 g carbohydrate; 0 g fiber; 1 g sugar; 237 mg phosphorus; 32 mg calcium; 84 mg sodium; 400 mg potassium; 123 IU vitamin A; 1 mg ATE vitamin E; 1 mg vitamin C; 105 mg cholesterol

Lamb Mock Kabobs

Classic Mediterranean-style lamb with onions and peppers, cubed and quickly cooked with simple flavorings.

1 cup (160 g) quartered onion

1 cup (150 g) 1-inch (2.5-cm) pieces red bell pepper

2 lemons, sliced

1½ pounds (680 g) leg of lamb, cut into 1-inch (2.5-cm) cubes

1 tablespoon (15 ml) olive oil

1 tablespoon (10 g) finely chopped onion

½ teaspoon freshly ground black pepper

Preheat the broiler and place the oven rack 6 inches (15 cm) below the heat source. Combine all the ingredients in a bowl, mixing well. Spread on a baking sheet and broil until the lamb is cooked through and the vegetables are crisp-tender, turning once, 6 to 8 minutes.

Yield: 6 servings

Per serving: 320 calories (52% from fat, 38% from protein, 10% from carbohydrate); 31 g protein; 19 g total fat; 7 g saturated fat; 9 g monounsaturated fat; 1 g polyunsaturated fat; 8 g carbohydrate; 3 g fiber; 2 g sugar; 240 mg phosphorus; 42 mg calcium; 79 mg sodium; 509 mg potassium; 789 IU vitamin A; 0 mg ATE vitamin E; 77 mg vitamin C; 104 mg cholesterol

Moroccan Lamb Mock Kabobs

Take a trip to Marrakesh with these tasty lamb bites, flavored with traditional Moroccan spices. They are great served on an appetizer tray as well.

1½ pounds (680 g) leg of lamb, cut into 1-inch (2.5-cm) cubes

3 tablespoons (45 ml) olive oil

2 tablespoons (12 g) coriander

1½ teaspoons minced garlic

2 teaspoons paprika

Preheat the broiler and place the oven rack 6 inches (15 cm) below the heat source. Combine all the ingredients in a bowl, mixing

(continued on page 142)

well. Spread on a baking sheet and broil until the lamb is cooked through, turning once, 6 to 8 minutes.

Yield: 6 servings

Per serving: 339 calories (63% from fat, 36% from protein, 1% from carbohydrate); 30 g protein; 23 g total fat; 8 g saturated fat; 12 g monounsaturated fat; 2 g polyunsaturated fat; 1 g carbohydrate; 0 g fiber; 0 g sugar; 227 mg phosphorus; 22 mg calcium; 78 mg sodium; 409 mg potassium; 439 IU vitamin A; 0 mg ATE vitamin E; 4 mg vitamin C; 104 mg cholesterol

9

15-Minute Fish and Seafood Dishes

There are so many good things to say about fish and seafood. First of all, fish is good for you. It is naturally low in sodium and harmful fats, while containing healthy omega-3 fatty acids. And when you are in a hurry, it's almost hard to find a fish recipe that doesn't take very little time to prepare. You can't go wrong having fish a couple of nights a week. Seafood such as shrimp and scallops also require short cooking times, although they do contain a bit more sodium than fish, so you may not want to have them as often.

Asian Grilled Salmon

In this dish a large salmon fillet is grilled with an Asian-flavored glaze. This is another one of those meals that looks like you put a lot of effort into it, even though it only takes 15 minutes. Serve with steamed vegetables and rice.

2 pounds (908 g) salmon fillets, boned but skin on

2 tablespoons (22 g) Dijon mustard

3 tablespoons (45 ml) Low-Sodium Soy Sauce (page 29)

6 tablespoons (90 ml) olive oil

½ teaspoon minced garlic

Prepare a grill for high heat. While the grill is heating, lay the salmon skin side down on a cutting board and cut it crosswise into 6 equal pieces. Whisk together the mustard, soy sauce, olive oil, and garlic in a small bowl. Drizzle half of the marinade onto the salmon. Place the salmon skin side down on the hot grill; discard the marinade the fish was sitting in. Grill for 4 to 5 minutes, depending on the thickness of the fish. Turn carefully with a wide spatula and grill for another 4 to 5 minutes, or until the fish flakes easily with a fork. Transfer the fish to a flat plate, remove the skin if desired, and spoon the reserved marinade on top. Serve warm, at room temperature, or chilled.

Yield: 6 servings

Per serving: 341 calories (59% from fat, 39% from protein, 1% from carbohydrate); 33 g protein; 22 g total fat; 4 g saturated fat; 13 g monounsaturated fat; 4 g polyunsaturated fat; 1 g carbohydrate; 0 g fiber; 0 g sugar; 549 mg phosphorus; 383 mg calcium; 192 mg sodium; 477 mg potassium; 99 IU vitamin A; 27 mg ATE vitamin E; 0 mg vitamin C; 59 mg cholesterol

Balsamic and Honey Salmon

This salmon is a nice change of pace, flavor-wise. The sweetness of the honey goes well with the natural sweetness of the fish.

¼ cup (60 ml) balsamic vinegar

¼ cup (60 ml) water

2 tablespoons (30 ml) olive oil

2 tablespoons (40 g) honey

¼ teaspoon garlic powder

8 ounces (225 g) salmon fillets, skinned

Combine the vinegar, water, oil, honey, and garlic in a large skillet over medium heat, stirring to combine. Add the salmon, cover, and cook until the fish flakes easily with a fork, about 10 minutes, turning once.

Yield: 2 servings

Per serving: 397 calories (58% from fat, 23% from protein, 19% from carbohydrate); 23 g protein; 26 g total fat; 4 g saturated fat; 14 g monounsaturated fat; 6 g polyunsaturated fat; 19 g carbohydrate; 0 g fiber; 19 g sugar; 269 mg phosphorus; 18 mg calcium; 69 mg sodium; 456 mg potassium; 57 IU vitamin A; 17 mg ATE vitamin E; 5 mg vitamin C; 67 mg cholesterol

Blackened Salmon

This Cajun-style salmon is pan seared and then finished in the oven.

2 cups (380 g) instant rice

12 ounces (336 g) frozen corn

2½ tablespoons (18 g) paprika

¾ teaspoon cayenne pepper

1 teaspoon dried thyme

½ teaspoon garlic powder

3½ tablespoons (50 g) unsalted butter, divided

2 tablespoons (30 ml) lemon juice

1½ pounds (680 g) salmon fillets, skinned

⅓ cup (20 g) finely chopped fresh parsley

1 lemon, cut into wedges

Preheat the oven to 400°F (200°C, or gas mark 6). Cook the rice according to the package directions. Cook the corn and drain. Meanwhile, in a shallow bowl, combine the paprika, cayenne, thyme, and garlic powder. In a saucepan over medium heat, melt 2½ tablespoons (35 g) of the butter, and then add the lemon juice. Working with 1 salmon fillet at a time, dip the top and bottom halves first in the lemon butter, then in the spices.

Heat a large ovenproof skillet over medium-high heat. Add the salmon and cook until blackened, 2 minutes per side. Transfer to the oven and bake for 8 minutes, or until the fish flakes easily with a fork. Stir the corn, parsley, and remaining 1 tablespoon (15 g) butter into the rice. Divide the salmon and rice among 4 individual plates and serve with the lemon wedges.

Yield: 4 servings

Per serving: 587 calories (46% from fat, 27% from protein, 28% from carbohydrate); 39 g protein; 30 g total fat; 10 g saturated fat; 10 g monounsaturated fat; 8 g polyunsaturated fat; 41 g carbohydrate; 5 g fiber; 3 g sugar; 520 mg phosphorus; 57 mg calcium; 118 mg sodium; 1009 mg potassium; 3243 IU vitamin A; 109 mg ATE vitamin E; 33 mg vitamin C; 127 mg cholesterol

Brown Sugar and Mustard–Glazed Salmon

You will enjoy a lot of flavor from just 4 ingredients. The mustard and brown sugar provide just the right amount of sweetness and spice. This is one of my favorite ways to cook salmon.

1½ pounds (680 g) salmon fillets, skinned

½ teaspoon freshly ground black pepper

¼ cup (60 g) packed light brown sugar

2 tablespoons (22 g) Dijon mustard

Preheat the broiler and set the oven rack 6 inches (15 cm) from the heat source; coat the rack of a broiler pan with cooking spray. Season the salmon with pepper and arrange on the prepared broiler pan. Whisk together the brown sugar and Dijon mustard in a small bowl; spoon the mixture evenly on top of the salmon fillets. Broil until the fish flakes easily with a fork, 10 to 12 minutes.

Yield: 4 servings

(continued on page 146)

Per serving: 369 calories (47% from fat, 38% from protein, 16% from carbohydrate); 34 g protein; 19 g total fat; 4 g saturated fat; 7 g monounsaturated fat; 7 g polyunsaturated fat; 14 g carbohydrate; 0 g fiber; 13 g sugar; 407 mg phosphorus; 40 mg calcium; 193 mg sodium; 678 mg potassium; 96 IU vitamin A; 26 mg ATE vitamin E; 7 mg vitamin C; 100 mg cholesterol

Creamy Mediterranean Salmon

Basted with a yogurt and herb sauce, this salmon will recall flavors or Spain, Greece, and North Africa. But wherever you say it's from, it's quick and good.

½ cup (120 g) low-fat plain yogurt

2 tablespoons (30 ml) lemon juice

1 tablespoon (15 ml) olive oil

½ teaspoon smashed garlic

1½ teaspoons coriander

1½ teaspoons ground cumin

¼ teaspoon freshly ground black pepper

1½ pounds salmon fillets, skinned

¼ cup (4 g) chopped fresh cilantro

Prepare a grill for medium-high heat and lightly oil the grate. Stir together the yogurt, lemon juice, olive oil, garlic, coriander, cumin, and pepper in a small bowl. Pour half of the sauce into a large resealable plastic bag; cover and refrigerate the remaining sauce. Add the salmon to the bag and turn to coat with the marinade. Remove the salmon from the marinade and blot off the excess yogurt with paper towels. Grill the salmon, turning once, until browned on the outside and opaque in the center, 4 to 6 minutes per side, depending on the thickness. Serve with the reserved yogurt sauce and garnish with the cilantro.

Yield: 4 servings

Per serving: 792 calories (55% from fat, 42% from protein, 4% from carbohydrate); 80 g protein; 47 g total fat; 9 g saturated fat; 18 g monounsaturated fat; 16 g polyunsaturated fat; 7 g carbohydrate; 0 g fiber; 6 g sugar; 964 mg phosphorus; 103 mg calcium; 253 mg sodium; 1538 mg potassium; 411 IU vitamin A; 63 mg ATE vitamin E; 22 mg vitamin C; 235 mg cholesterol

Caribbean Salmon

Spicy, but good, this salmon will cart you away to warmer climes, with its use of lime juice and cilantro. If it's too spicy for your liking, reduce the amount of cayenne.

2 tablespoons (30 ml) olive oil

2 tablespoons (30 ml) lime juice

½ teaspoon minced garlic

1 teaspoon ground cumin

1 teaspoon cayenne pepper

¼ cup (4 g) roughly chopped fresh cilantro

1½ pounds (680 g) salmon fillets, skinned

Prepare a grill for medium-high heat and lightly oil the grate. In a large bowl, whisk together the olive oil, lime juice, garlic, cumin, cayenne, and cilantro. Add the salmon and turn to coat. Let marinate for 5 minutes at room temperature. Grill the salmon, round side down, until marked on the bottom, about 4 minutes. Turn and continue grilling until marked on the other side and the fish is opaque in the center, 2 to 3 more minutes.

Yield: 4 servings

Per serving: 378 calories (62% from fat, 37% from protein, 2% from carbohydrate); 34 g protein; 25 g total fat; 5 g saturated fat; 12 g monounsaturated fat; 7 g polyunsaturated fat; 1 g carbohydrate; 0 g fiber; 0 g sugar; 403 mg phosphorus; 29 mg calcium; 103 mg sodium; 658 mg potassium; 455 IU vitamin A; 26 mg ATE vitamin E; 10 mg vitamin C; 100 mg cholesterol

Hawaiian Baked Salmon

A quick-to-prepare pineapple salsa, with enough ginger to give it a little bite, makes this salmon something special.

1 pound (454 g) salmon fillets, skinned

½ cup (80 g) crushed pineapple, juice reserved

2 tablespoons (18 g) Salt-Free Seasoning (page 27)

¼ cup (38 g) diced green bell pepper

¼ cup (38 g) diced red bell pepper

1 tablespoon (6 g) finely chopped fresh ginger

Preheat the oven to 375°F (190°C, or gas mark 5). Arrange the salmon on a lightly oiled baking sheet. Brush with 2 tablespoons (30 ml) of the reserved pineapple juice.

Sprinkle the fillets evenly with the seasoning. Bake in the middle of the oven for 10 to 12 minutes, or until the fish starts to flake slightly. Combine the pineapple, bell peppers, and ginger in a medium bowl. Serve the fish, spooning the fresh salsa alongside.

Yield: 4 servings

Per serving: 233 calories (49% from fat, 40% from protein, 11% from carbohydrate); 23 g protein; 12 g total fat; 3 g saturated fat; 4 g monounsaturated fat; 5 g polyunsaturated fat; 6 g carbohydrate; 1 g fiber; 5 g sugar; 273 mg phosphorus; 21 mg calcium; 68 mg sodium; 498 mg potassium; 397 IU vitamin A; 17 mg ATE vitamin E; 32 mg vitamin C; 67 mg cholesterol

Salmon with Basil Oil

Here's another way of cooking salmon. This one gets a real boost of Italian flavor from fresh basil. It's good with the Italian Barley Pilaf on page 208 and a simple vegetable such as steamed broccoli.

1½ pounds (680 g) salmon fillets, skinned

2 cups (40 g) fresh basil

½ cup (120 ml) olive oil

¼ teaspoon freshly ground black pepper

Preheat the broiler to high and place the oven rack 6 inches (15 cm) below the heat source. Bring a large pot of water to a boil. Fill a bowl halfway with ice water. Place the salmon on a foil-lined broiler pan and broil, without turning, until it is the same color throughout and

(continued on page 148)

flakes easily with a fork, 7 to 10 minutes, depending on the thickness. Transfer to plates. Meanwhile, add the basil to the pot of water and cook for 5 seconds. Using a slotted spoon, transfer it to the ice water. Drain, squeeze to remove excess water, place on a paper towel, and pat dry. Place the basil, oil, and pepper in a blender and purée until smooth. Drizzle the salmon with some of the basil oil and serve.

Yield: 4 servings

Per serving: 592 calories (69% from fat, 24% from protein, 7% from carbohydrate); 36 g protein; 46 g total fat; 7 g saturated fat; 27 g monounsaturated fat; 10 g polyunsaturated fat; 10 g carbohydrate; 7 g fiber; 0 g sugar; 479 mg phosphorus; 376 mg calcium; 107 mg sodium; 1194 mg potassium; 1660 IU vitamin A; 26 mg ATE vitamin E; 17 mg vitamin C; 100 mg cholesterol

Tip: If you don't use all the oil the remainder can be refrigerated, covered, for up to 2 weeks.

Salmon with Brown Butter and Almonds

I love salmon because it's so versatile, not to mention good for you. This version, paired with green beans, gets extra flavor from browned butter and almonds.

¼ cup (55 g) unsalted butter, divided

1¼ pounds (570 g) salmon fillets, cut into 4 pieces

½ teaspoon freshly ground black pepper

1 pound (454 g) fresh green beans, trimmed and cut in half

¼ cup (26 g) sliced almonds

Heat 1 tablespoon (14 g) of the butter in a large nonstick skillet over medium heat. Season the salmon with pepper. Cook the fish until opaque throughout, 3 to 5 minutes per side. Transfer to individual plates. Meanwhile, fill a second skillet with ½ inch (1.3 cm) of water and bring to a boil. Add the green beans to the second skillet, cover, and steam until just tender, 4 to 5 minutes. Drain and transfer to the plates. Wipe out the green bean skillet and heat the remaining 3 tablespoons (41 g) butter over medium heat. Add the almonds and cook, stirring frequently, until the almonds and the butter are golden brown (but not burned), 2 to 3 minutes. Spoon over the fish and beans.

Yield: 4 servings

Per serving: 457 calories (63% from fat, 28% from protein, 9% from carbohydrate); 33 g protein; 32 g total fat; 11 g saturated fat; 12 g monounsaturated fat; 7 g polyunsaturated fat; 10 g carbohydrate; 5 g fiber; 2 g sugar; 423 mg phosphorus; 92 mg calcium; 92 mg sodium; 825 mg potassium; 1209 IU vitamin A; 116 mg ATE vitamin E; 24 mg vitamin C; 114 mg cholesterol

Super Simple Salmon

This simple and super-quick pan-seared salmon is flavored with basil and garlic. Serve with pasta and steamed broccoli for a complete meal.

1 tablespoon (9 g) garlic powder

1 tablespoon (2.5 g) chopped fresh basil

1½ pounds (680 g) salmon fillets

2 tablespoons (28 g) unsalted butter

1 lemon, cut into wedges

Stir together the garlic powder and basil in a small bowl; rub in equal amounts onto the salmon fillets. Melt the butter in a skillet over medium heat; cook the salmon in the butter until browned and flaky, about 5 minutes per side. Serve each piece of salmon with a lemon wedge.

Yield: 4 servings

Per serving: 375 calories (59% from fat, 37% from protein, 3% from carbohydrate); 34 g protein; 24 g total fat; 7 g saturated fat; 8 g monounsaturated fat; 7 g polyunsaturated fat; 3 g carbohydrate; 1 g fiber; 1 g sugar; 412 mg phosphorus; 39 mg calcium; 102 mg sodium; 679 mg potassium; 315 IU vitamin A; 73 mg ATE vitamin E; 15 mg vitamin C; 116 mg cholesterol

Asian Tuna Steaks

Tuna steaks are great when you're in a hurry because they cook quickly. They are best when still pink on the inside so the don't dry out and get tough. This version gets additional flavor from an Asian-flavored orange glaze.

2 tablespoons (30 ml) orange juice

1 tablespoon (15 ml) sesame oil

1 tablespoon (8 g) sesame seeds

2 tablespoons (30 ml) Low-Sodium Soy Sauce (page 29)

2 teaspoons grated fresh ginger, or 1¼ teaspoons ground ginger

¼ cup (25 g) chopped scallion

1 pound (454 g) tuna steaks

Preheat the broiler and place the oven rack 6 inches (15 cm) below the heat source or prepare a grill for medium-high heat. In a resealable plastic bag, combine the juice, oil, sesame seeds, soy sauce, ginger, and scallion. Add the tuna, seal the bag, and shake well to coat. Broil or grill the tuna for 4 to 5 minutes per side, or until fish flakes easily with a fork, brushing frequently with the marinade.

Yield: 4 servings

Per serving: 202 calories (42% from fat, 55% from protein, 4% from carbohydrate); 27 g protein; 9 g total fat; 2 g saturated fat; 3 g monounsaturated fat; 3 g polyunsaturated fat; 2 g carbohydrate; 0 g fiber; 0 g sugar; 293 mg phosphorus; 15 mg calcium; 46 mg sodium; 330 mg potassium; 2545 IU vitamin A; 743 mg ATE vitamin E; 4 mg vitamin C; 43 mg cholesterol

Five-Spice Sesame Tuna and Avocado

Tuna steaks get a quick Asian treatment, producing a salad that you can be proud to serve to anyone. But don't wait: Try it with your family, too.

(continued on page 150)

2 avocados

1 tablespoon (15 ml) lime juice

⅓ cup (80 ml) balsamic vinegar

¼ cup (60 ml) Low-Sodium Soy Sauce
(page 29)

3 tablespoons (60 g) honey

2 tablespoons (30 ml) olive oil

1 pound (454 g) tuna steaks

2 teaspoons five-spice powder

½ cup (64 g) sesame seeds, toasted

¼ cup (12 g) snipped fresh chives

4 cups (220 g) shredded iceberg lettuce

Peel, pit, and thickly slice the avocados lengthwise and coat with the lime juice to prevent browning; set aside. In a small saucepan over medium-high heat, bring the vinegar, soy sauce, and honey to a low boil. Lower the heat and simmer until syrupy, 6 to 7 minutes. Set aside. Meanwhile, in a large skillet, heat the oil over high heat. Sprinkle the tuna with the five-spice powder. Place the tuna in the skillet and cook, turning once, until just browned, 1 to 2 minutes per side. Slice the tuna and top with the sesame seeds and chives. Divide the lettuce among 4 plates and top with the tuna and avocado. Drizzle with the dressing.

Yield: 4 servings

Per serving: 578 calories (54% from fat, 26% from protein, 19% from carbohydrate); 39 g protein; 36 g total fat; 6 g saturated fat; 19 g monounsaturated fat; 8 g polyunsaturated fat; 29 g carbohydrate; 9 g fiber; 16 g sugar; 553 mg phosphorus; 216 mg calcium; 110 mg sodium; 1031 mg potassium; 3539 IU vitamin A; 928 mg ATE vitamin E; 12 mg vitamin C; 54 mg cholesterol

Baked Tilapia Rockefeller

Named after the classic oyster dish containing spinach, this fish version cooks in minutes and has marvelous flavor.

1 pound (454 g) tilapia fillets

3 tablespoons (45 ml) olive oil, divided

8 ounces (225 g) frozen spinach, thawed,
drained, and patted dry

½ cup (80 g) diced onion

¼ cup (32 g) Salt-Free Seasoning (page 27)

Preheat the oven to 350°F (180°C, or gas mark 4). Rub the tilapia fillets with 1½ tablespoons (22 ml) of the olive oil. Toss the remaining 1½ tablespoons (22 ml) olive oil with the spinach and onion in a separate bowl. Sprinkle the seasoning evenly over each fillet. Place the spinach and onion mixture in 4 lines on a baking sheet lightly coated with cooking spray. Top each with a tilapia fillet. Bake for 5 to 7 minutes, or until fish flakes easily with a fork.

Yield: 4 servings

Per serving: 241 calories (49% from fat, 43% from protein, 8% from carbohydrate); 26 g protein; 13 g total fat; 2 g saturated fat; 8 g monounsaturated fat; 2 g polyunsaturated fat; 5 g carbohydrate; 2 g fiber; 1 g sugar; 285 mg phosphorus; 145 mg calcium; 117 mg sodium; 710 mg potassium; 7017 IU vitamin A; 53 mg ATE vitamin E; 3 mg vitamin C; 36 mg cholesterol

Tilapia Parmesan

Basil and Parmesan cheese in the creamy mayonnaise coating give these tilapia fillets an Italian flair. Serve with pasta and steamed veggies.

½ cup (40 g) shredded Parmesan cheese

¼ cup (55 g) unsalted butter, softened

3 tablespoons (42 g) mayonnaise

2 tablespoons (30 ml) lemon juice

¼ teaspoon dried basil

¼ teaspoon freshly ground black pepper

⅛ teaspoon onion powder

⅛ teaspoon celery seed

2 pounds (908 g) tilapia fillets

Preheat the broiler and set the oven rack about 6 inches (15 cm) from the heat source. Grease a broiling pan or line with aluminum foil. In a small bowl, mix together the Parmesan cheese, butter, mayonnaise, and lemon juice. Add the basil, pepper, onion powder, and celery seed. Mix well and set aside. Arrange the fillets in a single layer on the prepared pan. Broil for 2 to 3 minutes. Flip the fillets over and broil for 2 to 3 more minutes, until fish flakes easily with a fork. Remove the fillets from the oven and spread the Parmesan cheese mixture on top. Broil for 2 more minutes, or just until the topping is browned. Be careful not to overcook the fish.

Yield: 8 servings

Per serving: 216 calories (48% from fat, 50% from protein, 3% from carbohydrate); 26 g protein; 11 g total fat; 5 g saturated fat; 3 g monounsaturated fat; 2 g polyunsaturated fat; 2 g carbohydrate; 0 g fiber; 0 g sugar; 300 mg phosphorus; 126 mg calcium; 164 mg sodium; 527 mg potassium; 386 IU vitamin A; 108 mg ATE vitamin E; 2 mg vitamin C; 58 mg cholesterol

Spanish Mackerel

The fish is called Spanish mackerel and the preparation is also Spanish, featuring lemon and paprika.

1½ pounds (680 g) Spanish mackerel fillets

¼ cup (60 ml) olive oil

½ teaspoon paprika

½ teaspoon freshly ground black pepper

2 lemons, sliced

Preheat the broiler and set the oven rack about 6 inches (15 cm) from the heat source. Lightly grease a baking dish. Rub both sides of each mackerel fillet with olive oil and place skin side down in the prepared baking dish. Season each fillet with the paprika and pepper. Top each fillet with 2 lemon slices. Broil until the fish just begins to flake when tested with a fork, 5 to 7 minutes. Serve immediately.

Yield: 6 servings

Per serving: 245 calories (58% from fat, 35% from protein, 6% from carbohydrate); 22 g protein; 16 g total fat; 3 g saturated fat; 8 g monounsaturated fat; 3 g polyunsaturated fat; 4 g carbohydrate; 2 g fiber; 0 g sugar; 239 mg phosphorus; 36 mg calcium; 68 mg sodium; 565 mg potassium; 226 IU vitamin A; 34 mg ATE vitamin E; 30 mg vitamin C; 86 mg cholesterol

Creole Fish

Spicy Creole-style catfish cooks quickly in the microwave in a traditional tomato sauce with celery, onion, and green bell pepper, for a tender and very flavorful meal. Serve over rice.

1½ pounds (680 g) catfish fillets

1 cup (160 g) chopped onion

¼ cup (25 g) chopped celery

½ cup (75 g) chopped green bell pepper

½ teaspoon minced garlic

¼ cup (60 ml) olive oil

16 ounces (454 g) no-salt-added stewed tomatoes

3 ounces (84 g) mushrooms, sliced

¼ teaspoon hot pepper sauce

Arrange the fish in a microwave-safe dish. Combine the onion, celery, green pepper, garlic, and oil in a medium microwave-safe bowl and microwave on high for 3 minutes. Add the tomatoes, mushrooms, and hot pepper sauce, stir to combine, and pour over the fish. Microwave for 8 to 10 minutes, until the fish is opaque.

Yield: 4 servings

Per serving: 376 calories (64% from fat, 30% from protein, 6% from carbohydrate); 28 g protein; 27 g total fat; 5 g saturated fat; 16 g monounsaturated fat; 4 g polyunsaturated fat; 6 g carbohydrate; 1 g fiber; 3 g sugar; 379 mg phosphorus; 30 mg calcium; 101 mg sodium; 687 mg potassium; 193 IU vitamin A; 26 mg ATE vitamin E; 19 mg vitamin C; 80 mg cholesterol

Lemon-Pepper Catfish

Simple but very good, with just a little lemon juice and black pepper for seasoning, these fish fillets are a great start to a weekday meal. Steamed broccoli with a little more lemon juice squeezed over it, would be a great accompaniment.

3 tablespoons (45 ml) olive oil

1½ pounds (680 g) catfish fillets

¼ cup (60 ml) lemon juice, divided

½ teaspoon freshly ground black pepper, divided

Heat the oil in a large skillet over medium-high heat. Add the fish and drizzle 2 tablespoons (30 ml) of the lemon juice over the top. Sprinkle with ¼ teaspoon of the pepper. Cook for 4 minutes and turn. Drizzle with the remaining 2 tablespoons (30 ml) juice and sprinkle with the remaining ¼ teaspoon pepper. Cook for 4 to 6 minutes longer, until the fish flakes easily with a fork.

Yield: 4 servings

Per serving: 324 calories (65% from fat, 33% from protein, 2% from carbohydrate); 27 g protein; 23 g total fat; 4 g saturated fat; 14 g monounsaturated fat; 4 g polyunsaturated fat; 1 g carbohydrate; 0 g fiber; 0 g sugar; 345 mg phosphorus; 18 mg calcium; 91 mg sodium; 531 mg potassium; 89 IU vitamin A; 26 mg ATE vitamin E; 8 mg vitamin C; 80 mg cholesterol

Micro Fish Fillets

Not micro as in size, but micro as in microwave. Fish cooks quickly this way and gets nicely done without drying out. This recipe has simple seasonings, so it can be used with a variety of side dishes.

1½ pounds (680 g) haddock or other firm white fish

½ teaspoon lemon pepper

½ teaspoon paprika

1 teaspoon parsley (fresh or dried)

2 tablespoons (28 g) unsalted butter

In 7 × 12-inch (18 × 30.5-cm) glass baking dish, arrange the fish fillets with the thick edges toward the outside of the dish. Sprinkle with the lemon pepper, paprika, and parsley. Dot with the butter. Cover with waxed paper and microwave on high for 8 to 12 minutes, or until the fish is opaque and flakes easily with a fork.

Yield: 6 servings

Per serving: 134 calories (33% from fat, 67% from protein, 1% from carbohydrate); 22 g protein; 5 g total fat; 3 g saturated fat; 1 g monounsaturated fat; 0 g polyunsaturated fat; 0 g carbohydrate; 0 g fiber; 0 g sugar; 215 mg phosphorus; 40 mg calcium; 78 mg sodium; 362 mg potassium; 302 IU vitamin A; 51 mg ATE vitamin E; 0 mg vitamin C; 75 mg cholesterol

Italian Fish

This fish gets a flavor boost from typical Italian herbs. The fresh tomato sauce and fish both cook in the microwave in less than 15 minutes. Serve the sauce over pasta with the fish on the side.

2 cups (360 g) diced tomatoes

1 teaspoon dried basil

½ teaspoon dried oregano

½ teaspoon finely minced garlic

¼ teaspoon freshly ground black pepper

1½ pounds (680 g) tilapia fillets

Combine the tomatoes, basil, oregano, garlic, and pepper in a medium mixing bowl. Microwave on high, uncovered, for 4 to 5 minutes, until tomatoes are softened; keep warm. Place the fillets in shallow microwave-safe baking dish, with the thick edges toward the outside of the dish. Cover with plastic wrap; vent one side to allow steam to escape. Microwave on high for 3 to 6 minutes, or until the fish is slightly translucent in the center. Allow the fish to stand, covered, for 2 to 3 minutes to finish cooking. Drain. Top with the warm sauce and serve.

Yield: 6 servings

Per serving: 136 calories (19% from fat, 73% from protein, 8% from carbohydrate); 24 g protein; 3 g total fat; 0 g saturated fat; 1 g monounsaturated fat; 1 g polyunsaturated fat; 3 g carbohydrate; 1 g fiber; 0 g sugar; 264 mg phosphorus; 58 mg calcium; 66 mg sodium; 625 mg potassium; 501 IU vitamin A; 53 mg ATE vitamin E; 13 mg vitamin C; 36 mg cholesterol

White-Wine Poached Fish

It doesn't get any better than this. Not only does the fish cook in a few minutes, but also the wine-based poaching liquid adds a great flavor and becomes a sauce that you can serve over cooked rice.

1 can (14.5 ounces, or 411 g) no-salt-added stewed tomatoes

12 ounces (336 g) frozen corn

½ cup (120 ml) dry white wine

¼ teaspoon garlic powder

¼ teaspoon Salt-Free Seafood Seasoning (page 27)

8 ounces (56 g) catfish fillets

In a saucepan, combine the tomatoes, corn, wine, garlic, and seasoning, bring to a boil over high heat, and then reduce the heat to a simmer. Add the fish fillets, cover, and simmer for 2 to 3 minutes, until the fish is opaque and flakes easily with a fork.

Yield: 2 servings

Per serving: 381 calories (27% from fat, 27% from protein, 46% from carbohydrate); 25 g protein; 11 g total fat; 2 g saturated fat; 5 g monounsaturated fat; 3 g polyunsaturated fat; 42 g carbohydrate; 7 g fiber; 12 g sugar; 431 mg phosphorus; 83 mg calcium; 110 mg sodium; 1132 mg potassium; 689 IU vitamin A; 17 mg ATE vitamin E; 43 mg vitamin C; 53 mg cholesterol

Sesame Cod

Sesame seeds are often thought of in association with Asian dishes, but here they add flavor to an otherwise simple lemon and tarragon accented fish dish.

1½ pounds (680 g) cod fillets

1 teaspoon unsalted butter, melted

1 teaspoon lemon juice

1 teaspoon tarragon

Pinch of freshly ground black pepper

1 tablespoon (8 g) sesame seeds

Preheat the broiler and set the oven rack about 6 inches (15 cm) from the heat source. Line a broiler pan with aluminum foil. Place the cod fillets on the foil, and brush with the butter. Sprinkle with the lemon juice, tarragon, black pepper, and sesame seeds. Broil until the fish is opaque and white and flakes easily with a fork, about 10 minutes.

Yield: 6 servings

Per serving: 108 calories (19% from fat, 79% from protein, 2% from carbohydrate); 20 g protein; 2 g total fat; 1 g saturated fat; 1 g monounsaturated fat; 1 g polyunsaturated fat; 0 g carbohydrate; 0 g fiber; 0 g sugar; 240 mg phosphorus; 34 mg calcium; 62 mg sodium; 480 mg potassium; 70 IU vitamin A; 19 mg ATE vitamin E; 2 mg vitamin C; 50 mg cholesterol

Teriyaki Fish

This lightly breaded Asian-flavored catfish dish is perfect for those (like me) who love Chinese food. It has the traditional teriyaki flavor and goes well with rice and stir-fried vegetables.

¼ cup (60 g) all-purpose flour

⅛ teaspoon freshly ground black pepper

12 ounces (340 g) catfish fillets, cut into 1-inch (2.5-cm) cubes

2 tablespoons (30 ml) olive oil

¼ cup (60 ml) Low-Sodium Teriyaki Sauce (page 30)

¼ cup (60 g) packed brown sugar

½ teaspoon sesame oil

¼ cup (4 g) chopped fresh chives

Combine the flour and pepper in a resealable plastic bag. Add the fish and shake to coat. Heat the olive oil in a large skillet over medium heat, add the fish, and cook until the fish is opaque in the center and flakes easily with a fork, about 5 minutes per side. Remove from the skillet. And the teriyaki sauce and brown sugar to the pan. Cook, stirring, until the sugar is dissolved. Stir in the sesame oil. Add the fish and chives and stir to coat.

Yield: 3 servings

Per serving: 359 calories (47% from fat, 22% from protein, 31% from carbohydrate); 20 g protein; 19 g total fat; 3 g saturated fat; 11 g monounsaturated fat; 3 g polyunsaturated fat; 28 g carbohydrate; 0 g fiber; 18 g sugar; 270 mg phosphorus; 35 mg calcium; 121 mg sodium; 465 mg potassium; 231 IU vitamin A; 17 mg ATE vitamin E; 3 mg vitamin C; 53 mg cholesterol

Pasta with Fish and Vegetables

A combination of fish and vegetables makes a quick and flavorful topping for pasta.

2 tablespoons (30 ml) olive oil

12 ounces (340 g) salmon fillets, cubed

12 ounces (340 g) cod fillets, cubed

1 teaspoon minced garlic

½ cup (120 ml) white wine

½ teaspoon dried oregano

½ teaspoon dried rosemary

1 teaspoon dried parsley

½ cup (80 g) minced onion

1 cup (150 g) coarsely chopped red bell pepper

1 cup (150 g) coarsely chopped green bell pepper

1 cup (70 g) broccoli florets

8 ounces (225 g) spaghetti, cooked according to package directions

6 tablespoons (30 g) shredded Parmesan cheese

Heat the oil in a heavy skillet over medium heat. Add the fish and garlic and sauté for 1 to 2 minutes, until nearly cooked through. Add the wine, spices, and vegetables and continue

(continued on page 156)

cooking until the sauce has been reduced by about half, 3 to 4 minutes. Serve over the pasta, garnished with the Parmesan.

Yield: 6 servings

Per serving: 299 calories (41% from fat, 37% from protein, 21% from carbohydrate); 27 g protein; 13 g total fat; 3 g saturated fat; 6 g monounsaturated fat; 3 g polyunsaturated fat; 15 g carbohydrate; 3 g fiber; 3 g sugar; 353 mg phosphorus; 108 mg calcium; 167 mg sodium; 638 mg potassium; 1329 IU vitamin A; 23 mg ATE vitamin E; 82 mg vitamin C; 63 mg cholesterol

Curried Tuna

This dish has great curry flavor, with a bit of sweetness imparted by the unusual inclusion of pineapple. Serve over rice.

2 cups (470 ml) Condensed Cream of Mushroom Soup (page 31)

8¾ ounces (245 g) crushed pineapple, undrained

¼ cup (38 g) chopped green bell pepper

1 tablespoon (1 g) snipped fresh chives

1½ teaspoons curry powder

2 cans (5 ounces, or 142 g each) tuna, packed in water, drained, and broken into chunks

Combine the soup, undrained pineapple, green pepper, chives, and curry powder in a medium saucepan and bring to a boil over high heat, stirring. Add the tuna chunks, reduce the heat to medium, and cook until heated through, 1 to 2 minutes.

Yield: 6 servings

Per serving: 141 calories (21% from fat, 42% from protein, 37% from carbohydrate); 15 g protein; 3 g total fat; 1 g saturated fat; 1 g monounsaturated fat; 1 g polyunsaturated fat; 13 g carbohydrate; 1 g fiber; 7 g sugar; 173 mg phosphorus; 28 mg calcium; 46 mg sodium; 512 mg potassium; 84 IU vitamin A; 5 mg ATE vitamin E; 8 mg vitamin C; 27 mg cholesterol

Salade Niçoise

You can make an even more classic Niçoise salad if you have a few boiled potatoes and leftover green beans in the refrigerator. But even if you don't, it makes a filling and flavorful lunch or light dinner.

12 romaine lettuce leaves

2 cans (5 ounces, or 142 g each) tuna, packed in water, drained and crumbled

2 hard-cooked eggs, coarsely chopped

3 tablespoons (15 g) grated Parmesan cheese

¼ cup (60 ml) Caesar Salad Dressing (page 91)

¼ teaspoon freshly ground black pepper

Place 3 romaine lettuce leaves on each of 4 plates. Top with the tuna, hard-cooked eggs, and Parmesan. Drizzle with the Caesar dressing, sprinkle with the black pepper, and serve.

Yield: 4 servings

Per serving: 219 calories (39% from fat, 51% from protein, 10% from carbohydrate); 27 g protein; 9 g total fat; 3 g saturated fat; 3 g monounsaturated fat; 2 g polyunsaturated fat; 5 g carbohydrate; 0 g fiber; 5 g sugar; 292 mg phosphorus; 83 mg calcium; 163 mg sodium; 282 mg potassium; 268 IU vitamin A; 51 mg ATE vitamin E; 0 mg vitamin C; 165 mg cholesterol

Open-Faced Tuna Sandwiches

This is basically an open-faced version of the classic tuna-melt sandwich. It makes a great quick lunch or after school and work snack. And it is super-fast to fix.

1 can (5 ounces, or 142 g) tuna, packed in water, drained and crumbled

⅓ cup (75 g) mayonnaise

½ teaspoon celery seed

½ teaspoon onion powder

¼ teaspoon freshly ground black pepper

4 slices Low-Sodium Whole Wheat Bread (page 312), toasted

4 slices tomato

4 slices Swiss cheese

Combine the tuna and mayonnaise in a small bowl; season with the celery seed, onion powder, and pepper. Spread the tuna on the toast; top with a tomato slice. On a paper plate, microwave the sandwiches on medium for 2 minutes; top with the cheese. Microwave on medium for 1 to 2 minutes more, until the cheese is melted.

Yield: 2 servings

Per serving: 231 calories (39% from fat, 32% from protein, 29% from carbohydrate); 18 g protein; 10 g total fat; 4 g saturated fat; 3 g monounsaturated fat; 3 g polyunsaturated fat; 16 g carbohydrate; 1 g fiber; 2 g sugar; 238 mg phosphorus; 178 mg calcium; 58 mg sodium; 238 mg potassium; 281 IU vitamin A; 33 mg ATE vitamin E; 2 mg vitamin C; 38 mg cholesterol

Tuna Rice Muffins

These tasty tuna muffins can actually be picked up and eaten on the run if you are really in a hurry, but they are also good as the basis for a full meal.

2 cups (330 g) cooked rice

1 cup (110 g) shredded Swiss cheese

1 can (5 ounces, or 142 g) tuna, packed in water, drained and crumbled

1 tablespoon (10 g) minced onion

1 tablespoon (4 g) chopped fresh parsley

½ cup (125 g) egg substitute, or 2 eggs

2 tablespoons (30 ml) skim milk

Preheat the oven to 375°F (190°C, or gas mark 5). Combine all the ingredients in a medium bowl and mix thoroughly. Spray 6 muffin cups with nonstick cooking spray. Divide the mixture among the cups and bake for 12 minutes, or until eggs are completely set.

Yield: 3 servings

(continued on page 158)

Per serving: 427 calories (34% from fat, 34% from protein, 32% from carbohydrate); 35 g protein; 16 g total fat; 9 g saturated fat; 4 g monounsaturated fat; 2 g polyunsaturated fat; 33 g carbohydrate; 1 g fiber; 2 g sugar; 513 mg phosphorus; 485 mg calcium; 112 mg sodium; 422 mg potassium; 649 IU vitamin A; 103 mg ATE vitamin E; 3 mg vitamin C; 67 mg cholesterol

Angel Hair with Spicy Shrimp

Red pepper flakes add a bit of heat to the classic Italian white pasta sauce and lift the shrimp out of the ordinary.

12 ounces (340 g) angel hair pasta

1 pound (454 g) medium shrimp, peeled and deveined

1 tablespoon (15 ml) olive oil

½ teaspoon finely chopped garlic

¾ cup (180 ml) dry white wine

¼ teaspoon red pepper flakes

2 tablespoons (28 g) unsalted butter

Cook the pasta according to the package directions until al dente. Drain and return the pasta to the pot. Rinse the shrimp under cold water and pat dry with paper towels. Heat the oil in a large skillet over medium heat. Add the garlic and cook, stirring, for 1 minute (do not let it brown). Add the shrimp, wine, and red pepper flakes. Simmer until the shrimp are opaque, 2 to 3 minutes. Stir in the butter and cook until melted. Toss the pasta with the shrimp mixture and serve.

Yield: 4 servings

Per serving: 339 calories (34% from fat, 33% from protein, 33% from carbohydrate); 25 g protein; 12 g total fat; 5 g saturated fat; 4 g monounsaturated fat; 2 g polyunsaturated fat; 25 g carbohydrate; 4 g fiber; 0 g sugar; 306 mg phosphorus; 66 mg calcium; 171 mg sodium; 275 mg potassium; 436 IU vitamin A; 109 mg ATE vitamin E; 3 mg vitamin C; 188 mg cholesterol

Buffalo Shrimp

These spicy shrimp are especially for those who like it hot. For a classic combination serve them with celery sticks and the Peppercorn Ranch Dressing on page 35.

1 pound (454 g) medium shrimp, peeled and deveined

½ teaspoon paprika

¼ teaspoon cayenne pepper

5 tablespoons (70 g) unsalted butter

2 teaspoons minced garlic

¼ teaspoon red pepper flakes

¼ cup (4 g) coarsely chopped fresh cilantro

2 teaspoons lime juice

1 lime, cut into wedges

Rinse the shrimp under cold water and pat dry with paper towels. Add the shrimp, paprika, and cayenne to a resealable plastic bag and shake to coat. Heat the butter, garlic, and red pepper flakes in a large skillet over medium heat until the butter has melted. Raise the heat to medium-high; when the butter begins to pop and sizzle, add the shrimp to the pan. Cook and stir the shrimp until they are bright pink on the outside and opaque in the center, about 4 to 5 minutes. Do not overcook. Remove the pan from the heat and stir in the cilantro and lime juice. Garnish with the lime wedges and serve hot.

Yield: 4 servings

Per serving: 252 calories (59% from fat, 37% from protein, 3% from carbohydrate); 23 g protein; 16 g total fat; 9 g saturated fat; 4 g monounsaturated fat; 1 g polyunsaturated fat; 2 g carbohydrate; 0 g fiber; 0 g sugar; 241 mg phosphorus; 67 mg calcium; 170 mg sodium; 234 mg potassium; 892 IU vitamin A; 180 mg ATE vitamin E; 4 mg vitamin C; 210 mg cholesterol

Grilled Shrimp Salad

Perfect for a summer dinner, this shrimp and pasta salad gets a flavor boost from Mexican seasoning. Then the addition of grilled asparagus takes it to an even higher level.

8 ounces (225 g) medium shrimp, peeled and deveined

½ cup (65 g) frozen corn

2 ounces (54 g) orzo, uncooked

6 asparagus spears, trimmed

1 tablespoon (8 g) Salt-Free Mexican Seasoning (page 27)

½ cup (75 g) chopped red bell pepper

2 tablespoons (30 ml) white vinegar

1 tablespoon (15 ml) water

1 tablespoon (15 ml) olive oil

¼ teaspoon freshly ground black pepper

Prepare a grill for medium heat. Rinse the shrimp under cold water and pat dry with paper towels. Microwave the corn in a small bowl until cooked through, 1 to 2 minutes, then rinse under cold water. Cook the orzo according to package directions until al dente. Drain and rinse under cold water; set aside. Thread the asparagus spears onto 2 parallel metal or soaked wooden skewers. Rub the shrimp with the seasoning; thread onto 2 skewers. Grill the asparagus and shrimp, with the lid closed, for 5 to 6 minutes, or until the asparagus is crisp-tender and the shrimp are pink, turning once. Place the corn in a large bowl. Cut the asparagus into 1-inch (2.5-cm) pieces; add to the bowl. Add the shrimp, orzo, and bell pepper. In a small bowl, whisk together the vinegar, water, oil, and black pepper. Pour over the salad and toss to coat.

Yield: 2 servings

Per serving: 482 calories (22% from fat, 41% from protein, 37% from carbohydrate); 55 g protein; 13 g total fat; 2 g saturated fat; 6 g monounsaturated fat; 3 g polyunsaturated fat; 50 g carbohydrate; 16 g fiber; 7 g sugar; 782 mg phosphorus; 234 mg calcium; 204 mg sodium; 1984 mg potassium; 8456 IU vitamin A; 61 mg ATE vitamin E; 290 mg vitamin C; 172 mg cholesterol

Tip: Vary the seasonings and vegetables to create new options, such as Italian seasoning and zucchini.

Quick Skillet Gumbo

Do you want a little Cajun food, but not the long preparation time it often takes? Then try this quick shrimp gumbo. Even though the preparation is simple, the ingredients and taste are classic gumbo. To serve it the traditional way, put a scoop of cooked rice in a bowl, then ladle the gumbo over top.

12 ounces (340 g) medium shrimp, peeled and deveined

1 tablespoon (15 ml) olive oil

1 cup (160 g) chopped onion

10 ounces (280 g) frozen okra

1 can (14.5 ounces, or 411 g) no-salt-added tomatoes, broken up

1 cup (235 ml) Low-Sodium Chicken Broth (page 232)

1/8 teaspoon freshly ground black pepper

1 bay leaf

Rinse the shrimp under cold water and pat dry with paper towels. Heat the oil in a large skillet over medium heat, add the onion, and cook until soft, about 5 minutes. Add the shrimp, okra, tomatoes, broth, pepper, and bay leaf. Cover and bring to a boil over high heat. Reduce the heat to a simmer, uncover, and simmer for 10 minutes, or until the okra is tender, the shrimp are pink, and the liquid is slightly thickened. Discard the bay leaf before serving.

Yield: 4 servings

Per serving: 187 calories (25% from fat, 44% from protein, 31% from carbohydrate); 21 g protein; 5 g total fat; 1 g saturated fat; 3 g monounsaturated fat; 1 g polyunsaturated fat; 15 g carbohydrate; 4 g fiber; 5 g sugar; 267 mg phosphorus; 143 mg calcium; 161 mg sodium; 707 mg potassium; 553 IU vitamin A; 46 mg ATE vitamin E; 33 mg vitamin C; 129 mg cholesterol

Shrimp Newburg

A classic seafood dish made quick and simple. Small shrimp are best for this. Serve over rice.

12 ounces (340 g) small shrimp, peeled and deveined

1/4 cup (55 g) unsalted butter

1/4 cup (60 ml) all-purpose flour

1 1/2 cups (355 ml) skim milk

1/4 cup (60 ml) sherry

Pinch of paprika

1 tablespoon (20 g) no-salt-added tomato paste

Dash of Worcestershire sauce

Rinse the shrimp under cold water and pat dry with paper towels. Combine the butter and flour in a saucepan over medium heat. Cook for 2 minutes, then slowly pour in the milk and bring the mixture to a boil over high heat. Stir in the sherry, paprika, tomato paste, and Worcestershire sauce. Add the shrimp and cook until the shrimp are pink on the outside and opaque in the center, 4 to 6 minutes.

Yield: 4 servings

Per serving: 285 calories (45% from fat, 33% from protein, 22% from carbohydrate); 22 g protein;

13 g total fat; 8 g saturated fat; 3 g monounsaturated fat; 1 g polyunsaturated fat; 15 g carbohydrate; 0 g fiber; 2 g sugar; 294 mg phosphorus; 183 mg calcium; 187 mg sodium; 392 mg potassium; 757 IU vitamin A; 197 mg ATE vitamin E; 4 mg vitamin C; 162 mg cholesterol

Shrimp Scampi

This classic recipe of shrimp sautéed in garlic butter is naturally fast to fix. Serve over pasta.

1 pound (454 g) medium shrimp, peeled and deveined

½ cup (112 g) unsalted butter

1 teaspoon minced garlic

¼ cup (40 g) minced onion

½ teaspoon dried oregano

1 teaspoon dried parsley

Rinse the shrimp under cold water and pat dry with paper towels. Heat the butter in a large skillet over medium heat. Add the garlic, onion, oregano, parsley, and shrimp and sauté for about 5 minutes, until the shrimp are pink on the outside and opaque in the center.

Yield: 4 servings

Per serving: 329 calories (69% from fat, 29% from protein, 3% from carbohydrate); 23 g protein; 25 g total fat; 15 g saturated fat; 6 g monounsaturated fat; 2 g polyunsaturated fat; 2 g carbohydrate; 0 g fiber; 0 g sugar; 243 mg phosphorus; 72 mg calcium; 172 mg sodium; 238 mg potassium; 948 IU vitamin A; 252 mg ATE vitamin E; 4 mg vitamin C; 233 mg cholesterol

Angel Hair Pasta with Shrimp

Sun-dried tomatoes give this shrimp and pasta recipe a little extra spark. It is a great family recipe as well as one that is fancy enough for guests.

1 pound (454 g) medium shrimp, peeled and deveined

1 pound (454 g) angel hair pasta

2 tablespoons (30 ml) olive oil

3 tablespoons (42 g) unsalted butter, cut into small pieces

1 teaspoon crushed garlic

¼ teaspoon freshly ground black pepper

1 cup (235 ml) Low-Sodium Chicken Broth (page 232)

½ cup chopped oil-packed sun-dried tomatoes

¼ cup (15 g) chopped or snipped fresh parsley

Rinse the shrimp under cold water and pat dry with paper towels. Cook the pasta according to package directions until al dente. Drain the pasta. Meanwhile, heat the oil and butter in a large skillet over medium heat. When the butter has melted, add the crushed garlic and cook for 2 minutes. Add the shrimp and pepper and cook until the shrimp are pink on the outside and opaque in the center, 2 to 3 minutes. Add the broth and sun-dried tomatoes and bring to a boil over high heat. When the liquid boils, remove the skillet from the heat, add the pasta, and toss to combine. Sprinkle with the parsley and serve.

(continued on page 162)

Yield: 4 servings

Per serving: 441 calories (40% from fat, 27% from protein, 33% from carbohydrate); 28 g protein; 21 g total fat; 7 g saturated fat; 9 g monounsaturated fat; 2 g polyunsaturated fat; 37 g carbohydrate; 6 g fiber; 0 g sugar; 362 mg phosphorus; 79 mg calcium; 226 mg sodium; 540 mg potassium; 1028 IU vitamin A; 133 mg ATE vitamin E; 22 mg vitamin C; 195 mg cholesterol

Shrimp with Arugula Couscous

This is exactly the kind of thing I look for on busy evenings: something quick to fix, full of healthy ingredients, and delicious.

1 pound (454 g) medium shrimp, peeled and deveined

1 cup (175 g) couscous

3 tablespoons (45 ml) olive oil, divided

½ teaspoon thinly sliced garlic

5 ounces (140 g) arugula

⅛ teaspoon freshly ground black pepper, divided

1 lemon, quartered

Rinse the shrimp under cold water and pat dry with paper towels. Prepare the couscous according to the package directions and fluff with a fork. Meanwhile, heat 2 tablespoons (30 ml) of the oil in a large skillet over medium heat. Add the garlic and cook until aromatic, about 1 minute. Add the arugula and cook until just wilted, about 1 minute. Transfer the arugula and the couscous to a large bowl, season with half the pepper, and toss gently. In the same skillet, heat the remaining 1 tablespoon (15 ml) oil over medium-high heat. Add the shrimp and the remaining pepper and cook for 2 minutes on each side, until pink on the outside and opaque in the center. Serve the shrimp over the couscous with a squeeze of lemon.

Yield: 4 servings

Per serving: 268 calories (42% from fat, 38% from protein, 20% from carbohydrate); 26 g protein; 12 g total fat; 2 g saturated fat; 8 g monounsaturated fat; 2 g polyunsaturated fat; 13 g carbohydrate; 2 g fiber; 1 g sugar; 263 mg phosphorus; 124 mg calcium; 180 mg sodium; 387 mg potassium; 1048 IU vitamin A; 61 mg ATE vitamin E; 16 mg vitamin C; 172 mg cholesterol

Shrimp with Lemon and Zucchini

Fresh ginger gives this shrimp and zucchini dish a nice little bit of zing. This dish is proof positive that you can fix a fancy meal and still get it on the table in 15 minutes. (Letting everyone peel his or her own shrimp helps.) With a slice of bread, this is a complete meal.

1½ pounds (680 g) medium shrimp, unpeeled

½ cup (120 ml) olive oil, divided

1 tablespoon (8 g) grated fresh ginger

1 teaspoon paprika

½ teaspoon freshly ground black pepper

1 lemon, thinly sliced

2 cups (240 g) zucchini, cut into 2½ × ½-inch (6.4 × 1.3-cm) sticks

¼ cup (15 g) chopped fresh parsley

Preheat the broiler and place the oven rack 6 inches (15 cm) below the heat source. Use a sharp knife to make a slit through the shell along the back of each shrimp. Rinse and pat dry, and then transfer to a large bowl. Whisk ¼ cup (60 ml) of the olive oil, ginger, paprika, and pepper in a bowl. Add half of the dressing to the bowl with the shrimp and toss. Add the lemon and zucchini to the remaining dressing and toss, and then spread on a large foil-lined baking sheet. Broil until the lemon and zucchini begin to brown, 5 to 7 minutes. Add the shrimp and broil until the shells are pink, about 3 minutes. Turn the shrimp, lemon, and zucchini and broil for 3 to 4 more minutes. Whisk the remaining ¼ cup (60 ml) olive oil and the parsley in a small bowl. Divide the shrimp, lemon, and zucchini among 4 plates and drizzle with the parsley oil.

Yield: 4 servings

Per serving: 441 calories (62% from fat, 32% from protein, 6% from carbohydrate); 36 g protein; 30 g total fat; 4 g saturated fat; 20 g monounsaturated fat; 4 g polyunsaturated fat; 7 g carbohydrate; 2 g fiber; 2 g sugar; 381 mg phosphorus; 111 mg calcium; 262 mg sodium; 553 mg potassium; 1055 IU vitamin A; 92 mg ATE vitamin E; 27 mg vitamin C; 259 mg cholesterol

Spicy Sautéed Shrimp

This one is a little on the hot side, but still extremely good. These shrimp can also be served as an appetizer.

1½ pounds (680 g) medium shrimp, peeled and deveined

2 tablespoons (28 g) unsalted butter

¼ cup (60 ml) olive oil

2 teaspoons minced garlic

¼ teaspoon cayenne pepper, or to taste

¼ cup (60 ml) white wine

¼ teaspoon freshly ground black pepper

3 tablespoons (21 g) sweet paprika

Rinse the shrimp under cold water and pat dry with paper towels. Heat the butter and olive oil in a large skillet over medium heat. Stir in the garlic and cayenne pepper, and cook until fragrant, about 1 minute. Increase the heat to high, and add the shrimp and white wine. Bring to a boil, and cook until the shrimp are pink on the outside and opaque in the center, about 3 minutes. Season with the pepper and sweet paprika before serving.

Yield: 6 servings

Per serving: 252 calories (56% from fat, 39% from protein, 6% from carbohydrate); 24 g protein; 15 g total fat; 4 g saturated fat; 8 g monounsaturated fat; 2 g polyunsaturated fat; 3 g carbohydrate; 1 g fiber; 0 g sugar; 249 mg phosphorus; 69 mg calcium; 171 mg sodium; 306 mg potassium; 2173 IU vitamin A; 93 mg ATE vitamin E; 5 mg vitamin C; 183 mg cholesterol

Asian Lemon Herb Shrimp

A flavorful soy and lemon sauce livens up this quick stir-fry of shrimp, spinach, and snow peas.

1 cup (190 g) rice

1 pound (454 g) medium shrimp, peeled and deveined

¼ cup (60 ml) Low-Sodium Soy Sauce (page 29)

3 tablespoons (45 ml) lemon juice

1½ tablespoons (15 g) minced garlic

1½ tablespoons (20 g) sugar

1½ tablespoons (4 g) chopped fresh basil

1½ tablespoons (1.5 g) chopped fresh cilantro

2½ tablespoons (38 ml) olive oil, divided

6 ounces (170 g) snow pea pods

2 tablespoons (30 ml) water

6 ounces (170 g) fresh spinach

Cook the rice as desired. Rinse the shrimp under cold water and pat dry with paper towels. In a small bowl, combine the soy sauce, lemon juice, garlic, and sugar and stir until the sugar dissolves. Add the basil and cilantro. Set aside. Heat a wok or large skillet over high heat. Add 2 tablespoons (30 ml) of the oil and heat for 30 seconds. Add the shrimp and stir-fry until pink on the outside and opaque in the center, 3 to 4 minutes. Transfer to a plate. Wipe out the pan. Reduce the heat to medium-high, add the remaining ½ tablespoon (8 ml) oil, and heat for 30 seconds. Add the pea pods and water. Cover partially and cook, stirring occasionally, until bright green, about 1 minute. Add the spinach and the reserved sauce. When it starts to bubble, return the shrimp to the pan. Stir-fry until warmed through, about 1 minute. Serve immediately over the rice.

Yield: 4 servings

Per serving: 310 calories (31% from fat, 36% from protein, 33% from carbohydrate); 28 g protein; 11 g total fat; 2 g saturated fat; 7 g monounsaturated fat; 2 g polyunsaturated fat; 26 g carbohydrate; 3 g fiber; 7 g sugar; 320 mg phosphorus; 150 mg calcium; 245 mg sodium; 634 mg potassium; 4796 IU vitamin A; 61 mg ATE vitamin E; 47 mg vitamin C; 172 mg cholesterol

Shrimp and Chicken Paella

Paella can be a long and involved process, but I've shortened it here. Chicken and shrimp sauté quickly and using couscous instead of rice further reduces the cooking time. But the flavor is still exactly what you would expect.

1 pound (454 g) medium shrimp, peeled and deveined

¼ cup (60 ml) olive oil

12 ounces (340 g) boneless skinless chicken breasts, cut into bite-size pieces

1 bay leaf

2 tablespoons (5 g) fresh thyme sprigs

1 cup (160 g) chopped onion

½ teaspoon red pepper flakes

1 teaspoon grated or chopped garlic

½ cup (90 g) chopped roasted red bell pepper

1 teaspoon turmeric

½ teaspoon freshly ground black pepper

2 cups (470 ml) Low-Sodium Chicken Broth (page 232)

2 cups (350 g) couscous

1 cup (130 g) no-salt-added frozen peas

1 teaspoon lemon zest

¼ cup (15 g) chopped fresh parsley

Rinse the shrimp under cold water and pat dry. Heat the oil in a deep skillet over medium-high heat (be sure to choose a pan with a tight-fitting lid). Add the chicken, bay leaf, thyme, and onion. Cook for 2 minutes to start softening the onion; then, add the shrimp, red pepper flakes, garlic, red pepper, and turmeric and cook until the shrimp are almost cooked through, about 3 minutes. Season with the pepper; then, add the chicken broth. Bring to a boil over high heat, and boil for about 1 minute. Stir in the couscous, peas, and lemon zest. Cover and turn off the heat. Let stand for 5 minutes, then fluff with a fork. Remove the bay leaf and thyme stems, sprinkle with the chopped parsley, and serve.

Yield: 4 servings

Per serving: 431 calories (35% from fat, 35% from protein, 31% from carbohydrate); 37 g protein; 17 g total fat; 3 g saturated fat; 11 g monounsaturated fat; 2 g polyunsaturated fat; 33 g carbohydrate; 5 g fiber; 5 g sugar; 368 mg phosphorus; 102 mg calcium; 196 mg sodium; 649 mg potassium; 1988 IU vitamin A; 29 mg ATE vitamin E; 51 mg vitamin C; 118 mg cholesterol

Shrimp and Corn Chowder

This great soup is a traditional chowder and can be a full meal with just a slice of bread. And you won't toil over a hot stove to fix it.

8 ounces (225 g) medium shrimp, peeled and deveined

1 tablespoon (14 g) unsalted butter

1 cup (160 g) diced onion

1 cup (235 ml) Low-Sodium Chicken Broth (page 232)

¼ teaspoon dried thyme

12 ounces (336 g) frozen corn

1 medium red potato, boiled and diced

1 cup (235 ml) skim milk

¼ teaspoon paprika

1 teaspoon fresh parsley

Rinse the shrimp under cold water and pat dry with paper towels. Heat the butter in a large, heavy-bottomed pot over medium heat, add the onion, and cook until lightly browned, 3 to 4 minutes. Add the broth, thyme, corn, and diced cooked potato. Reduce the heat to low and simmer for 5 minutes. Add the shrimp and cook until pink on the outside and opaque in the center, 3 to 4 minutes. Add the milk and heat through, 1 to 2 minutes. Sprinkle with the paprika and parsley and serve.

Yield: 3 servings

Per serving: 353 calories (18% from fat, 29% from protein, 54% from carbohydrate); 26 g protein; 7 g total fat; 3 g saturated fat; 2 g

(continued on page 166)

monounsaturated fat; 1 g polyunsaturated fat; 49 g carbohydrate; 5 g fiber; 7 g sugar; 442 mg phosphorus; 185 mg calcium; 209 mg sodium; 1235 mg potassium; 631 IU vitamin A; 123 mg ATE vitamin E; 25 mg vitamin C; 127 mg cholesterol

Arugula and Scallop Salad

The spicy taste of arugula goes well with mild-flavored things such as seafood. In this salad it is topped with simple sautéed scallops.

1 pound (454 g) scallops

¼ cup (60 ml) olive oil, divided

¼ teaspoon freshly ground black pepper

2 Portobello mushrooms, thinly sliced

5 cups (100 g) arugula

½ cup (60 g) thinly sliced celery

¼ cup (40 g) thinly sliced red onion

1 teaspoon lemon juice

Rinse the scallops under cold water and pat dry. Heat 2 tablespoons (30 ml) of the oil a large stainless steel skillet over medium heat until smoking hot. Season the scallops with pepper, and add them to the hot skillet one by one. Cook the scallops until golden in color, about 3 to 4 minutes per side. In a large mixing bowl, combine the sliced mushrooms, arugula, celery, onion, and lemon juice. Drizzle with the remaining 2 tablespoons (30 ml) oil. Toss to coat. Arrange the veggies on the center of a platter. Arrange the scallops on top of the salad and serve.

Yield: 4 servings

Per serving: 232 calories (57% from fat, 34% from protein, 9% from carbohydrate); 20 g protein; 15 g total fat; 2 g saturated fat; 10 g monounsaturated fat; 2 g polyunsaturated fat; 5 g carbohydrate; 1 g fiber; 1 g sugar; 268 mg phosphorus; 76 mg calcium; 202 mg sodium; 514 mg potassium; 718 IU vitamin A; 17 mg ATE vitamin E; 9 mg vitamin C; 37 mg cholesterol

Broiled Scallops

A simple preparation results in simple perfection, as only garlic butter, and lemon are added to these tasty scallops.

1 pound (454 g) scallops

1 tablespoon (9 g) garlic powder

2 tablespoons (28 g) unsalted butter, melted

2 tablespoons (30 ml) lemon juice

Preheat the broiler and place the oven rack 6 inches (15 cm) below the heat source. Rinse the scallops under cold water and pat dry. Place in a shallow baking pan, sprinkle with the garlic powder, melted butter, and lemon juice, and broil for 6 to 8 minutes, turning once, or until golden.

Yield: 3 servings

Per serving: 213 calories (38% from fat, 50% from protein, 12% from carbohydrate); 26 g protein; 9 g total fat; 5 g saturated fat; 2 g monounsaturated fat; 1 g polyunsaturated fat; 6 g carbohydrate; 0 g fiber; 1 g sugar; 346 mg phosphorus; 42 mg calcium; 245 mg sodium;

533 mg potassium; 314 IU vitamin A; 86 mg ATE vitamin E; 10 mg vitamin C; 70 mg cholesterol

Salmon Mock Kabobs

Simple and fast, flavored with dill, these chunks of salmon can be served as is or as a great topper for a Caesar salad.

1½ pounds (680 g) salmon, cut into 1-inch (2.5-cm) cubes
2 tablespoons (30 ml) olive oil
1½ tablespoons (6 g) dried dill

Preheat the broiler and place the oven rack 6 inches (15 cm) below the heat source. Combine all the ingredients in a bowl. Spread on a lightly oiled baking sheet and broil for 4 to 6 minutes, turning once, until the salmon flakes easily with a fork.

Yield: 6 servings

Per serving: 202 calories (49% from fat, 50% from protein, 1% from carbohydrate); 24 g protein; 11 g total fat; 2 g saturated fat; 6 g monounsaturated fat; 2 g polyunsaturated fat; 0 g carbohydrate; 0 g fiber; 0 g sugar; 406 mg phosphorus; 296 mg calcium; 87 mg sodium; 366 mg potassium; 115 IU vitamin A; 20 mg ATE vitamin E; 0 mg vitamin C; 44 mg cholesterol

Greek Shrimp Mock Kabobs

If you like shrimp as much as I do, this is a special treat, full of the great taste of the Mediterranean region, yet easy to fix. And I don't miss trying to thread shrimp onto skewers at all.

1½ pounds (680 g) medium shrimp, peeled and deveined
24 cherry tomatoes
2 lemons, sliced
2 tablespoons (30 ml) olive oil
1½ teaspoons dried marjoram
1 tablespoon (6 g) dried dill
1½ teaspoons crushed garlic

Preheat the broiler and place the oven rack 6 inches (15 cm) below the heat source. Rinse the shrimp under cold water and pat dry with paper towels. Combine all the ingredients in a bowl. Spread on a lightly oiled baking sheet and broil for 4 to 6 minutes, turning once, until the shrimp are pink on the outside and opaque in the center.

Yield: 6 servings

Per serving: 184 calories (32% from fat, 50% from protein, 18% from carbohydrate); 24 g protein; 7 g total fat; 1 g saturated fat; 4 g monounsaturated fat; 1 g polyunsaturated fat; 9 g carbohydrate; 3 g fiber; 0 g sugar; 242 mg phosphorus; 98 mg calcium; 170 mg sodium; 435 mg potassium; 680 IU vitamin A; 61 mg ATE vitamin E; 44 mg vitamin C; 172 mg cholesterol

Sesame Shrimp Mock Kabobs

This Asian-inspired shrimp dish is perfect with plain white rice and steamed broccoli.

1½ pounds (680 g) medium shrimp, peeled and deveined

2 tablespoons (30 ml) olive oil

1 teaspoon sesame oil

2 tablespoons (30 ml) rice vinegar

2 tablespoons (30 ml) Low-Sodium Soy Sauce (page 29)

3 tablespoons (24 g) sesame seeds

Preheat the broiler and place the oven rack 6 inches (15 cm) below the heat source. Rinse the shrimp under cold water and pat dry with paper towels. Combine all the ingredients in a bowl. Spread on a lightly oiled baking sheet and broil for 4 to 6 minutes, turning once, until the shrimp are pink on the outside and opaque in the center.

Yield: 6 servings

Per serving: 196 calories (44% from fat, 50% from protein, 6% from carbohydrate); 24 g protein; 9 g total fat; 1 g saturated fat; 5 g monounsaturated fat; 3 g polyunsaturated fat; 3 g carbohydrate; 1 g fiber; 0 g sugar; 267 mg phosphorus; 104 mg calcium; 182 mg sodium; 245 mg potassium; 205 IU vitamin A; 61 mg ATE vitamin E; 2 mg vitamin C; 172 mg cholesterol

10

15-Minute Vegetarian Dishes

Because most vegetables do not contain as much natural sodium as animal products do, their sodium contents can be very low. And vegetables typically do not require long cooking times; in fact, they taste better and contain more nutrients if cooked just until crisp-tender. This chapter's assortment of vegetarian pasta dishes, sandwiches, and soups are sure to please even the meat eaters in your family.

Green Spaghetti (But No Ham)

This sauce of a different color may look and sound a little funny, but trust me, it tastes great. The fresh herbs take this to a whole new level. It is the kind of simple, yet incredibly full-flavored meal that can make vegetarian options so good.

1 cup (60 g) fresh parsley

¼ cup (10 g) fresh basil

½ teaspoon pressed garlic

½ cup (120 ml) olive oil

16 ounces (454 g) spaghetti

¼ cup (25 g) grated Parmesan cheese

Combine the parsley, basil, and garlic in a blender. Pulse until finely chopped. Slowly add the oil until it reaches a thick, but moist, state. Cook the spaghetti according to package directions until al dente; drain. Pour the sauce over the pasta and toss to combine. Sprinkle the Parmesan cheese over the top and serve.

Yield: 6 servings

Per serving: 278 calories (61% from fat, 8% from protein, 30% from carbohydrate); 6 g protein; 20 g total fat; 3 g saturated fat; 14 g monounsaturated fat; 2 g polyunsaturated fat; 22 g carbohydrate; 4 g fiber; 1 g sugar; 111 mg phosphorus; 102 mg calcium; 73 mg sodium; 143 mg potassium; 994 IU vitamin A; 5 mg ATE vitamin E; 14 mg vitamin C; 4 mg cholesterol

Spaghetti with Spicy Red Pepper Sauce

This is similar to a number of spicy red pepper sauces on the market, based primarily on fresh red peppers and sour cream. It has great flavor and much lower in sodium than store-bought varieties.

12 ounces (340 g) spaghetti

1½ cups (225 g) julienned red bell pepper

1 teaspoon minced garlic

¾ teaspoon cayenne pepper

1 cup (230 g) reduced-fat sour cream

¾ cup (180 ml) Low-Sodium Vegetable Broth (page 232)

½ cup (50 g) grated Parmesan cheese

Cook the spaghetti according to package directions until al dente; drain. Meanwhile, coat a large skillet with cooking spray and sauté the red bell pepper, garlic, and cayenne pepper over medium heat for 3 to 5 minutes, until peppers are softened. Stir in the sour cream and broth; simmer, uncovered, for 5 minutes. Remove from the heat and stir in the cheese. Pour the sauce over the pasta and toss to combine.

Yield: 4 servings

Per serving: 265 calories (38% from fat, 18% from protein, 43% from carbohydrate); 13 g protein; 12 g total fat; 7 g saturated fat; 3 g monounsaturated fat; 1 g polyunsaturated fat; 30 g carbohydrate; 5 g fiber; 3 g sugar; 254 mg phosphorus; 222 mg calcium; 233 mg sodium; 297 mg potassium; 2170 IU vitamin A; 75 mg ATE vitamin E; 107 mg vitamin C; 35 mg cholesterol

Spinach Spaghetti

This is a totally painless way to eat spinach. Combined with chicken broth and yogurt, the result is a creamy sauce that even spinach haters will like.

16 ounces (454 g) spaghetti

10 ounces (280 g) fresh spinach

¼ cup (60 ml) Low-Sodium Vegetable Broth (page 232)

½ cup (50 g) grated Parmesan cheese

½ cup (115 g) low-fat plain yogurt

Cook the spaghetti according to package directions until al dente; drain. Steam or sauté the fresh spinach until just wilted, 2 to 3 minutes. Put the spinach into a blender, add the broth, and blend until liquefied. Stir in the cheese and yogurt. Pour the sauce over the pasta and toss to combine.

Yield: 5 servings

Per serving: 195 calories (17% from fat, 22% from protein, 61% from carbohydrate); 12 g protein; 4 g total fat; 2 g saturated fat; 1 g monounsaturated fat; 0 g polyunsaturated fat; 31 g carbohydrate; 5 g fiber; 6 g sugar; 212 mg phosphorus; 215 mg calcium; 217 mg sodium; 422 mg potassium; 5373 IU vitamin A; 14 mg ATE vitamin E; 16 mg vitamin C; 10 mg cholesterol

Quick Fresh Tomato Sauce

This sauce of fresh tomatoes and basil has so much flavor you won't want to add meat to it. This sauce is best made in summer, when the best sun-ripened fresh plum or Roma tomatoes and basil are in season. You'll love it over your favorite pasta.

1⅔ pounds (754 g) Roma tomatoes

¼ cup (60 ml) olive oil

1 teaspoon finely chopped garlic

½ cup (20 g) finely chopped fresh basil

1½ teaspoons dried oregano

Bring a large saucepan of water to a boil over high heat. With a small, sharp knife, remove the core of each tomato. Blanch the tomatoes in the water for 30 seconds, then lift them out with a slotted spoon. Peel off the skins. Cut each in half horizontally and scoop out and discard the seeds. Coarsely chop the tomato pulp. In a large skillet, heat the olive oil over medium heat. Add the garlic and sauté for about 1 minute. Add the tomatoes, raise the heat to medium-high, and sauté just until the juices thicken, about 5 minutes. Add the herbs and simmer for about 1 minute more.

Yield: 4 servings, about 2 cups total

Per serving: 166 calories (71% from fat, 5% from protein, 23% from carbohydrate); 2 g protein; 14 g total fat; 2 g saturated fat; 10 g monounsaturated fat; 2 g polyunsaturated fat; 10 g carbohydrate; 4 g fiber; 5 g sugar; 68 mg phosphorus; 115 mg calcium; 11 mg sodium; 601 mg potassium; 1994 IU vitamin A; 0 mg ATE vitamin E; 27 mg vitamin C; 0 mg cholesterol

Veggie and Cheese Pitas

A generous assortment of vegetables combine with Swiss cheese to create this quick and easy lunch that packs a lot of nutrition and enough bulk to hold you through the afternoon.

¼ cup (18 g) chopped broccoli

¼ cup (25 g) chopped cauliflower

¼ cup (18 g) sliced mushrooms

¼ cup (40 g) thinly sliced red onion

¼ cup (45 g) sliced tomato

1 whole wheat pita, cut in half

1 ounce (28 g) Swiss cheese

Stuff all of the vegetables into the pita bread. Top with the cheese and warm in the microwave until the cheese melts, about 1 minute.

Yield: 2 servings

Per serving: 160 calories (26% from fat, 20% from protein, 54% from carbohydrate); 8 g protein; 5 g total fat; 3 g saturated fat; 1 g monounsaturated fat; 1 g polyunsaturated fat; 23 g carbohydrate; 4 g fiber; 2 g sugar; 173 mg phosphorus; 154 mg calcium; 181 mg sodium; 225 mg potassium; 307 IU vitamin A; 30 mg ATE vitamin E; 23 mg vitamin C; 13 mg cholesterol

Black Bean Quesadillas

Black beans, tomatoes, and cheese fill these quesadillas, making you forget that there is no meat in there. I usually add a bit more cilantro because I like the flavor (and I'm the cook, so I can). You can use either salt-free canned beans or dried ones cooked in advance.

2 cups (512 g) black beans, drained

¼ cup (45 g) chopped tomato

3 tablespoons (3 g) chopped cilantro

8 tortillas, 6 inches (15 cm)

4 ounces (112 g) Swiss cheese, shredded

¼ cup (65 g) Low-Sodium Salsa (page 232)

Preheat the oven to 350°F (180°C, or gas mark 4). In a medium bowl, mash the beans with a fork, then stir in the tomato and cilantro. Spread evenly onto 4 tortillas. Sprinkle with the cheese and salsa. Top with the remaining 4 tortillas. Bake on an ungreased cookie sheet for 12 minutes, until lightly browned and cheese is melted. Cut into wedges and serve.

Yield: 4 servings

Per serving: 309 calories (26% from fat, 23% from protein, 51% from carbohydrate); 18 g protein; 9 g total fat; 5 g saturated fat; 2 g monounsaturated fat; 1 g polyunsaturated fat; 40 g carbohydrate; 10 g fiber; 1 g sugar; 416 mg phosphorus; 368 mg calcium; 136 mg sodium; 461 mg potassium; 556 IU vitamin A; 60 mg ATE vitamin E; 4 mg vitamin C; 26 mg cholesterol

Eggplant Burgers

Vegetarian burgers are often made with portobello mushrooms or a soy protein mixture. These use eggplant, for a delicious flavor difference. They are prepared simply but provide a great change of pace from the usual lunch or dinner fare.

1 eggplant, peeled and sliced into six ¾-inch (2-cm) rounds

1 tablespoon (14 g) unsalted butter

6 slices (½ ounce, or 14 g each) Swiss cheese

6 hamburger buns, split

Place the eggplant slices on a microwave-safe plate, and microwave for about 5 minutes, or until the centers are cooked through. Melt the butter in a large skillet over medium-high heat. Fry the eggplant slices until lightly toasted on each side, 1 to 2 minutes, turn, then place 1 slice of cheese on each one. Cook until the cheese has melted, 1 minute or less, and remove from the skillet. Place the eggplant on the hamburger buns, and allow each person to top as desired. Top with your favorite burger toppings such as lettuce, tomato, or red onion slices.

Yield: 6 servings

Per serving: 202 calories (37% from fat, 17% from protein, 46% from carbohydrate); 9 g protein; 9 g total fat; 4 g saturated fat; 3 g monounsaturated fat; 1 g polyunsaturated fat; 24 g carbohydrate; 4 g fiber; 5 g sugar; 158 mg phosphorus; 185 mg calcium; 201 mg sodium; 261 mg potassium; 196 IU vitamin A; 46 mg ATE vitamin E; 2 mg vitamin C; 18 mg cholesterol

Barbecued Tofu

If you believe that tofu can only be used in Asian dishes, you should give these tofu-based barbecue sandwiches a try. It will make a convert out of you.

12 ounces (340 g) firm tofu

3 tablespoons (45 ml) olive oil

1 cup (160 g) thinly sliced onion

1½ cups (375 g) Barbecue Sauce (page 30)

6 hamburger buns, split

Drain the tofu between paper towels until most of the water has been squeezed out. Slice into ¼-inch (6-mm)-thick slices. Heat the oil in a large skillet over medium heat, add the tofu strips, and sauté until golden brown on both sides, 1 to 2 minutes per side. Add the onion and cook for a few minutes, until softened. Pour in the barbecue sauce. Reduce the heat to low and cook for 5 minutes. Divide the mixture among the buns and serve.

Yield: 6 servings

Per serving: 345 calories (28% from fat, 10% from protein, 61% from carbohydrate); 9 g protein; 11 g total fat; 2 g saturated fat; 7 g monounsaturated fat; 2 g polyunsaturated fat; 54 g carbohydrate; 2 g fiber; 28 g sugar; 111 mg phosphorus; 65 mg calcium; 238 mg sodium; 217 mg potassium; 1 IU vitamin A; 0 mg ATE vitamin E; 2 mg vitamin C; 0 mg cholesterol

Glazed Tofu

This tofu is coated with a glaze made of maple syrup and pineapple juice, flavored with soy sauce and mustard. It makes a nice addition to some stir-fried vegetables for a meatless meal.

½ cup (120 ml) maple syrup

½ cup (120 ml) pineapple juice

1 teaspoon Low-Sodium Soy Sauce (page 29)

2 tablespoons (22 g) Dijon mustard

1 tablespoon (15 ml) olive oil

8 ounces (225 g) firm tofu, drained and cubed

Whisk together the maple syrup, pineapple juice, soy sauce, and mustard in a small bowl. Set aside. Heat the olive oil in a large skillet over medium-high heat and stir in the tofu. Cook and stir until the tofu is evenly browned, 2 to 3 minutes. Stir in the syrup mixture and continue to cook until the glaze has reduced to about half, 3 to 4 minutes.

Yield: 2 servings

Per serving: 387 calories (24% from fat, 9% from protein, 67% from carbohydrate); 9 g protein; 11 g total fat; 1 g saturated fat; 6 g monounsaturated fat; 3 g polyunsaturated fat; 67 g carbohydrate; 1 g fiber; 58 g sugar; 125 mg phosphorus; 114 mg calcium; 231 mg sodium; 497 mg potassium; 24 IU vitamin A; 0 mg ATE vitamin E; 7 mg vitamin C; 0 mg cholesterol

Tip: Serve over rice.

Grilled Cheese with Vegetables

Bored with plain grilled cheese sandwiches? Then try these with tomato, bell pepper, and basil. Still bored? Swap some Anaheim or serrano chile peppers for the bell peppers to take the flavor to the next level.

2 tablespoons (28 g) unsalted butter

8 slices Low-Sodium Bread (pages 312 to 324)

4 slices (½ ounce, or 14 g each) Swiss cheese

4 slices tomato

1 green bell pepper, seeded and thinly sliced

2 teaspoons dried basil

Preheat a griddle over medium heat. Butter one side of each slice of bread, and place 4 of the slices butter side down on the griddle. On each piece of bread, place 1 slice of cheese, 1 slice of tomato, and a few slices of pepper. Sprinkle the dried basil on top. Top each sandwich with a slice of buttered bread, butter side up. Grill the sandwiches until golden brown, about 2 to 3 minutes per side.

Yield: 4 servings

Per serving: 249 calories (42% from fat, 15% from protein, 43% from carbohydrate); 9 g protein; 12 g total fat; 7 g saturated fat; 3 g monounsaturated fat; 1 g polyunsaturated fat; 27 g carbohydrate; 3 g fiber; 5 g sugar; 181 mg phosphorus; 205 mg calcium; 24 mg sodium; 283 mg potassium; 774 IU vitamin A; 78 mg ATE vitamin E; 35 mg vitamin C; 28 mg cholesterol

Open-Faced Broiled Tomato Sandwiches

These may be the best tomato sandwiches I've ever had. And that's saying a lot, because I live on tomato sandwiches in the summer when the garden is producing. Marinating the tomatoes in a balsamic vinegar dressing before pairing them with an herb-flavored mayonnaise and Parmesan cheese just pushes them over the top.

2 tablespoons (30 ml) olive oil

2 tablespoons (30 ml) balsamic vinegar

2 tomatoes, sliced

3 tablespoons (42 g) mayonnaise

½ teaspoon dried parsley

¼ teaspoon dried oregano

¼ teaspoon freshly ground black pepper

3 tablespoons (20 g) grated Parmesan cheese, divided

4 slices Low-Sodium Bread (pages 312 to 324), lightly toasted

Preheat the broiler. In a shallow bowl, whisk together the olive oil and vinegar. Marinate the tomatoes in the mixture, stirring occasionally, for 5 minutes. Meanwhile, in a small bowl, combine the mayonnaise, parsley, oregano, black pepper, and 4 teaspoons (7 g) of the Parmesan cheese. Spread the mixture on each slice of toasted bread. Place the marinated tomatoes on 2 slices and sprinkle with the remaining 8 teaspoons (13 g) Parmesan cheese on the other two slices. Place on a baking sheet and broil for 5 minutes, or until the cheese turns golden brown and tomatoes are warmed. Combine tomato and cheese halves to make a sandwich.

Yield: 2 servings

Per serving: 373 calories (53% from fat, 10% from protein, 37% from carbohydrate); 10 g protein; 23 g total fat; 5 g saturated fat; 13 g monounsaturated fat; 4 g polyunsaturated fat; 35 g carbohydrate; 4 g fiber; 4 g sugar; 181 mg phosphorus; 169 mg calcium; 198 mg sodium; 467 mg potassium; 1005 IU vitamin A; 11 mg ATE vitamin E; 39 mg vitamin C; 13 mg cholesterol

Tip: Make these with the Sun-Dried Tomato Bread on page 319.

Tortilla Spinwheels

Although originally intended as an appetizer, these make a great quick meal. They are filled with black beans and cheese and taste great no matter when you eat them.

4 ounces (112 g) cream cheese, softened

½ cup (115 g) sour cream

1 cup (110 g) shredded Swiss cheese

¼ cup (40 g) chopped red onion

⅛ teaspoon garlic powder

2 cups (512 g) black beans, drained and rinsed

6 (8-inch, or 20-cm, diameter) flour tortillas

Combine the cream cheese and sour cream; mix until well blended. Stir in the Swiss

(continued on page 176)

cheese, onion, and garlic powder. Spread thin layer of the cream cheese mixture onto each tortilla. Purée the beans in a food processor or blender. Starting in the middle of each tortilla, spread a layer of beans, covering half of the tortilla. Roll up the tortilla, starting with the end that has the beans, and slice.

Yield: 6 servings

Per serving: 134 calories (56% from fat, 15% from protein, 29% from carbohydrate); 5 g protein; 8 g total fat; 5 g saturated fat; 3 g monounsaturated fat; 0 g polyunsaturated fat; 10 g carbohydrate; 2 g fiber; 0 g sugar; 89 mg phosphorus; 89 mg calcium; 1 mg iron; 146 mg sodium; 113 mg potassium; 256 IU vitamin A; 65 mg ATE vitamin E; 0 mg vitamin C; 23 mg cholesterol

Cheesy Vegetable Soup

This is a creamy vegetable soup full of potatoes and an assortment of other vegetables, topped off by the flavor of Swiss cheese. It's the sort of meal that goes down perfectly on a cold day.

2 tablespoons (30 ml) olive oil

1 cup (100 g) sliced celery

1 cup (160 g) chopped onion

⅔ cup (80 g) all-purpose flour

4 cups (940 ml) Low-Sodium Vegetable Broth (page 232)

¼ teaspoon freshly ground black pepper

2 cups (300 g) frozen broccoli, cauliflower, and carrot

1 cup (115 g) frozen hash browns

3 cups (705 ml) skim milk

1½ cups (165 g) shredded Swiss cheese

Heat the oil in a large kettle over medium heat, add the celery and onion, and cook until tender, 5 minutes. Add the flour and stir until smooth. Gradually add the broth and stir to combine, and then add the black pepper, vegetables, and hash browns. Increase the heat to high and bring to a boil. Reduce the heat to a simmer, cover, and simmer for 10 minutes. Add the milk and cheese and cook, stirring, until the cheese melts and the soup is heated through, being careful not to boil.

Yield: 5 servings

Per serving: 433 calories (44% from fat, 22% from protein, 34% from carbohydrate); 24 g protein; 22 g total fat; 10 g saturated fat; 9 g monounsaturated fat; 2 g polyunsaturated fat; 37 g carbohydrate; 2 g fiber; 3 g sugar; 517 mg phosphorus; 623 mg calcium; 181 mg sodium; 740 mg potassium; 737 IU vitamin A; 174 mg ATE vitamin E; 7 mg vitamin C; 9 mg cholesterol

Quick Summer Vegetable Soup

This super quick soup is chock-full of fresh vegetables and herbs, giving it amazing depth of flavor for something that cooks so quickly.

3 cups (705 ml) Low-Sodium Vegetable Broth (page 232)

½ cup (55 g) shredded carrot

½ cup (60 g) shredded zucchini

½ cup (35 g) shredded cabbage

½ cup (75 g) shredded green bell pepper

2 cups (60 g) chopped spinach

1 can (14.5 ounces, or 411 g) no-salt-added tomatoes

⅓ cup (30 g) egg noodles

½ teaspoon minced garlic

½ cup (30 g) chopped fresh parsley

Bring the broth to a boil in a kettle over high heat. Add the carrot, zucchini, cabbage, bell pepper, spinach, and tomatoes. Bring to a boil again and simmer for 5 minutes. Add the noodles, bring to a boil again, and simmer for another 5 minutes. Add the garlic and parsley, remove from the heat, and serve immediately.

Yield: 4 servings

Per serving: 86 calories (15% from fat, 27% from protein, 59% from carbohydrate); 6 g protein; 2 g total fat; 0 g saturated fat; 1 g monounsaturated fat; 0 g polyunsaturated fat; 14 g carbohydrate; 3 g fiber; 5 g sugar; 114 mg phosphorus; 85 mg calcium; 98 mg sodium; 713 mg potassium; 4242 IU vitamin A; 1 mg ATE vitamin E; 53 mg vitamin C; 3 mg cholesterol

Cream of Broccoli Soup

There are only 3 ingredients, but don't let that fool you. This soup is full of the kind of flavor you can't get out of a can. It is perfect when you are looking for a snack or a quick lunch, but want something that also has some nutrition in it.

12 ounces (336g) frozen broccoli

2 cups (470 ml) Low-Sodium Vegetable Broth (page 232)

12 ounces (340 g) nonfat evaporated milk

Combine the broccoli and broth in a saucepan over medium heat and cook for 5 minutes. Add the milk and cook until heated through, 1 to 2 minutes. Do not boil.

Yield: 2 servings

Per serving: 219 calories (9% from fat, 37% from protein, 54% from carbohydrate); 22 g protein; 2 g total fat; 1 g saturated fat; 1 g monounsaturated fat; 0 g polyunsaturated fat; 32 g carbohydrate; 4 g fiber; 22 g sugar; 497 mg Phosphorus; 570 mg calcium; 274 mg sodium; 1219 mg potassium; 1606 IU vitamin A; 201 mg ATE vitamin E; 128 mg vitamin C; 7 mg cholesterol

Not Just Your Ordinary Tomato Soup

Tomato soup can be kind of bland, but not this one, with the added flavor and nutrition boost of celery, onions, and green peppers. This quick soup is the kind of thing you can put together for a lunch in a jiffy and not feel like you are sacrificing anything.

1 can (14.5 ounces, or 411 g) no-salt-added tomatoes

½ cup (50 g) chopped celery

¼ cup (40 g) sliced onion

½ cup (75 g) chopped green bell pepper

(continued on page 178)

2 cups (470 ml) Low-Sodium Beef Broth
  (page 231)

1½ cups (355 ml) water

2 tablespoons (28 g) unsalted butter

2 tablespoons (15 g) all-purpose flour

½ teaspoon sugar

1 teaspoon dried basil

⅛ teaspoon paprika

In a saucepan over medium heat, combine the tomatoes, celery, onion, and bell pepper and simmer for 10 minutes. Add the beef broth and water. Meanwhile, in a small skillet over medium heat, melt the butter. Stir in the flour to form a roux and cook for 5 minutes, until lightly browned. Add to the tomato mixture and stir to combine. Stir in the sugar, basil, and paprika and simmer until slightly thickened, 2 to 3 minutes. Transfer to a blender and purée until smooth, if desired.

Yield: 4 servings

Per serving: 109 calories (49% from fat, 12% from protein, 39% from carbohydrate); 3 g protein; 6 g total fat; 4 g saturated fat; 2 g monounsaturated fat; 0 g polyunsaturated fat; 13 g carbohydrate; 2 g fiber; 5 g sugar; 55 mg phosphorus; 61 mg calcium; 98 mg sodium; 437 mg potassium; 525 IU vitamin A; 48 mg ATE vitamin E; 33 mg vitamin C; 15 mg cholesterol

Quick and Easy Gazpacho

This is a fairly typical gazpacho recipe, featuring pureed fresh tomatoes, cucumbers, and peppers in a slightly spicy, slightly sour broth. It can be used as either a light meal or an appetizer.

2 ripe tomatoes, blanched in boiling water for
  30 seconds and peeled

1 cucumber, peeled

¼ cup (38 g) diced bell pepper

¼ cup (40 g) diced onion

1 cup (235 ml) tomato juice

2 tablespoons (30 ml) olive oil

1½ teaspoons vinegar (red wine is best)

Dash of hot pepper sauce

Garlic powder, to taste

Freshly ground black pepper, to taste

Combine all the ingredients in a blender. Process to the desired texture. Serve at room temperature or chilled.

Yield: 4 servings

Per serving: 82 calories (71% from fat, 4% from protein, 25% from carbohydrate); 1 g protein; 7 g total fat; 1 g saturated fat; 5 g monounsaturated fat; 1 g polyunsaturated fat; 5 g carbohydrate; 1 g fiber; 4 g sugar; 29 mg phosphorus; 18 mg calcium; 8 mg sodium; 252 mg potassium; 352 IU vitamin A; 0 mg ATE vitamin E; 13 mg vitamin C; 0 mg cholesterol

Tip: Garnish with a celery stick or low-sodium croutons.

Teriyaki Tofu Mock Kabobs

This is the tofu that even tofu haters like. It only contains three ingredients, but the teriyaki sauce and sesame oil impart a flavor that makes you forget you didn't like tofu.

1 pound (454 g) firm tofu

¼ cup (60 ml) Low-Sodium Teriyaki Sauce (page 30)

2 tablespoons (30 ml) sesame oil

Drain and cube the tofu. Preheat the broiler and place the oven rack 6 inches (15 cm) below the heat source. Combine all the ingredients in a bowl. Spread on a baking sheet and broil until the tofu is golden brown and nicely glazed, turning once, 4 to 6 minutes.

Yield: 6 servings

Per serving: 101 calories (62% from fat, 21% from protein, 17% from carbohydrate); 5 g protein; 7 g total fat; 1 g saturated fat; 2 g monounsaturated fat; 3 g polyunsaturated fat; 4 g carbohydrate; 0 g fiber; 3 g sugar; 70 mg phosphorus; 25 mg calcium; 133 mg sodium; 152 mg potassium; 0 IU vitamin A; 0 mg ATE vitamin E; 0 mg vitamin C; 0 mg cholesterol

11

15-Minute Salads

Salads are an obvious choice for quick, healthy meals. The vegetables are packed with nutrients and if you have a few Low-Sodium Salad Dressings (pages 34 to 37) in the refrigerator, you can throw one together in a few minutes using whatever is handy in your vegetable bin. But there are other kinds of salads, too, as this chapter shows. They are still fast to prepare, but are the kind of thing to prepare when you are looking for something a little more interesting. This chapter contains hot salads, pasta salads, and an assortment of main dish salads that can be on the table in minutes.

Broccoli Salad

Kidney beans, red onion, and sesame seeds lift this salad above the ordinary. I've used several different dressings with this salad, but my favorite is ranch. Any of the Dressings on pages 34 to 37 may be used.

1 cup (70 g) broccoli florets

¼ cup (40 g) chopped red onion

½ cup (125 g) no-salt-added kidney beans

¼ cup (38 g) unsalted sunflower seeds

½ cup (120 ml) Dressing (pages 34 to 37)

Combine all the ingredients in a bowl and toss to mix.

Yield: 4 servings

Per serving: 83 calories (41% from fat, 19% from protein, 40% from carbohydrate); 4 g protein; 4 g total fat; 0 g saturated fat; 1 g monounsaturated fat; 3 g polyunsaturated fat; 9 g carbohydrate; 3 g fiber; 1 g sugar; 137 mg phosphorus; 31 mg calcium; 6 mg sodium; 233 mg potassium; 535 IU vitamin A; 0 mg ATE vitamin E; 18 mg vitamin C; 0 mg cholesterol

Carrot Salad

This is as simple and traditional as you can get. Still, it's something everyone likes and it's a cinch to fix, so go for it.

3 cups (330 g) shredded carrots

1 cup (145 g) raisins

½ cup (75 g) chopped cashews

½ cup (112 g) mayonnaise

Combine all the ingredients in a bowl and toss to mix.

Yield: 4 servings

Per serving: 326 calories (35% from fat, 6% from protein, 59% from carbohydrate); 5 g protein; 14 g total fat; 3 g saturated fat; 6 g monounsaturated fat; 4 g polyunsaturated fat; 52 g carbohydrate; 5 g fiber; 30 g sugar; 159 mg phosphorus; 60 mg calcium; 104 mg sodium; 716 mg potassium; 11555 IU vitamin A; 0 mg ATE vitamin E; 7 mg vitamin C; 7 mg cholesterol

Classic Cucumber Salad

You've seen these cucumbers in sour cream on every buffet you've ever gone to. But that's a reason to have them, not a reason not to. If they are that popular, they must be good. And they certainly are easy.

8 ounces (225 g) sour cream

¼ cup (40 g) thinly sliced onion

2 tablespoons (30 ml) lemon juice

2 tablespoons (30 ml) cider vinegar

¼ teaspoon freshly ground black pepper

3 cups (360 g) peeled and thinly sliced cucumber

In a bowl, combine the sour cream, onion, lemon juice, vinegar, and pepper. Add the cucumbers and mix well.

Yield: 6 servings

(continued on page 182)

Per serving: 64 calories (61% from fat, 9% from protein, 29% from carbohydrate); 2 g protein; 5 g total fat; 3 g saturated fat; 1 g monounsaturated fat; 0 g polyunsaturated fat; 5 g carbohydrate; 0 g fiber; 2 g sugar; 51 mg phosphorus; 50 mg calcium; 17 mg sodium; 147 mg potassium; 197 IU vitamin A; 38 mg ATE vitamin E; 5 mg vitamin C; 15 mg cholesterol

Creamed Pea Salad

I was never all that fond of the creamed peas my mom used to make, basically just peas covered in white sauce. But this pea salad with additional vegetables and creamy ranch dressing is an entirely different story.

4 cups (520 g) no-salt-added frozen peas, cooked according to package directions

1 cup (150 g) chopped red bell pepper

½ cup (80 g) chopped red onion

⅓ cup (75 g) mayonnaise

⅓ cup (80 ml) Ranch Dressing (page 34)

Rinse the peas under cold water to chill. Drain well and pour into a bowl. Add the red pepper, red onion, mayonnaise, and ranch dressing. Gently stir to combine.

Yield: 8 servings

Per serving: 131 calories (35% from fat, 13% from protein, 51% from carbohydrate); 5 g protein; 5 g total fat; 1 g saturated fat; 1 g monounsaturated fat; 3 g polyunsaturated fat; 17 g carbohydrate; 5 g fiber; 6 g sugar; 72 mg

phosphorus; 24 mg calcium; 74 mg sodium; 144 mg potassium; 2285 IU vitamin A; 1 mg ATE vitamin E; 44 mg vitamin C; 5 mg cholesterol

It's Easy Being Greens

Those of you who aren't familiar with Kermit the Frog of the Muppets won't get the title, but thats all right, you'll still get this salad. Get the flavor of long-cooked Southern greens without the long cooking time, and get fantastic nutrition at the same time.

8 cups (240 g) spinach or other greens

3 tablespoons (45 ml) olive oil

1 tablespoon (15 ml) cider vinegar

1 teaspoon Dijon mustard

½ teaspoon Italian seasoning

½ teaspoon onion powder

Place the spinach in a salad bowl. Combine the oil, vinegar, mustard, seasoning, and onion powder in a jar with a tight-fitting lid; shake well. Pour over the spinach and toss to coat.

Yield: 8 servings

Per serving: 53 calories (84% from fat, 6% from protein, 10% from carbohydrate); 1 g protein; 5 g total fat; 1 g saturated fat; 4 g monounsaturated fat; 1 g polyunsaturated fat; 1 g carbohydrate; 1 g fiber; 0 g sugar; 16 mg phosphorus; 32 mg calcium; 31 mg sodium; 173 mg potassium; 2818 IU vitamin A; 0 mg ATE vitamin E; 9 mg vitamin C; 0 mg cholesterol

Mushroom Salad

This quick and easy salad is flavored with lemon juice and Swiss cheese, It's great with steak or chicken instead of sautéed mushrooms.

3 tablespoons (45 ml) lemon juice

3 tablespoons (45 ml) olive oil

¼ teaspoon freshly ground black pepper

16 ounces (454 g) mushrooms, sliced

½ cup (55 g) shredded Swiss cheese

½ cup (30 g) chopped fresh parsley

In a large bowl, combine the lemon juice, oil, and pepper. Add the mushrooms, cheese, and parsley and toss.

Yield: 4 servings

Per serving: 182 calories (70% from fat, 18% from protein, 12% from carbohydrate); 8 g protein; 15 g total fat; 4 g saturated fat; 9 g monounsaturated fat; 1 g polyunsaturated fat; 6 g carbohydrate; 2 g fiber; 3 g sugar; 201 mg phosphorus; 174 mg calcium; 12 mg sodium; 432 mg potassium; 769 IU vitamin A; 35 mg ATE vitamin E; 18 mg vitamin C; 15 mg cholesterol

Quickie Coleslaw

It doesn't get any easier than this. Use your SaladShooter or food processor to shred the cabbage for this traditional vinegar-based cole slaw and you can be done in about 3 minutes.

2 cups (140 g) shredded cabbage

3 tablespoons (38 g) sugar

2 tablespoons (30 ml) canola oil

3 tablespoons (45 ml) vinegar

¼ teaspoon celery seed

Place the cabbage in a large serving bowl. Combine the sugar, oil, vinegar, and celery seed in a jar with a tight-fitting lid; shake well. Pour over the cabbage and toss to coat.

Yield: 4 servings

Per serving: 110 calories (54% from fat, 2% from protein, 44% from carbohydrate); 1 g protein; 7 g total fat; 0 g saturated fat; 4 g monounsaturated fat; 2 g polyunsaturated fat; 13 g carbohydrate; 1 g fiber; 12 g sugar; 12 mg phosphorus; 24 mg calcium; 8 mg sodium; 123 mg potassium; 76 IU vitamin A; 0 mg ATE vitamin E; 14 mg vitamin C; 0 mg cholesterol

Sesame Slaw

This is not exactly your usual down-home slaw, unless home happens to be in Asia. Asian ingredients such as napa cabbage, rice vinegar, and sesame seeds give it a unique flavor, but it is extraordinarily tasty and easy to fix.

6 cups thinly sliced napa cabbage

1 cup (16 g) fresh cilantro

¼ cup (60 ml) orange juice

2 tablespoons (30 ml) olive oil

2 tablespoons (30 ml) rice vinegar

2 teaspoons sesame seeds

1 tablespoon (20 g) honey

(continued on page 184)

In a large bowl, combine the cabbage and cilantro. Combine the orange juice, oil, vinegar, sesame seeds, and honey in a jar with a tight-fitting lid; shake well. Pour over the cabbage and cilantro and toss to coat.

Yield: 6 servings

Per serving: 76 calories (57% from fat, 8% from protein, 35% from carbohydrate); 2 g protein; 5 g total fat; 1 g saturated fat; 4 g monounsaturated fat; 1 g polyunsaturated fat; 7 g carbohydrate; 0 g fiber; 3 g sugar; 33 mg phosphorus; 48 mg calcium; 17 mg sodium; 165 mg potassium; 765 IU vitamin A; 0 mg ATE vitamin E; 10 mg vitamin C; 0 mg cholesterol

Tip: Great with pork chops brushed with teriyaki sauce.

Spinach Salad

Parts of this salad, such as hard-cooked eggs and mandarin oranges, are typical to many spinach salads. Other things, such as bean sprouts and water chestnuts, are not. The dressing is a simple vinaigrette based on red wine vinegar. For a little different flavor substitute balsamic vinegar.

12 ounces (280 g) fresh spinach

4 ounces (112 g) bean sprouts

4 ounces (112 g) sliced water chestnuts

2 hard-cooked eggs, sliced

6 ounces (170 g) mandarin orange segments

½ cup (120 ml) olive oil

¼ cup (50 g) sugar

¼ cup (60 ml) red wine vinegar

2 tablespoons (30 g) no-salt-added ketchup

½ cup (80 g) finely chopped red onion

2 teaspoons Worcestershire sauce

Combine the spinach, bean sprouts, water chestnuts, eggs, and orange segments in a salad bowl. Combine the oil, sugar, vinegar, ketchup, onion, and Worcestershire sauce in a jar with a tight-fitting lid; shake well. Pour over the salad and toss to coat.

Yield: 6 servings

Per serving: 433 calories (41% from fat, 5% from protein, 54% from carbohydrate); 5 g protein; 21 g total fat; 3 g saturated fat; 14 g monounsaturated fat; 2 g polyunsaturated fat; 61 g carbohydrate; 2 g fiber; 53 g sugar; 90 mg phosphorus; 79 mg calcium; 100 mg sodium; 590 mg potassium; 5725 IU vitamin A; 30 mg ATE vitamin E; 38 mg vitamin C; 70 mg cholesterol

Tip: Add some leftover chicken for a complete meal.

Vegetable Dip Salad

This salad tastes like vegetable dip, because it's really just fresh vegetables and ranch dressing over lettuce. It is popular with kids and adults alike. To make it even quicker, cut up vegetables ahead of time and store in sealed bags in the refrigerator.

1 cup (125 g) cauliflower florets

1 cup (70 g) broccoli florets

1 cup (130 g) sliced carrot

½ cup (50 g) sliced celery

½ cup (120 ml) Ranch Dressing (page 34)

1½ cups (83 g) chopped lettuce

Combine the cauliflower, broccoli, carrot, and celery in a medium bowl. Pour the ranch dressing over and toss to coat. Divide the lettuce among 6 plates, and top with the vegetables.

Yield: 6 servings

Per serving: 98 calories (59% from fat, 5% from protein, 36% from carbohydrate); 1 g protein; 7 g total fat; 1 g saturated fat; 2 g monounsaturated fat; 4 g polyunsaturated fat; 9 g carbohydrate; 2 g fiber; 3 g sugar; 34 mg phosphorus; 27 mg calcium; 42 mg sodium; 193 mg potassium; 2799 IU vitamin A; 2 mg ATE vitamin E; 24 mg vitamin C; 5 mg cholesterol

Wilted Lettuce Salad

This is another one of those classic salads, with its warm sweet and sour bacon dressing, that people don't seem to fix very often at home, but it doesn't take much time, so give it a try.

4 cups (220 g) chopped lettuce

½ cup (80 g) sliced onion

¼ cup (29 g) sliced radishes

3 slices low-sodium bacon, diced

2 tablespoons (30 ml) vinegar

1 teaspoon packed brown sugar

¼ teaspoon dry mustard powder

⅛ teaspoon freshly ground black pepper

In a large salad bowl, combine the lettuce, onion, and radishes; set aside. In a skillet over medium heat, cook the bacon until crisp, 4 to 5 minutes; remove with a slotted spoon to drain on paper towels. To the drippings, add the vinegar, brown sugar, mustard, and pepper and simmer for 5 minutes. Pour over the lettuce and toss; sprinkle with the bacon. Serve immediately.

Yield: 4 servings

Per serving: 56 calories (40% from fat, 22% from protein, 37% from carbohydrate); 3 g protein; 3 g total fat; 1 g saturated fat; 1 g monounsaturated fat; 0 g polyunsaturated fat; 5 g carbohydrate; 1 g fiber; 3 g sugar; 56 mg phosphorus; 29 mg calcium; 82 mg sodium; 201 mg potassium; 4153 IU vitamin A; 1 mg ATE vitamin E; 13 mg vitamin C; 7 mg cholesterol

Italian Tomato Salad

This is a simple salad, but sometimes those are the best kind. In this case you should get very ripe tomatoes, fresh off the vine if possible, to combine with the cucumber, fresh mozzarella, and red onion.

4 cups (220 g) torn romaine lettuce

1 o 2 tomatoes, cut into wedges

¾ cup (90 g) sliced cucumber

½ cup (80 g) thinly sliced red onion

½ cup (60 g) cubed fresh mozzarella

½ cup (120 ml) Italian Dressing (page 35)

(continued on page 186)

Combine all the ingredients in a bowl and toss to mix.

Yield: 4 servings

Per serving: 98 calories (45% from fat, 23% from protein, 32% from carbohydrate); 6 g protein; 5 g total fat; 2 g saturated fat; 1 g monounsaturated fat; 1 g polyunsaturated fat; 8 g carbohydrate; 2 g fiber; 3 g sugar; 126 mg phosphorus; 151 mg calcium; 20 mg sodium; 320 mg potassium; 3594 IU vitamin A; 22 mg ATE vitamin E; 25 mg vitamin C; 11 mg cholesterol

Pasta Salad in a Hurry

If you don't have time to spend chopping vegetables, then this is the pasta salad for you. Instead of chopping, just thaw frozen vegetables and you are ready to go.

1 pound (454 g) pasta, such as elbows or shells

12 ounces (340 g) frozen broccoli and cauliflower mix, thawed

¾ cup (180 ml) Italian Dressing (page 35)

¼ cup (25 g) grated Parmesan cheese

Cook the pasta according to package directions until al dente; drain. Place the pasta and vegetables in a large bowl. Mix well. Pour the dressing over the salad and toss. Sprinkle with the Parmesan cheese before serving.

Yield: 6 servings

Per serving: 336 calories (12% from fat, 16% from protein, 73% from carbohydrate); 13 g protein;

4 g total fat; 1 g saturated fat; 1 g monounsaturated fat; 1 g polyunsaturated fat; 61 g carbohydrate; 4 g fiber; 2 g sugar; 180 mg phosphorus; 86 mg calcium; 87 mg sodium; 294 mg potassium; 667 IU vitamin A; 5 mg ATE vitamin E; 39 mg vitamin C; 5 mg cholesterol

Tip: Turn this into a main dish by adding chunks of chicken, tuna, or another protein.

Asian Vegetable Salad

This can be thrown together in a jiffy because it's easy to keep all the ingredients on hand and the frozen vegetables mean less preparation work. It goes well with any grilled meat brushed with an Asian-style sauce.

20 ounces (560 g) frozen Oriental vegetable mix, thawed

5 ounces (140 g) sliced water chestnuts

2 tablespoons (30 ml) Ranch Dressing Mix (page 34)

2 tablespoons (28 g) mayonnaise

Combine all the ingredients in a bowl and toss to mix.

Yield: 4 servings

Per serving: 172 calories (28% from fat, 10% from protein, 61% from carbohydrate); 5 g protein; 6 g total fat; 1 g saturated fat; 1 g monounsaturated fat; 3 g polyunsaturated fat; 27 g carbohydrate; 7 g fiber; 6 g sugar; 97 mg phosphorus; 41 mg calcium; 94 mg sodium; 449 mg potassium; 6082 IU vitamin A; 6 mg ATE vitamin E; 6 mg vitamin C; 3 mg cholesterol

Hot Bean and Onion Salad

As the weather gets colder, I become fonder of hot salads. This is sort of a quickie three-bean salad, with the traditional flavor, but without several kinds of beans or the need for time to cool.

18 ounces (504 g) frozen green beans

¾ cup (120 g) sliced onion, separated into rings

3 tablespoons (45 ml) olive oil

3 tablespoons (45 ml) red wine vinegar

½ teaspoon dried oregano

⅛ teaspoon freshly ground black pepper

Cook the beans according to package directions; drain. Combine the beans and onion in a salad bowl. Combine the oil, vinegar, oregano, and pepper in a jar with a tight-fitting lid; shake well. Pour over the hot bean mixture and toss to coat.

Yield: 4 servings

Per serving: 144 calories (60% from fat, 7% from protein, 33% from carbohydrate); 3 g protein; 10 g total fat; 1 g saturated fat; 7 g monounsaturated fat; 1 g polyunsaturated fat; 13 g carbohydrate; 5 g fiber; 4 g sugar; 58 mg phosphorus; 57 mg calcium; 9 mg sodium; 323 mg potassium; 893 IU vitamin A; 0 mg ATE vitamin E; 23 mg vitamin C; 0 mg cholesterol

Waldorf Salad

Waldorf salad is one of those classic dishes that look like it takes a lot of time to prepare. But don't be misled, a little quick chopping is really all that is required.

3 apples, peeled, cored, and chopped

½ cup (50 g) chopped celery

¼ cup (38 g) raisins

¼ cup (25 g) unsalted walnuts

1 teaspoon cider vinegar

⅓ cup (75 g) mayonnaise

Combine all the ingredients in a bowl and toss to mix.

Yield: 4 servings

Per serving: 247 calories (64% from fat, 3% from protein, 33% from carbohydrate); 2 g protein; 19 g total fat; 3 g saturated fat; 4 g monounsaturated fat; 11 g polyunsaturated fat; 23 g carbohydrate; 2 g fiber; 16 g sugar; 55 mg phosphorus; 27 mg calcium; 117 mg sodium; 242 mg potassium; 157 IU vitamin A; 15 mg ATE vitamin E; 5 mg vitamin C; 7 mg cholesterol

Tip: Serve over lettuce.

Southeast Asian Rice Noodle Salad

I'm not sure if this is more typically Thai or Vietnamese or maybe just something vaguely Asian, but wherever it comes from it is good. It is a varied combination of ingredients and

(continued on page 188)

flavors that gets a bit of heat from the jalapeno and some cooling effect from the mint and the lime juice.

1 clove garlic

1 cup (16 g) chopped fresh cilantro

½ jalapeño pepper, seeded and minced

¼ cup (60 ml) lime juice

3 tablespoons (38 g) sugar

12 ounces (340 g) rice noodles

1 cup (130 g) julienned carrot

1 cup (120 g) chopped cucumber

¼ cup (24 g) chopped fresh mint

½ cup (45 g) chopped napa cabbage

¼ cup (38 g) unsalted peanuts

4 sprigs fresh mint

Finely mince the garlic with the cilantro and the jalapeño. Transfer the mixture to a bowl, add the lime juice and sugar, and stir well. Let the sauce sit for 5 minutes. Meanwhile, bring a large pot of water to a boil. Add the rice noodles and boil for 2 minutes. Drain well. Rinse the noodles under cold water until cool. Let them drain again. Combine the sauce, noodles, carrot, cucumber, mint, and cabbage in a large serving bowl. Toss well and serve the salad garnished with the peanuts and mint sprigs.

Yield: 6 servings

Per serving: 252 calories (3% from fat, 2% from protein, 95% from carbohydrate); 1 g protein; 1 g total fat; 0 g saturated fat; 0 g monounsaturated fat; 0 g polyunsaturated fat; 60 g carbohydrate; 2 g fiber; 8 g sugar; 45 mg phosphorus; 43 mg

calcium; 47 mg sodium; 184 mg potassium; 3248 IU vitamin A; 0 mg ATE vitamin E; 9 mg vitamin C; 0 mg cholesterol

Tip: Rice noodles are available in the Asian section of large supermarkets or from an Asian market.

Chicken Chef's Salad

This is a fairly traditional combination of greens, vegetables, and chicken, producing a light, main dish salad that is good with just about any dressing from chapter 3.

4 cups (220 g) mixed salad greens

¼ cup (32 g) sliced carrot

1 or 2 tomatoes, cut into wedges

¼ cup (38 g) sliced red bell pepper

4 ounces (112 g) mushrooms, sliced

4 ounces (112 g) chicken breast, cooked and sliced

2 ounces (56 g) Swiss cheese, cut into strips

2 hard-cooked eggs, sliced

¼ cup (60 ml) Salad Dressing (pages 34 to 37)

Layer the veggies and other ingredients in about the order described. Drizzle with the dressing and serve.

Yield: 2 servings

Per serving: 342 calories (43% from fat, 43% from protein, 14% from carbohydrate); 37 g protein; 16 g total fat; 8 g saturated fat; 5 g monounsaturated fat; 2 g polyunsaturated fat; 13 g carbohydrate; 5 g fiber; 7 g sugar; 522 mg

phosphorus; 364 mg calcium; 153 mg sodium; 976 mg potassium; 5919 IU vitamin A; 144 mg ATE vitamin E; 74 mg vitamin C; 320 mg cholesterol (That appears to be a glitch in the software. It says that ½ cup of salad greens has 565 units, but a serving here has over 6500. I've manually
adjusted it.

Chunky Chicken Salad

Avocado, pineapple, and pecans make this more than the usual chicken salad. It makes a fancy enough salad to serve for a luncheon or party. But don't wait for that—treat yourself to it anytime.

1 avocado, divided

1 tablespoon (15 ml) lemon juice, divided

2 cups (110 g) coarsely chopped Boston lettuce, plus 3 whole leaves, for serving

1⅓ cups (186 g) cooked and cubed chicken breast

8 ounces (225 g) pineapple chunks, drained

1 apple, cut into ¾-inch (2-cm) chunks

¼ cup (36 g) chopped pecans

⅓ cup (75 g) mayonnaise

Peel the avocado; cut in half lengthwise and remove the pit. Slice half of the avocado and brush with half of the lemon juice. Chop the remaining avocado and toss with the remaining lemon juice. In a large bowl, gently combine the chopped lettuce, chopped avocado, chicken, pineapple, apple, pecans, and mayonnaise. Place the lettuce leaves on 3 plates, top with the salad, and fan the sliced avocado on top.

Yield: 3 servings

Per serving: 370 calories (53% from fat, 23% from protein, 24% from carbohydrate); 22 g protein; 23 g total fat; 3 g saturated fat; 11 g monounsaturated fat; 6 g polyunsaturated fat; 23 g carbohydrate; 6 g fiber; 11 g sugar; 218 mg phosphorus; 50 mg calcium; 81 mg sodium; 720 mg potassium; 1363 IU vitamin A; 4 mg ATE vitamin E; 16 mg vitamin C; 59 mg cholesterol

Tip: for a really nice presentation chop the chicken and avocado into large pieces about the same size as the pineapple.

Hot Chicken Salad

With the mushroom soup and melted cheese, this is almost more of a sauce than a salad. It is good in a number of ways. You can use it as a sandwich filling, over greens, or just as the main part of a meal.

4 cups (560 g) cooked and sliced chicken breast

½ cup (112 g) mayonnaise

¾ cup (180 ml) Condensed Cream of Mushroom Soup (page 31)

4 hard-cooked eggs, diced

2 cups chopped (200 g) celery

1 tablespoon (10 g) finely chopped onion

1 cup (110 g) shredded Swiss cheese

Preheat the oven to 400°F (200°C, or gas mark 6). In a baking dish, combine the chicken, mayonnaise, soup, eggs, celery, and onion and mix well. Top with the cheese. Bake

(continued on page 190)

for 10 to 12 minutes, until heated through and the cheese is melted.

Yield: 8 servings

Per serving: 331 calories (59% from fat, 36% from protein, 5% from carbohydrate); 30 g protein; 22 g total fat; 6 g saturated fat; 6 g monounsaturated fat; 7 g polyunsaturated fat; 4 g carbohydrate; 1 g fiber; 1 g sugar; 331 mg phosphorus; 200 mg calcium; 208 mg sodium; 404 mg potassium; 492 IU vitamin A; 95 mg ATE vitamin E; 1 mg vitamin C; 186 mg cholesterol

Chicken Fiesta Salad

Full of the flavors of Mexico, this simple, but flavorful, main dish salad is good for warmer evenings or for lunch.

¼ cup (60 ml) olive oil, divided

2 tablespoons (30 ml) lime juice

2 tablespoons (30 ml) lemon juice

1 teaspoon minced garlic

1 teaspoon ground cumin

½ teaspoon dried oregano

2 boneless skinless chicken breasts, thinly sliced

8 cups (440 g) torn romaine lettuce

16 cherry tomatoes, cut in half

2 avocados, peeled, pitted, and sliced

¼ cup (27 g) shredded Swiss cheese

1 cup (50 g) Crumbled Baked Tortilla Chips (page 37)

¼ cup (60 g) fat-free sour cream

½ cup (130 g) Low-Sodium Salsa (page 232)

Combine 2 tablespoons (30 ml) oil, lime and lemon juices, garlic, cumin, and oregano in a resealable plastic bag. Add the chicken and toss to coat. Heat the remaining 2 tablespoons (30 ml) oil in a skillet over medium heat. Add the chicken and sauté until no longer pink in the center, about 5 minutes. Divide the lettuce among 4 plates. Top with the tomatoes, avocado, and chicken. Sprinkle with the cheese and tortilla chips. Combine the sour cream and salsa in a small bowl and spoon over the top.

Yield: 4 servings

Per serving: 461 calories (61% from fat, 15% from protein, 25% from carbohydrate); 17 g protein; 33 g total fat; 6 g saturated fat; 20 g monounsaturated fat; 4 g polyunsaturated fat; 31 g carbohydrate; 11 g fiber; 3 g sugar; 277 mg phosphorus; 194 mg calcium; 258 mg sodium; 1129 mg potassium; 7380 IU vitamin A; 20 mg ATE vitamin E; 59 mg vitamin C; 30 mg cholesterol

Roast Beef and Apple Salad

This salad is a great use of leftover roast beef and the pairing with the apple makes a memorable impression. Even with the simple vinaigrette dressing, this is the kind of thing you could serve at a luncheon without having to apologize for "low-sodium" stuff. It tastes so good no one will know the difference.

3 cups (450 g) diced apple

4 ounces (112 g) cooked roast beef, julienned

1 cup (100 g) thinly sliced celery

¼ cup (25 g) thinly sliced scallion

¼ cup (15 g) minced fresh parsley

⅓ cup (80 ml) olive oil

2 tablespoons (30 ml) cider vinegar

½ teaspoon minced garlic

¼ teaspoon freshly ground black pepper

2 cups (110 g) chopped lettuce

In a bowl, combine the apple, roast beef, celery, scallion, and parsley. In a small bowl, combine the oil, vinegar, garlic, and pepper; mix well. Pour over the apple mixture; toss to coat. Place ½ cup (55 g) lettuce on each of 4 plates and top with the salad.

Yield: 4 servings

Per serving: 265 calories (67% from fat, 13% from protein, 20% from carbohydrate); 9 g protein; 20 g total fat; 3 g saturated fat; 14 g monounsaturated fat; 2 g polyunsaturated fat; 13 g carbohydrate; 2 g fiber; 10 g sugar; 79 mg phosphorus; 39 mg calcium; 46 mg sodium; 317 mg potassium; 2624 IU vitamin A; 0 mg ATE vitamin E; 16 mg vitamin C; 24 mg cholesterol

Shrimp Salad

This delicious salad contains shrimp, tomato and hard-cooked egg in a creamy dressing. It has a little more sodium than many recipes here, due to the shrimp and mayonnaise, so be careful with portion control. Serve on crackers for an appetizer or on a bed of lettuce for a salad.

1 pound (454 g) small shrimp, peeled and deveined

1 cup (180 g) diced tomato

¼ cup (25 g) finely chopped celery

2 hard-cooked eggs

¼ cup (40 g) finely chopped red onion

½ teaspoon freshly ground black pepper

½ teaspoon Salt-Free Seasoning (page 27)

¼ cup (56 g) mayonnaise

Combine all the ingredients in a bowl and toss to mix.

Yield: 4 servings

Per serving: 270 calories (54% from fat, 39% from protein, 7% from carbohydrate); 27 g protein; 16 g total fat; 3 g saturated fat; 4 g monounsaturated fat; 7 g polyunsaturated fat; 5 g carbohydrate; 1 g fiber; 1 g sugar; 298 mg phosphorus; 82 mg calcium; 300 mg sodium; 366 mg potassium; 688 IU vitamin A; 117 mg ATE vitamin E; 14 mg vitamin C; 283 mg cholesterol

Fruity Tuna Salad

Like many tuna salads this one starts with canned tuna and mayonnaise. But that's where the similarity ends. This one also includes less common ingredients such as grapes, pineapple, and almonds. It makes a great quick lunch or light dinner.

1 can (5 ounces, or 142 g) tuna, packed in water, drained and crumbled

½ cup (80 g) diced pineapple

(continued on page 192)

½ cup (75 g) sliced seedless green grapes

½ cup (50 g) chopped celery

½ cup (55 g) unsalted sliced almonds

½ cup (112 g) mayonnaise

6 cups (330 g) lettuce leaves

Combine the tuna, pineapple, grapes, celery, almonds, and mayonnaise in a bowl; mix lightly. Place 1 cup (55 g) lettuce on each of 6 plates and top with the salad.

Yield: 6 servings

Per serving: 248 calories (72% from fat, 16% from protein, 12% from carbohydrate); 11 g protein; 21 g total fat; 3 g saturated fat; 8 g monounsaturated fat; 10 g polyunsaturated fat; 8 g carbohydrate; 2 g fiber; 4 g sugar; 146 mg phosphorus; 62 mg calcium; 146 mg sodium; 333 mg potassium; 4265 IU vitamin A; 16 mg ATE vitamin E; 12 mg vitamin C; 19 mg cholesterol

12

15-Minute Side Dishes

Like salads, many side dishes can easily be made in a short amount of time. Most frozen or fresh vegetables can be prepared in less than 15 minutes without any special considerations. You can make instant rice, instant mashed potatoes, quick-cooking barley, microwaved baked potatoes, and any number of other starches in very little time, too. But again, there may be times when you want something just a little different. One of the reasons I started developing low-sodium recipes to begin with was that I was bored with meals of plain steamed or microwaved vegetables and plain pasta, rice, or potatoes. This chapter will help you satisfy the need for variety without spending long periods of time in the kitchen. There are flavorful vegetables as well as pasta, potato, and rice dishes to perk up your meals in a jiffy.

Broccoli with Orange Sauce

Bored with broccoli? Brighten it up with this orange-flavored sauce. Both orange juice and orange zest contribute to the subtle, yet distinct flavor.

20 ounces (560 g) frozen broccoli

¼ cup (112 g) unsalted butter

1 teaspoon cornstarch

½ cup (120 ml) orange juice

1 tablespoon (6 g) orange zest

Cook the broccoli according to package directions. Meanwhile, in a small saucepan over medium heat, melt the butter. Add the cornstarch and whisk until smooth. Gradually stir in the orange juice and then the orange zest. Increase the heat to high and bring to a boil; cook and stir for 2 minutes, or until thickened. Drain the broccoli, transfer to a large bowl, drizzle with the sauce, and toss to coat.

Yield: 4 servings

Per serving: 168 calories (60% from fat, 10% from protein, 30% from carbohydrate); 4 g protein; 12 g total fat; 7 g saturated fat; 3 g monounsaturated fat; 1 g polyunsaturated fat; 14 g carbohydrate; 4 g fiber; 2 g sugar; 101 mg phosphorus; 76 mg calcium; 49 mg sodium; 514 mg potassium; 1321 IU vitamin A; 95 mg ATE vitamin E; 139 mg vitamin C; 31 mg cholesterol

Key West Broccoli

One step up from the previous orange broccoli we find this enticing combination. Lemon and lime flavors replace the orange, and onions and pimentos add even more flavor. You'll never want to go back to plain broccoli again.

3 pounds (1362 g) fresh broccoli, cut into florets

¼ cup (112 g) unsalted butter

2 tablespoons (20 g) diced onion

2 tablespoons (12.5 g) diced pimentos

4 teaspoons lime juice

2 teaspoons lemon zest

½ teaspoon Salt-Free Seasoning (page 27)

Pinch of freshly ground black pepper

Pour 1 inch (2.5 cm) of water into a large saucepan, add the broccoli, and bring to a boil over high heat. Reduce the heat to a simmer, cover, and cook for 5 to 8 minutes, or until crisp-tender. Meanwhile, melt the butter in a small saucepan over medium heat; stir in the onion, pimentos, lime juice, lemon zest, seasoning, and pepper. Cook for 5 minutes, until vegetables are softened. Drain the broccoli, transfer to a large bowl, add the butter mixture, and toss to coat.

Yield: 8 servings

Per serving: 111 calories (46% from fat, 16% from protein, 38% from carbohydrate); 5 g protein; 6 g total fat; 4 g saturated fat; 2 g monounsaturated fat; 0 g polyunsaturated fat; 12 g

carbohydrate; 5 g fiber; 3 g sugar; 115 mg phosphorus; 83 mg calcium; 57 mg sodium; 551 mg potassium; 1381 IU vitamin A; 48 mg ATE vitamin E; 156 mg vitamin C; 15 mg cholesterol

Lemon-Garlic Broccoli

Broccoli seems to go with just about everything. This is why I'm often looking for something a little different to flavor it with, so it isn't the same thing several nights a week. In this case lemon and garlic add flavor to plain broccoli, turning it into something special. The combination works well with Italian meals.

1 pound (454 g) fresh broccoli, cut into spears

2 tablespoons (30 ml) olive oil

1 tablespoon (15 ml) lemon juice

½ teaspoon minced garlic

⅛ teaspoon freshly ground black pepper

Place the broccoli in a saucepan with a small amount of water; cover and cook over medium heat until crisp-tender, about 5 minutes. Meanwhile, combine the oil, lemon juice, garlic, and pepper in a jar with a tight-fitting lid; shake to combine. Drain the broccoli and place in a serving dish; add the lemon mixture and toss to coat.

Yield: 6 servings

Per serving: 62 calories (61% from fat, 14% from protein, 26% from carbohydrate); 2 g protein; 5 g total fat; 1 g saturated fat; 3 g monounsaturated

fat; 0 g polyunsaturated fat; 4 g carbohydrate; 2 g fiber; 1 g sugar; 38 mg phosphorus; 26 mg calcium; 9 mg sodium; 112 mg potassium; 846 IU vitamin A; 0 mg ATE vitamin E; 32 mg vitamin C; 0 mg cholesterol

Taste of Italy Broccoli

This is an all-the-way Italian treatment for broccoli. Sun-dried tomatoes and Italian dressing perk up the flavor. It's perfect with pasta and other Italian dishes, but It's also good with just plain chicken or beef.

12 ounces (340 g) frozen broccoli florets, cooked according to package directions

2 tablespoons (22 g) chopped oil-packed sun-dried tomatoes

¼ cup (60 ml) Italian Dressing (page 35)

Stir the prepared broccoli, sun-dried tomatoes, and salad dressing together in a bowl until the vegetables are well coated.

Yield: 4 servings

Per serving: 40 calories (25% from fat, 24% from protein, 51% from carbohydrate); 3 g protein; 1 g total fat; 0 g saturated fat; 0 g monounsaturated fat; 0 g polyunsaturated fat; 6 g carbohydrate; 0 g fiber; 1 g sugar; 64 mg phosphorus; 44 mg calcium; 63 mg sodium; 347 mg potassium; 2568 IU vitamin A; 0 mg ATE vitamin E; 80 mg vitamin C; 1 mg cholesterol

Bourbon Carrots

Southern-style carrots with a glaze of bourbon, butter, and brown sugar. Try this with pork for a real treat.

3 cups (705 ml) water

1½ pounds (680 g) baby carrots

1 tablespoon (12 g) granulated sugar

2 tablespoons (28 g) unsalted butter

3 tablespoons (45 g) packed brown sugar

2 tablespoons (30 ml) bourbon

Bring the water to a boil in a 3-quart (3-L) saucepan; add the carrots and granulated sugar. Return to a boil and cook for 5 minutes. Meanwhile, melt the butter and brown sugar in a large skillet over medium-high heat. Stir in the carrots and cook, stirring occasionally, for 2 to 3 minutes, or until well coated. Add the bourbon and cook, stirring occasionally, for 3 more minutes.

Yield: 6 servings

Per serving: 126 calories (31% from fat, 4% from protein, 66% from carbohydrate); 1 g protein; 4 g total fat; 2 g saturated fat; 1 g monounsaturated fat; 0 g polyunsaturated fat; 20 g carbohydrate; 3 g fiber; 14 g sugar; 43 mg phosphorus; 47 mg calcium; 84 mg sodium; 388 mg potassium; 13767 IU vitamin A 32 mg ATE vitamin E; 7 mg vitamin C; 10 mg cholesterol

Candied Carrots

Butter and orange marmalade glaze these carrots to sweet perfection. Kind of the same idea as candied sweet potatoes, only with carrots.

2 cups (260 g) baby carrots

1 tablespoon (14 g) unsalted butter

2 tablespoons (40 g) orange marmalade

In a medium saucepan, bring a ½ inch (1.3 cm) of water to a boil over high heat, add the carrots, and cook for 10 minutes; drain in a colander. In the same saucepan, melt the butter over medium heat. Add the carrots and orange marmalade. Cook and stir for 2 to 3 minutes, or until the carrots are tender and glazed.

Yield: 4 servings

Per serving: 76 calories (34% from fat, 3% from protein, 63% from carbohydrate); 1 g protein; 3 g total fat; 2 g saturated fat; 1 g monounsaturated fat; 0 g polyunsaturated fat; 13 g carbohydrate; 2 g fiber; 9 g sugar; 24 mg phosphorus; 26 mg calcium; 50 mg sodium; 209 mg potassium; 7798 IU vitamin A; 24 mg ATE vitamin E; 4 mg vitamin C; 8 mg cholesterol

Honey-Glazed Carrots

This simple recipe with just butter and sweeteners brings out the natural sweetness of carrots and is perfect with a simple piece of chicken or a pork chop.

2 cups (260 g) sliced carrots

2 tablespoons (28 g) unsalted butter

1 teaspoon packed brown sugar

2 tablespoons (40 g) honey

In a medium saucepan, bring a ½ inch (1.3 cm) of water to a boil over high heat, add the carrots, and cook for 10 minutes; drain in a colander. Melt the butter in a medium skillet, add the sugar and honey, and stir to blend. Add the carrots and cook over low heat, stirring, until each carrot is glazed, 1 to 2 minutes.

Yield: 4 servings

Per serving: 114 calories (44% from fat, 2% from protein, 53% from carbohydrate); 1 g protein; 6 g total fat; 4 g saturated fat; 1 g monounsaturated fat; 0 g polyunsaturated fat; 16 g carbohydrate; 2 g fiber; 13 g sugar; 25 mg phosphorus; 24 mg calcium; 86 mg sodium; 216 mg potassium; 7880 IU vitamin A; 48 mg ATE vitamin E; 4 mg vitamin C; 15 mg cholesterol

Green Beans with Tomatoes

These green beans with a bit of Italian flair from tomatoes, garlic, and oregano go well with grilled Italian meats. But they are also good with other kinds of meals such as Mexican or just plain American.

12 ounces (340 g) frozen green beans, thawed

1 can (14.5 ounces, or 411 g) no-salt-added tomatoes, drained

1 tablespoon (14 g) unsalted butter

1 teaspoon minced garlic

½ teaspoon dried oregano

Combine the green beans, tomatoes, butter, garlic, and oregano in a 2-quart (1.8-L) nonstick saucepan. Cook over medium heat until heated through, 4 to 5 minutes.

Yield: 4 servings

Per serving: 72 calories (35% from fat, 13% from protein, 53% from carbohydrate); 3 g protein; 3 g total fat; 2 g saturated fat; 1 g monounsaturated fat; 0 g polyunsaturated fat; 11 g carbohydrate; 4 g fiber; 4 g sugar; 53 mg phosphorus; 65 mg calcium; 16 mg sodium; 409 mg potassium; 814 IU vitamin A; 24 mg ATE vitamin E; 28 mg vitamin C; 8 mg cholesterol

Italian Green Beans

Unlike the previous recipe, this one gets the full Italian treatment. Italian dressing mix perks up the flavor of green beans. They are good with pasta or grilled meat. And they are also good chilled in a salad, so you might want to plan on having enough for leftovers.

1 pound (454 g) fresh or frozen green beans

2 tablespoons (30 ml) olive oil

2 tablespoons (16 g) Italian Dressing Mix (page 35)

Steam the green beans in a steamer over boiling water until tender, about 6 to 8 minutes. Drizzle with the olive oil and sprinkle

(continued on page 198)

the dressing mix over the top. Toss together and serve hot.

Yield: 6 servings

Per serving: 63 calories (60% from fat, 8% from protein, 32% from carbohydrate); 1 g protein; 5 g total fat; 1 g saturated fat; 3 g monounsaturated fat; 0 g polyunsaturated fat; 5 g carbohydrate; 3 g fiber; 1 g sugar; 29 mg phosphorus; 28 mg calcium; 5 mg sodium; 158 mg potassium; 522 IU vitamin A; 0 mg ATE vitamin E; 12 mg vitamin C; 0 mg cholesterol

Really Sweet Corn

Do you like your sweet corn even sweeter? Or maybe you are just a fan of honey. Either way, this honey-lemon corn is for you.

12 ounces (340 g) frozen corn kernels, cooked according to package directions

1 tablespoon (14 g) unsalted butter

1 tablespoon (20 g) honey

2 teaspoons lemon juice

1 teaspoon parsley flakes

Combine the cooked corn, butter, honey, lemon juice, and parsley together in a bowl and toss until the butter melts and the kernels are well coated.

Yield: 4 servings

Per serving: 116 calories (27% from fat, 9% from protein, 64% from carbohydrate); 3 g protein; 4 g total fat; 2 g saturated fat; 1 g monounsaturated fat; 1 g polyunsaturated fat; 21 g carbohydrate; 2 g fiber; 7 g sugar; 77 mg phosphorus; 5 mg calcium;

14 mg sodium; 241 mg potassium; 101 IU vitamin A; 24 mg ATE vitamin E; 7 mg vitamin C; 8 mg cholesterol

Avocado-Stuffed Tomatoes

Avocados are the primary ingredient in these uncooked stuffed tomatoes. A little bell pepper and Southwestern herbs and spices complete the picture. These are particularly good as an appetizer or a side dish for a Mexican meal.

4 tomatoes

1 avocado, peeled and pitted

¼ teaspoon lemon juice

¼ cup (38 g) chopped green bell pepper

½ teaspoon chili powder

1 teaspoon parsley

¼ teaspoon coriander

Cut the tops off the tomatoes and scoop out the insides; save the insides for another dish. Mash the avocado and mix with the lemon juice, bell pepper, and seasonings. Stuff into the tomato shells.

Yield: 4 servings

Per serving: 91 calories (51% from fat, 8% from protein, 41% from carbohydrate); 2 g protein; 6 g total fat; 1 g saturated fat; 3 g monounsaturated fat; 1 g polyunsaturated fat; 11 g carbohydrate; 4 g fiber; 0 g sugar; 57 mg phosphorus; 15 mg calcium; 1 mg Iron; 20 mg sodium; 529 mg potassium; 1134 IU vitamin A; 0 mg ATE vitamin E; 50 mg vitamin C; 0 mg cholesterol

Quick Broiled Tomatoes

A little olive oil and Parmesan cheese are the only additions to these tomatoes, so you would do well do find some full-flavored ones fresh off the vine. By the time the broiler gets completely heated up they will be finished. And they taste wonderful.

2 medium tomatoes, cut in half

1 teaspoon olive oil

½ teaspoon freshly ground black pepper

2 tablespoons (12.5 g) grated Parmesan cheese

Preheat the broiler. Place the tomatoes, cut side up, on a baking sheet. Drizzle with the oil and sprinkle with the pepper. Broil until tender, 2 to 3 minutes. Sprinkle with the Parmesan and serve.

Yield: 2 servings

Per serving: 72 calories (52% from fat, 18% from protein, 30% from carbohydrate); 3 g protein; 4 g total fat; 1 g saturated fat; 2 g monounsaturated fat; 0 g polyunsaturated fat; 6 g carbohydrate; 1 g fiber; 0 g sugar; 73 mg phosphorus; 77 mg calcium; 106 mg sodium; 263 mg potassium; 725 IU vitamin A; 7 mg ATE vitamin E; 29 mg vitamin C; 6 mg cholesterol

Veggie-Stuffed Tomatoes

When you are looking for a really simple meal, this is the only side dish you'll need, since it contains pasta and lots of vegetables, all held together with a creamy dressing. I like it with a grilled piece of meat.

1½ cups (150 g) pasta, cooked and drained

¼ cup (56 g) mayonnaise

½ cup (115 g) sour cream

1 cup (120 g) chopped zucchini

¾ cup (75 g) chopped celery

¾ cup (83 g) shredded carrot

½ cup (75 g) chopped green bell pepper

1 cup (120 g) chopped cucumber

12 ounces (336 g) frozen corn kernels, cooked and cooled

½ teaspoon celery seed

½ teaspoon onion powder

4 large tomatoes

2 cups (220 g) lettuce

Mix together the pasta, mayonnaise, sour cream, veggies, and spices. Remove the stems and hard centers from the tomatoes. Cut almost through in both directions, leaving 4 wedges. Divide the lettuce among each of 4 plates, fan a tomato on top, and scoop the salad in the middle.

Yield: 4 servings

Per serving: 395 calories (35% from fat, 10% from protein, 54% from carbohydrate); 11 g protein; 16 g total fat; 4 g saturated fat; 4 g monounsaturated fat; 7 g polyunsaturated fat; 57 g carbohydrate; 7 g fiber; 9 g sugar; 295 mg phosphorus; 96 mg calcium; 153 mg sodium; 988 mg potassium; 4629 IU vitamin A; 41 mg ATE vitamin E; 48 mg vitamin C; 17 mg cholesterol

Tip: To make a whole lunch or light meal of it, add a can of water-packed tuna, drained and crumbled.

Imitation Crab Cakes

These zucchini cakes are flavored with seafood seasoning. They make a great side dish with seafood or fish or can be eaten as a vegetarian main dish.

1 cup (120 g) shredded zucchini

1 cup (115 g) Italian-Style Bread Crumbs (page 33)

¼ cup (62 g) egg substitute, or 1 egg, beaten

1 teaspoon mayonnaise

1 teaspoon Salt-Free Seafood Seasoning (page 28)

2 tablespoons (30 ml) olive oil

Combine the zucchini, bread crumbs, egg, mayonnaise, and seasoning in a bowl and mix thoroughly. Shape into 6 patties. Heat the oil in a skillet over medium heat, add the patties, and fry until golden brown, about 4 to 5 minutes. Flip over and cook the other side until golden brown, about 4 to 5 minutes. Transfer to a paper towel–lined plate to drain.

Yield: 6 servings

Per serving: 88 calories (20% from fat, 18% from protein, 62% from carbohydrate); 4 g protein; 2 g total fat; 0 g saturated fat; 0 g monounsaturated fat; 1 g polyunsaturated fat; 14 g carbohydrate; 1 g fiber; 2 g sugar; 50 mg phosphorus; 42 mg calcium; 25 mg sodium; 124 mg potassium; 81 IU vitamin A; 1 mg ATE vitamin E; 4 mg vitamin C; 0 mg cholesterol

Sautéed Zucchini and Mushrooms

A little different take on a side dish. Simple ingredients and preparation, but a surprising amount of flavor. Pair these with a steak in place of the more common onions and mushrooms for a different taste and better nutrition.

2 tablespoons (28 g) unsalted butter

1½ cups (180 g) grated zucchini

8 ounces (225 g) fresh mushrooms, sliced

¼ teaspoon freshly ground black pepper

Melt the butter in a skillet over medium heat. Add the zucchini and mushrooms and sauté, stirring, for 5 minutes, until the vegetables are wilted but still crisp and very hot. Season with the pepper and serve.

Yield: 6 servings

Per serving: 47 calories (70% from fat, 12% from protein, 18% from carbohydrate); 2 g protein; 4 g total fat; 2 g saturated fat; 1 g monounsaturated fat; 0 g polyunsaturated fat; 2 g carbohydrate; 1 g fiber; 1 g sugar; 45 mg phosphorus; 7 mg calcium; 5 mg sodium; 201 mg potassium; 184 IU vitamin A; 32 mg ATE vitamin E; 6 mg vitamin C; 10 mg cholesterol

Zippy Zucchini

This zucchini is not exactly Asian in flavor, but the flavor goes well with Asian as well as other meals. Sesame seeds and garlic turn otherwise boring zucchini into something different and flavorful.

2 tablespoons (30 ml) olive oil

4 cups (480 g) thinly sliced zucchini

2 tablespoons (16 g) sesame seeds

½ teaspoon garlic powder

Heat the oil in a skillet over medium heat, add the zucchini, sesame seeds, and garlic powder, and sauté for 2 to 3 minutes, or until the zucchini is crisp-tender.

Yield: 6 servings

Per serving: 71 calories (73% from fat, 8% from protein, 19% from carbohydrate); 2 g protein; 6 g total fat; 1 g saturated fat; 4 g monounsaturated fat; 1 g polyunsaturated fat; 4 g carbohydrate; 1 g fiber; 1 g sugar; 51 mg phosphorus; 42 mg calcium; 9 mg sodium; 233 mg potassium; 166 IU vitamin A; 0 mg ATE vitamin E; 14 mg vitamin C; 0 mg cholesterol

Zucchini with Peas

It may be called zucchini and peas, but the thyme is the real star here, adding just the right amount of interesting taste. If you get tired of the same old vegetables, you might like this combination. And if you get tired of this, it's also great if you use rosemary instead of thyme.

2 tablespoons (30 ml) olive oil

4 cups (480 g) shredded zucchini

½ teaspoon minced garlic

1 cup (130 g) no-salt-added frozen peas, thawed

1 tablespoon (2.5 g) chopped fresh thyme

Heat the oil in a large skillet over medium heat, then add the zucchini and garlic. Cook, stirring occasionally, until the zucchini is softened, about 5 minutes. Add the peas and thyme, toss well, and cook until heated through, 1 to 2 minutes.

Yield: 6 servings

Per serving: 76 calories (53% from fat, 12% from protein, 35% from carbohydrate); 2 g protein; 5 g total fat; 1 g saturated fat; 3 g monounsaturated fat; 1 g polyunsaturated fat; 7 g carbohydrate; 3 g fiber; 3 g sugar; 53 mg phosphorus; 29 mg calcium; 28 mg sodium; 251 mg potassium; 744 IU vitamin A; 0 mg ATE vitamin E; 17 mg vitamin C; 0 mg cholesterol

Tip: Be careful when buying frozen peas, because many brands have added salt.

Stir-Fried Cabbage

Cabbage tends to get ignored as a vegetable because it just seems so plain. A simple addition of sesame seeds helps to perk up the flavor here. Stir-frying not only allows it to cook quickly but also to stay crisp and retain its bright color.

2 tablespoons (30 ml) olive oil

6 cups (540 g) sliced cabbage

3 tablespoons (45 ml) water

½ teaspoon sesame seeds

(continued on page 202)

Heat the oil in a large skillet over medium heat. Add the cabbage, water, and sesame seeds, and cook, uncovered, for 5 to 7 minutes, or until crisp-tender, stirring occasionally.

Yield: 4 servings

Per serving: 94 calories (63% from fat, 8% from protein, 30% from carbohydrate); 2 g protein; 7 g total fat; 1 g saturated fat; 5 g monounsaturated fat; 1 g polyunsaturated fat; 8 g carbohydrate; 3 g fiber; 5 g sugar; 33 mg phosphorus; 67 mg calcium; 24 mg sodium; 330 mg potassium; 228 IU vitamin A; 0 mg ATE vitamin E; 43 mg vitamin C; 0 mg cholesterol

Tip: For a German flavor, substitute caraway seeds for the sesame seeds.

Sautéed Asparagus

As if asparagus weren't good enough on its own, this recipe makes it even better. A little lemon and pepper enhance the natural flavor, and almonds provide a crunchy counterpoint.

2 pounds (908 g) fresh asparagus

2 tablespoons (28 g) unsalted butter

1 tablespoon (15 ml) lemon juice

¾ cup (83 g) slivered almonds, toasted

¼ teaspoon freshly ground black pepper

Snap off the tough ends of the asparagus. Place the asparagus in a pot, add water to cover, and bring to a boil over high heat. Cook for 3 minutes, or until crisp-tender; drain.

Plunge the asparagus into an ice water bath to stop the cooking process; drain. Melt the butter in a large skillet over medium heat, add the asparagus, and sauté for 3 to 5 minutes, until tender. Add the lemon juice, almonds, and pepper and stir to combine.

Yield: 6 servings

Per serving: 168 calories (64% from fat, 16% from protein, 20% from carbohydrate); 7 g protein; 13 g total fat; 3 g saturated fat; 7 g monounsaturated fat; 2 g polyunsaturated fat; 9 g carbohydrate; 5 g fiber; 4 g sugar; 164 mg phosphorus; 83 mg calcium; 4 mg sodium; 439 mg potassium; 1266 IU vitamin A; 32 mg ATE vitamin E; 10 mg vitamin C; 10 mg cholesterol

Sautéed Spinach

The flavorings in this dish are typical Southern greens, with bacon and red pepper flakes. But the preparation leaves it still slightly crisp and dark green. It has a little more sodium than most side dishes because it contains bacon, spinach, and Dijon mustard, all of which have a fair amount of sodium. Pair it with meat that doesn't have added sodium, such as grilled pork chops.

2 slices low-sodium bacon, cut into 1-inch (2.5-cm) pieces

10 ounces (280 g) fresh spinach

1 tablespoon (14 g) unsalted butter

1 tablespoon (11 g) Dijon mustard

¼ teaspoon red pepper flakes

In a very large skillet, cook the bacon over medium heat until crisp, about 4 to 5 minutes. Remove the bacon to drain on paper towels, reserving 1 tablespoon (15 ml) of the drippings in the skillet. Gradually add the spinach to the skillet, stirring frequently with metal tongs. Cook for 2 to 3 minutes, or until the spinach is just wilted. Transfer to a colander, hold over the sink, and press lightly with a spoon to drain. In the same skillet, melt the butter over medium heat; stir in the mustard and red pepper flakes. Add the drained spinach; toss to coat and reheat the spinach if necessary. Sprinkle with the cooked bacon and serve immediately.

Yield: 3 servings

Per serving: 88 calories (62% from fat, 21% from protein, 17% from carbohydrate); 5 g protein; 7 g total fat; 3 g saturated fat; 2 g monounsaturated fat; 1 g polyunsaturated fat; 4 g carbohydrate; 2 g fiber; 1 g sugar; 81 mg phosphorus; 100 mg calcium; 189 mg sodium; 569 mg potassium; 9050 IU vitamin A; 32 mg ATE vitamin E; 27 mg vitamin C; 16 mg cholesterol

Curried Fresh Vegetables

Curries are often long-cooked dishes, but this recipe proves that they don't need to be. Fresh vegetables cook quickly, taking on the deep curry flavor. It can be served as is for a side dish or over rice or pasta as an accompaniment to a meat course.

3 cups (540 g) chopped tomatoes

1 cup (160 g) coarsely chopped onion

1½ cups (180 g) cubed zucchini

1 cup (150 g) chopped green bell pepper

¼ teaspoon garlic powder

1 tablespoon (6 g) curry powder

Combine all the ingredients in a saucepan. Cook over medium heat, stirring, until the vegetables are softened, about 10 minutes.

Yield: 4 servings

Per serving: 61 calories (10% from fat, 14% from protein, 77% from carbohydrate); 2 g protein; 1 g total fat; 0 g saturated fat; 0 g monounsaturated fat; 0 g polyunsaturated fat; 14 g carbohydrate; 3 g fiber; 3 g sugar; 69 mg phosphorus; 33 mg calcium; 18 mg sodium; 519 mg potassium; 943 IU vitamin A; 0 mg ATE vitamin E; 70 mg vitamin C; 0 mg cholesterol

Southwestern Pasta

Just a simple change in the spices in the sauce gives this pasta a decidedly Southwestern flavor, rather than Italian. Meaning you can use it with a whole different set of meats.

16 ounces (454 g) pasta, such as elbows or shells

2 cups (360 g) cubed tomatoes

1 teaspoon chopped fresh cilantro

⅛ teaspoon dried basil

2 teaspoons sugar

(continued on page 204)

½ teaspoon dried oregano

⅓ cup (80 ml) olive oil

2 tablespoons (12.5 g) grated Parmesan
cheese

Cook the pasta according to package
directions until al dente; drain. In a large bowl,
combine the tomatoes, cilantro, basil, sugar,
and oregano; mix well, and then add the olive
oil. Mix well. Pour the sauce over the pasta
and toss to coat. Sprinkle with the cheese
and serve.

Yield: 6 servings

Per serving: 412 calories (31% from fat, 11%
from protein, 59% from carbohydrate); 11 g protein;
14 g total fat; 2 g saturated fat; 9 g
monounsaturated fat; 2 g polyunsaturated fat; 60 g
carbohydrate; 2 g fiber; 1 g sugar; 141 mg
phosphorus; 41 mg calcium; 42 mg sodium;
238 mg potassium; 336 IU vitamin A; 2 mg ATE
vitamin E; 13 mg vitamin C; 2 mg cholesterol

Spaghetti Alfredo

Spaghetti and broccoli in Alfredo sauce goes
together quickly and is filling enough to be a
hearty side dish or a whole meal in itself.

12 ounces (340 g) spaghetti

3 cups (210 g) broccoli florets

1½ cups (355 ml) skim milk

1 tablespoon (14 g) unsalted butter

1 tablespoon (8 g) all-purpose flour

½ cup (50 g) grated Parmesan cheese

Cook the pasta according to the package
directions until al dente; drain. Meanwhile,
bring a pot of water to a boil and cook the
broccoli until tender, 3 minutes. Drain. Heat
the milk and butter in a large saucepan over
low heat and slowly whisk in the flour. Simmer
until slightly thickened, whisking constantly, 1
to 2 minutes. Remove from the heat and stir
in the Parmesan. Add the pasta and broccoli,
return to the heat, and cook, stirring, over low
heat until heated through, 2 to 3 minutes.

Yield: 4 servings

Per serving: 147 calories (41% from fat, 28%
from protein, 31% from carbohydrate); 11 g protein;
7 g total fat; 4 g saturated fat; 2 g
monounsaturated fat; 0 g polyunsaturated fat; 12 g
carbohydrate; 2 g fiber; 1 g sugar; 241 mg
phosphorus; 303 mg calcium; 268 mg sodium;
395 mg potassium; 767 IU vitamin A; 95 mg ATE
vitamin E; 60 mg vitamin C; 20 mg cholesterol

Summer Pasta with Fresh Tomato Sauce

Here's a quick and easy pasta dish with a
great sauce made with fresh tomatoes,
mozzarella, and basil. The effect is similar to
brushcetta, but served over pasta instead of
on bread. Serve it as a side dish or make a
meal of it.

16 ounces (454 g) pasta, such as elbows or
spirals

1 cup (180 g) chopped Roma tomatoes

4 ounces (112 g) fresh mozzarella cheese,
shredded

⅓ cup (13 g) chopped fresh basil

1 teaspoon minced garlic

¼ cup (60 ml) olive oil

½ teaspoon garlic powder

¼ teaspoon freshly ground black pepper

Cook the pasta according to the package directions until al dente; drain. Meanwhile, combine the tomatoes, cheese, basil, garlic, olive oil, garlic powder, and black pepper in a serving bowl. Add the pasta and toss to combine.

Yield: 6 servings

Per serving: 428 calories (31% from fat, 14% from protein, 56% from carbohydrate); 14 g protein; 15 g total fat; 4 g saturated fat; 8 g monounsaturated fat; 2 g polyunsaturated fat; 59 g carbohydrate; 3 g fiber; 1 g sugar; 197 mg phosphorus; 152 mg calcium; 126 mg sodium; 265 mg potassium; 510 IU vitamin A; 33 mg ATE vitamin E; 5 mg vitamin C; 15 mg cholesterol

Asian Sesame Pasta

This is sort of a lo mien, especially if you make it with spaghetti or angel hair pasta. It can also be made with any other shape and still taste as good. The flavors are typically Asian, with the sesame oil providing the crowning touch.

8 ounces (225 g) pasta

1 tablespoon (15 ml) sesame oil

½ teaspoon Low-Sodium Soy Sauce (page 29)

¼ cup (25 g) chopped scallion

¾ cup (38 g) bean sprouts

Pinch of cayenne pepper

Pinch of white pepper

Pinch of garlic powder

1 tablespoon (8 g) sesame seeds, toasted

Cook the pasta according to package directions until al dente; drain and rinse. Heat the oil in skillet or wok over medium heat. Add the soy sauce, scallion, bean sprouts, cayenne, pepper, garlic powder, and pasta. Stir and cook for 2 to 3 minutes, until heated through and well combined. Transfer to serving plates and garnish with the toasted sesame seeds.

Yield: 4 servings

Per serving: 258 calories (19% from fat, 13% from protein, 68% from carbohydrate); 8 g protein; 5 g total fat; 1 g saturated fat; 2 g monounsaturated fat; 2 g polyunsaturated fat; 44 g carbohydrate; 2 g fiber; 0 g sugar; 107 mg phosphorus; 39 mg calcium; 7 mg sodium; 126 mg potassium; 72 IU vitamin A; 0 mg ATE vitamin E; 2 mg vitamin C; 0 mg cholesterol

Cranberry Couscous

Couscous is just SO plain. And I get bored so easily. So I like to add things to it. In this case, cranberries and scallion. This makes a great base for a curry or the Moroccan stew on page 249.

2 cups (470 ml) Low-Sodium Chicken Broth (page 232)

1 tablespoon (14 g) unsalted butter

(continued on page 206)

1½ cups (263 g) couscous

¼ cup (38 g) dried cranberries

3 tablespoons (18 g) chopped scallion

In a large saucepan, bring the broth and butter to a boil over high heat. Stir in the couscous, cranberries, and scallion. Remove from the heat, cover, and let stand for 5 minutes, or until the liquid has been absorbed. Fluff with a fork before serving.

Yield: 6 servings

Per serving: 77 calories (28% from fat, 16% from protein, 55% from carbohydrate); 3 g protein; 2 g total fat; 1 g saturated fat; 1 g monounsaturated fat; 0 g polyunsaturated fat; 11 g carbohydrate; 1 g fiber; 0 g sugar; 35 mg phosphorus; 10 mg calcium; 27 mg sodium; 105 mg potassium; 93 IU vitamin A; 16 mg ATE vitamin E; 1 mg vitamin C; 5 mg cholesterol

Vegetable Flecked Couscous

Couscous can be used as a base for curries, tomato-based sauces, or any number of stews, or it can be served by itself as a side dish. This variation adds a few veggies for flavor, color, and nutrition.

1 tablespoon (15 ml) olive oil

¼ cup (40 g) finely chopped onion

¼ cup (38 g) finely chopped red bell pepper

¼ cup (25 g) finely chopped celery

1½ cups (355 ml) Low-Sodium Chicken Broth (page 232)

1 cup (175 g) couscous

Heat the oil in a large skillet over medium heat. Add the vegetables and sauté until tender, about 5 minutes. In a saucepan, bring the broth to a boil. Stir in the couscous and veggies, cover, and let stand for 5 minutes, or until the liquid has been absorbed. Fluff with a fork before serving.

Yield: 4 servings

Per serving: 88 calories (36% from fat, 13% from protein, 51% from carbohydrate); 3 g protein; 3 g total fat; 0 g saturated fat; 3 g monounsaturated fat; 0 g polyunsaturated fat; 11 g carbohydrate; 1 g fiber; 1 g sugar; 32 mg phosphorus; 16 mg calcium; 59 mg sodium; 153 mg potassium; 325 IU vitamin A; 0 mg ATE vitamin E; 19 mg vitamin C; 0 mg cholesterol

Noodles Romanoff

I don't know why Romanoff—it just sounded good. And these noodles are good too, creamy with cottage cheese and sour cream and topped with cheese. And the good thing is they are done in about the time it would have taken to reheat plain noodles.

3 cups (420 g) cooked egg noodles

1 cup (225 g) cottage cheese

1 cup (230 g) sour cream

¼ cup (40 g) finely chopped onion

½ teaspoon crushed garlic

1½ teaspoons Worcestershire sauce

A few drops hot pepper sauce

½ cup (55 g) shredded Swiss cheese

Grease an 8-inch (20-cm) square microwave-safe baking dish. Combine the noodles, cottage cheese, sour cream, onion, garlic, Worcestershire sauce, and hot pepper sauce in a bowl; pour into the prepared dish. Sprinkle the Swiss cheese over the top and microwave, uncovered, for 8 to 10 minutes, or until heated through and the cheese has melted.

Yield: 6 servings

Per serving: 193 calories (41% from fat, 23% from protein, 35% from carbohydrate); 11 g protein; 9 g total fat; 5 g saturated fat; 2 g monounsaturated fat; 1 g polyunsaturated fat; 17 g carbohydrate; 1 g fiber; 1 g sugar; 174 mg phosphorus; 163 mg calcium; 38 mg sodium; 137 mg potassium; 261 IU vitamin A; 69 mg ATE vitamin E; 3 mg vitamin C; 46 mg cholesterol

Ranch Noodles

Ranch dressing adds flavor to noodles without adding time to the recipe. Sour cream and Parmesan cheese complete the conversion. You can also make ranch spaghetti or pasta this same way.

8 ounces (225 g) egg noodles

¼ cup (112 g) unsalted butter

½ cup (115 g) sour cream

½ cup (120 ml) Ranch Dressing (page 34)

¼ cup (25 g) grated Parmesan cheese

Cook the egg noodles according to package directions until al dente; drain and return to the pot. Add the butter, sour cream, dressing, and cheese, and stir to combine. Serve immediately.

Yield: 4 servings

Per serving: 500 calories (52% from fat, 9% from protein, 39% from carbohydrate); 12 g protein; 29 g total fat; 13 g saturated fat; 8 g monounsaturated fat; 7 g polyunsaturated fat; 49 g carbohydrate; 2 g fiber; 3 g sugar; 207 mg phosphorus; 126 mg calcium; 136 mg sodium; 186 mg potassium; 594 IU vitamin A; 146 mg ATE vitamin E; 0 mg vitamin C; 109 mg cholesterol

Spaetzle

These tender German-style egg noodles take only minutes to make, but they add a whole new demission to a meal.

2 cups (240 g) all-purpose flour

1 cup (225 g) egg substitute, or 4 eggs, lightly beaten

⅓ cup (80 ml) skim milk

1 tablespoon (14 g) unsalted butter

In a large bowl, stir together the flour, eggs, and milk until smooth (the dough will be sticky). In a large saucepan, bring 8 cups (1880 ml) water to a boil. Coat a colander or spaetzle maker with cooking spray, place the dough in it, and place over the boiling water. With a spoon, press down on the dough until small pieces drop into the boiling water. Cook

(continued on page 208)

for 2 minutes, or until the noodles are tender and float to the top. Remove with a slotted spoon and toss with the butter.

Yield: 6 servings

Per serving: 209 calories (16% from fat, 19% from protein, 64% from carbohydrate); 10 g protein; 4 g total fat; 2 g saturated fat; 1 g monounsaturated fat; 1 g polyunsaturated fat; 33 g carbohydrate; 1 g fiber; 0 g sugar; 111 mg phosphorus; 49 mg calcium; 76 mg sodium; 208 mg potassium; 237 IU vitamin A; 24 mg ATE vitamin E; 0 mg vitamin C; 6 mg cholesterol

Seasoned Fries

Store-bought seasoned fried have lots of sodium. You can make your own just as easily with much less. In this case Italian seasoning provides the flavor, but you could also use any of the seasoning mixes on pages 34 to 35.

10 ounces (280 g) frozen shoestring potatoes

¼ cup (25 g) grated Parmesan cheese

2 teaspoons Italian seasoning

Preheat the oven to 450°F (230°C, or gas mark 8). Spread the potatoes on a foil-lined baking sheet and bake for 8 minutes. Combine the cheese and seasoning in a small cup, sprinkle over the potatoes, and mix gently. Bake for 4 to 5 minutes longer, or until the potatoes are browned and crisp.

Yield: 3 servings

Per serving: 244 calories (37% from fat, 10% from protein, 53% from carbohydrate); 6 g protein;

20 g total fat; 5 g saturated fat; 4 g monounsaturated fat; 1 g polyunsaturated fat; 33 g carbohydrate; 3 g fiber; 0 g sugar; 124 mg phosphorus; 112 mg calcium; 170 mg sodium; 476 mg potassium; 83 IU vitamin A; 10 mg ATE vitamin E; 9 mg vitamin C; 7 mg cholesterol

Tip: Make sure you get frozen fries without salt added.

Italian Barley Pilaf

Barley provides excellent nutrition; Italian flavor makes it something that is much more than just plain starch.

1 cup (185 g) quick-cooking barley

1 tablespoon (15 ml) olive oil

½ teaspoon minced garlic

1 tablespoon (2.5 g) chopped fresh basil, or 1 teaspoon dried

⅛ teaspoon freshly ground black pepper

½ cup (90 g) chopped tomato

½ cup (75 g) chopped green bell pepper

Cook the barley according to package directions. Heat the oil in a large saucepan over medium heat, add the garlic, and sauté for about 30 seconds. Add the basil and pepper, mixing well. Stir in the barley, tomato, and bell pepper; mix well. Cook for about 3 minutes, or until heated through.

Yield: 4 servings

Per serving: 202 calories (20% from fat, 12% from protein, 69% from carbohydrate); 6 g protein;

5 g total fat; 1 g saturated fat; 3 g monounsaturated fat; 1 g polyunsaturated fat; 36 g carbohydrate; 9 g fiber; 1 g sugar; 133 mg phosphorus; 31 mg calcium; 7 mg sodium; 304 mg potassium; 286 IU vitamin A; 0 mg ATE vitamin E; 18 mg vitamin C; 0 mg cholesterol

Spanish Rice

This recipe adds the traditional tomatoes, onions and peppers to cooked rice and makes an easy side dish that can be used with any kind of meat.

1 tablespoon (15 ml) olive oil

¾ cup (120 g) chopped onion

½ cup (75 g) chopped green bell pepper

1 can (14.5 ounces, or 411 g) no-salt-added tomatoes

1 can (8 ounces, or 225 g) no-salt-added tomato sauce

1½ cups (250 g) cooked rice

½ teaspoon freshly ground black pepper

Heat the oil in a skillet over medium heat, add the onion and bell pepper, and sauté until softened, about 5 minutes. Add the tomatoes, tomato sauce, rice, and black pepper and mix well. Cook until heated through, about 5 minutes.

Yield: 4 servings

Per serving: 138 calories (3% from fat, 11% from protein, 86% from carbohydrate); 4 g protein; 1 g total fat; 0 g saturated fat; 0 g monounsaturated fat; 0 g polyunsaturated fat; 30 g carbohydrate; 3 g fiber; 8 g sugar; 79 mg phosphorus; 59 mg calcium; 20 mg sodium; 583 mg potassium; 424 IU vitamin A; 0 mg ATE vitamin E; 41 mg vitamin C; 0 mg cholesterol

Tip: Make it a meal by adding 1 pound (454 g) of ground beef with the onion and pepper. Drain off the fat before continuing with the recipe.

Cajun Rice

Spice up your meal with some Cajun-style rice. If you want it really New Orleans hot, increase the Cajun seasoning or add a little cayenne pepper to taste. This is great with fish or seafood.

2 tablespoons (28 g) unsalted butter

1 teaspoon Salt-Free Cajun Seasoning (page 29)

⅛ teaspoon freshly ground black pepper

2 cups (330 g) cooked long-grain rice

In a small saucepan over medium heat, melt the butter, then add the Cajun seasoning and black pepper. Cook for 3 minutes. Stir in the rice, cover, and cook until heated through, 2 to 3 minutes.

Yield: 4 servings

Per serving: 389 calories (15% from fat, 7% from protein, 78% from carbohydrate); 7 g protein; 6 g total fat; 4 g saturated fat; 2 g monounsaturated fat; 0 g polyunsaturated fat; 74 g carbohydrate; 1 g fiber; 0 g sugar; 108 mg phosphorus; 28 mg calcium; 5 mg sodium; 109 mg potassium; 177 IU vitamin A; 48 mg ATE vitamin E; 0 mg vitamin C; 15 mg cholesterol

Instant Mexican Rice

Mexican or Spanish-style rice adds spark to a meal. In this recipe the use of traditional Mexican seasonings such as chili powder and cumin give it that authentic taste. The use of instant rice makes it quick and easy to prepare.

1 medium onion

1 tablespoon (15 ml) olive oil

½ teaspoon minced garlic

1 cup (245 g) no-salt-added stewed tomatoes

½ cup (120 ml) Low-Sodium Chicken Broth (page 232)

½ teaspoon chili powder

⅛ teaspoon ground cumin

1 cup (180 g) instant rice

Cut the onion in half. Finely chop one half. Cut other half into very thin slices. Heat the oil in a medium saucepan over medium heat, add the chopped onion and the garlic, and cook until the onion is tender, about 5 minutes. Add the stewed tomatoes, chicken broth, chili powder, and cumin. Mash the tomatoes with a masher or the back of a spoon. Bring the mixture to a boil over high heat, then stir in the rice and the sliced onion. Remove from the heat, cover, and let stand for 5 minutes, or until the liquid has been absorbed.

Yield: 4 servings

Per serving: 116 calories (29% from fat, 9% from protein, 62% from carbohydrate); 3 g protein; 4 g total fat; 1 g saturated fat; 3 g monounsaturated fat; 0 g polyunsaturated fat; 18 g carbohydrate; 1 g fiber; 3 g sugar; 50 mg phosphorus; 34 mg calcium; 20 mg sodium; 242 mg potassium; 173 IU vitamin A; 0 mg ATE vitamin E; 11 mg vitamin C; 0 mg cholesterol

Apple Rice

Apple-flavored rice makes a tasty and healthy side dish that goes great with pork.

1 cup (235 ml) water

1 cup (245 g) applesauce

1 teaspoon unsalted butter

¼ teaspoon ground cinnamon

1½ cups (270 g) instant rice

½ cup (75 g) chopped apple

Bring the water, applesauce, butter, and cinnamon to a boil in a medium saucepan over high heat. Stir in the rice and return to a boil. Remove from the heat and stir in the apple. Cover and let stand for 5 minutes, or until the liquid has been absorbed.

Yield: 6 servings

Per serving: 94 calories (8% from fat, 5% from protein, 87% from carbohydrate); 1 g protein; 1 g total fat; 0 g saturated fat; 0 g monounsaturated fat; 0 g polyunsaturated fat; 21 g carbohydrate; 1 g fiber; 8 g sugar; 21 mg phosphorus; 8 mg calcium; 3 mg sodium; 49 mg potassium; 28 IU vitamin A; 5 mg ATE vitamin E; 1 mg vitamin C; 2 mg cholesterol

Marinated Veggies Mock Kabobs

A simple vegetable mixture flavored with Mediterranean spices such as rosemary and thyme is a nice addition to any meal.

2 tablespoons (30 ml) olive oil

1 teaspoon dried thyme

1 teaspoon dried rosemary

½ teaspoon minced garlic

1 cup (120 g) sliced zucchini

1 cup (82 g) peeled and cubed eggplant

1 cup (150 g) 1-inch (2.5-cm) pieces green
  bell pepper

Preheat the broiler and place the oven rack about 6 inches (15 cm) from the heat source. Combine the oil, thyme, rosemary, and garlic in a large bowl. Add the vegetables and toss to coat. Spread on a baking sheet and broil until crisp-tender, about 4 minutes.

Yield: 6 servings

Per serving: 52 calories (75% from fat, 5% from protein, 20% from carbohydrate); 1 g protein; 5 g total fat; 1 g saturated fat; 3 g monounsaturated fat; 0 g polyunsaturated fat; 3 g carbohydrate; 1 g fiber; 1 g sugar; 17 mg phosphorus; 11 mg calcium; 3 mg sodium; 132 mg potassium; 146 IU vitamin A; 0 mg ATE vitamin E; 24 mg vitamin C; 0 mg cholesterol

Veggie Souvlaki Mock Kabobs

This mixture of traditional Greek vegetables such as eggplant and zucchini is seasoned with Mediterranean flavorings such as coriander, garlic, and cumin. It is great with lamb or chicken.

¾ teaspoon crushed garlic

1 tablespoon (6 g) coriander

1 tablespoon (15 ml) olive oil

1 teaspoon ground cumin

1 teaspoon paprika

1 cup (120 g) sliced zucchini

1 cup (82 g) peeled and cubed eggplant

1 cup (150 g) 1-inch (2.5-cm) pieces green
  bell pepper

Preheat the broiler and place the oven rack about 6 inches (15 cm) from the heat source. In a small bowl, mash the garlic, coriander, oil, cumin, and paprika into a paste. Brush on the zucchini, eggplant, and bell pepper. Spread on a baking sheet and broil until crisp-tender, about 4 minutes.

Yield: 6 servings

Per serving: 35 calories (58% from fat, 8% from protein, 34% from carbohydrate); 1 g protein; 2 g total fat; 0 g saturated fat; 2 g monounsaturated fat; 0 g polyunsaturated fat; 3 g carbohydrate; 1 g fiber; 1 g sugar; 21 mg phosphorus; 15 mg calcium; 5 mg sodium; 159 mg potassium; 361 IU vitamin A; 0 mg ATE vitamin E; 26 mg vitamin C; 0 mg cholesterol

Curried Cauliflower Mock Kabobs

Curried cauliflower will add a taste treat to any meal. Particularly great with chicken or fish.

3 cups (300 g) cauliflower florets

2 tablespoons (30 ml) olive oil

2 teaspoons curry powder

Preheat the broiler and place the oven rack about 6 inches (15 cm) from the heat source. Combine the cauliflower, oil, and curry in a bowl and toss until the cauliflower is coated with curry powder. Spread on a baking sheet and broil until crisp-tender, about 4 to 6 minutes.

Yield: 6 servings

Per serving: 59 calories (67% from fat, 10% from protein, 23% from carbohydrate); 2 g protein; 5 g total fat; 1 g saturated fat; 3 g monounsaturated fat; 1 g polyunsaturated fat; 4 g carbohydrate; 3 g fiber; 1 g sugar; 24 mg phosphorus; 19 mg calcium; 17 mg sodium; 136 mg potassium; 16 IU vitamin A; 0 mg ATE vitamin E; 28 mg vitamin C; 0 mg cholesterol

13

15-Minute Desserts and Sweet Things

Many traditional desserts can take a long time to prepare. So what do you do when you want a little something sweet to finish off a meal, or maybe for a bedtime snack, but you don't want to spend a big chunk of time preparing it? In this chapter, I have some recipes that you might think are more obvious as quick desserts, like fruit salads. But I also have other things that you might think are more difficult, like cookies; or how about a two-minute chocolate cake for two? Got that, too! To round it all out, there are a couple of very tasty punch recipes.

Ambrosia

This is a lighter dessert, the sort of refreshing end you might want after a heavy or spicy meal. It contains only fresh fruit, garnished with pecans and coconut.

4 cups (600 g) orange sections

2 cups (300 g) sliced bananas

1 cup (110 g) coarsely chopped pecans

2 ounces (56 g) shredded coconut

½ cup (120 ml) orange juice (optional)

In a large glass bowl, arrange alternate layers of the orange sections, bananas, pecans, and coconut. Sprinkle 2 tablespoons (30 ml) of orange juice between layers, if desired. Repeat the layers until all the ingredients are used.

Yield: 8 servings

Per serving: 218 calories (47% from fat, 5% from protein, 48% from carbohydrate); 3 g protein; 12 g total fat; 3 g saturated fat; 6 g monounsaturated fat; 3 g polyunsaturated fat; 28 g carbohydrate; 5 g fiber; 16 g sugar; 70 mg phosphorus; 49 mg calcium; 2 mg sodium; 443 mg potassium; 246 IU vitamin A; 0 mg ATE vitamin E; 53 mg vitamin C; 0 mg cholesterol

Fruit Crisp

Fruit crisps often take time to prepare, what with slicing the fruit and baking in the oven. But this quick and easy dessert uses canned pie filling and is cooked in a skillet! The only hard part is picking what flavor you want. For an even more special treat, serve it with a scoop of ice cream or whipped topping.

1 can (21 ounces, or 588 g) peach, apple, or cherry pie filling

1 tablespoon (15 ml) lemon juice

1 cup (55 g) shredded wheat cereal

1 tablespoon (14 g) unsalted butter

1 tablespoon (12 g) sugar

¼ teaspoon ground cinnamon

In a medium skillet over medium heat, heat the pie filling and lemon juice for 5 minutes, or until bubbly, stirring occasionally. Meanwhile, place the cereal in a resealable plastic bag; crush slightly with a rolling pin. In another skillet, melt the butter over medium heat. Stir in the cereal, sugar, and cinnamon; cook and stir for 2 to 3 minutes, until heated through. Sprinkle over the fruit mixture. Serve warm.

Yield: 4 servings

Per serving: 235 calories (12% from fat, 2% from protein, 86% from carbohydrate); 1 g protein; 3 g total fat; 2 g saturated fat; 1 g monounsaturated fat; 0 g polyunsaturated fat; 53 g carbohydrate; 3 g fiber; 36 g sugar; 47 mg phosphorus; 11 mg calcium; 68 mg sodium; 116 mg potassium; 90 IU vitamin A; 24 mg ATE vitamin E; 2 mg vitamin C; 8 mg cholesterol

Microwave Baked Apple

Stuffed with brown sugar and cinnamon, you get all the nutrition of an apple, but in an even sweeter and better form, all done in minutes. What more could you want in a dessert?

1 medium apple (any variety)

1 teaspoon packed brown sugar

¼ teaspoon ground cinnamon

1 teaspoon unsalted butter

Peel and core the apple completely and place on a microwave-safe dish. Combine the sugar and cinnamon in a small bowl, then spoon into the apple. Place the butter on top. Microwave for 2 to 2½ minutes, until apple is soft.

Yield: 1 serving

Per serving: 114 calories (29% from fat, 1% from protein, 69% from carbohydrate); 0 g protein; 4 g total fat; 2 g saturated fat; 1 g monounsaturated fat; 0 g polyunsaturated fat; 21 g carbohydrate; 2 g fiber; 17 g sugar; 17 mg phosphorus; 18 mg calcium; 2 mg sodium; 135 mg potassium; 168 IU vitamin A; 32 mg ATE vitamin E; 5 mg vitamin C; 10 mg cholesterol

Peanut and Raisin Stuffed Apple

Looking for dessert that is healthy, but afraid that just handing people an apple won't go over well? Then take a minute and make that apple something everyone will like. The peanut butter and honey combination is always a winner and here it is paired with raisins to make it even better. Choose an apple that is good for cooking such as Granny Smith, Fuji, or Winesap.

2 tablespoons (32 g) no-salt-added peanut butter

1 tablespoon (9 g) raisins

1 teaspoon honey

1 apple, peeled and cored

In a small bowl, combine the peanut butter, raisins, and honey. Spoon into the center of the apple.

Yield: 1 serving

Per serving: 304 calories (45% from fat, 10% from protein, 45% from carbohydrate); 8 g protein; 16 g total fat; 3 g saturated fat; 8 g monounsaturated fat; 5 g polyunsaturated fat; 37 g carbohydrate; 4 g fiber; 27 g sugar; 127 mg phosphorus; 25 mg calcium; 7 mg sodium; 437 mg potassium; 49 IU vitamin A; 0 mg ATE vitamin E; 5 mg vitamin C; 0 mg cholesterol

Nutty Apple Wedges

Fix your family a dessert that not only is quick and good for them but also tastes great. Choose an apple that is good eaten fresh such as Gala, McIntosh, or Golden Delicious.

1 apple, unpeeled

½ cup (130 g) no-salt-added peanut butter

1 cup (55 g) cornflakes, crushed

Cut the apple into 12 wedges. Spread the peanut butter on the cut sides, then roll in the cornflakes.

Yield: 3 servings

(continued on page 216)

Per serving: 307 calories (59% from fat, 14% from protein, 27% from carbohydrate); 11 g protein; 22 g total fat; 4 g saturated fat; 10 g monounsaturated fat; 6 g polyunsaturated fat; 22 g carbohydrate; 3 g fiber; 8 g sugar; 145 mg phosphorus; 23 mg calcium; 8 mg sodium; 366 mg potassium; 33 IU vitamin A; 0 mg ATE vitamin E; 2 mg vitamin C; 0 mg cholesterol

Pear Crisp

This tasty dessert is full of shortcut ingredients, starting with canned pears and added vanilla wafers and whipped topping. But don't get the impression that it suffers in taste because of this. The combination hits just the right balance, pleasing both young and old.

1 can (19 ounces, or 532 g) pear slices, drained
½ cup (25 g) coarsely crushed vanilla wafers
½ cup whipped topping, such as Cool Whip
⅛ teaspoon ground cinnamon

Divide the pears among 4 dessert bowls. Sprinkle with the wafer crumbs. Combine the whipped topping and cinnamon, then spoon evenly over the desserts.

Yield: 4 servings

Per serving: 143 calories (17% from fat, 3% from protein, 80% from carbohydrate); 1 g protein; 3 g total fat; 1 g saturated fat; 1 g monounsaturated fat; 0 g polyunsaturated fat; 30 g carbohydrate; 4 g fiber; 18 g sugar; 32 mg phosphorus; 24 mg calcium; 39 mg sodium; 180 mg potassium; 41 IU

vitamin A; 1 mg ATE vitamin E; 6 mg vitamin C; 5 mg cholesterol

Tip: Any other canned fruit can be substituted.

Quick and Cool Fruit Salad

This delightful dessert is full of both flavor and nutrition. But the use of prepared ingredients means that it can be prepared and served in less than 10 minutes, which is a good thing if you have family members waiting.

1 8-ounce (225 g) container whipped topping, such as Cool Whip
1 cup (230 g) sour cream
3 ounces (84 g) sugar-free orange-flavored gelatin
16 ounces (454 g) fruit cocktail, drained

Combine the whipped topping and sour cream in a serving bowl. Add the gelatin, mix well, and then add the drained fruit cocktail and stir to combine.

Yield: 6 servings

Per serving: 197 calories (37% from fat, 8% from protein, 54% from carbohydrate); 5 g protein; 9 g total fat; 7 g saturated fat; 2 g monounsaturated fat; 0 g polyunsaturated fat; 31 g carbohydrate; 1 g fiber; 17 g sugar; 258 mg phosphorus; 73 mg calcium; 168 mg sodium; 161 mg potassium; 399 IU vitamin A; 38 mg ATE vitamin E; 2 mg vitamin C; 15 mg cholesterol

Orange Fluff

This is a cool and refreshing dessert after a heavy meal. It is packed with a double punch of orange flavor and well as pineapple, but they are subdued to just the right level by the cottage cheese.

16 ounces (454 g) cottage cheese

3 ounces (84 g) sugar-free orange-flavored gelatin

11 ounces (308 g) mandarin oranges, drained

15 ounces (420 g) crushed pineapple, drained

1 16 ounce container (454 g) whipped topping, such as Cool Whip

Combine the cottage cheese and gelatin in a serving bowl. Add the drained oranges and pineapple, then fold in the whipped topping.

Yield: 6 servings

Per serving: 289 calories (31% from fat, 22% from protein, 47% from carbohydrate); 16 g protein; 10 g total fat; 9 g saturated fat; 1 g monounsaturated fat; 0 g polyunsaturated fat; 35 g carbohydrate; 1 g fiber; 33 g sugar; 158 mg phosphorus; 94 mg calcium; 77 mg sodium; 244 mg potassium; 548 IU vitamin A; 7 mg ATE vitamin E; 23 mg vitamin C; 7 mg cholesterol

Chocolate Coconut Bananas

Looking for a quick, tasty dessert that isn't just empty calories? Get the vitamins and potassium of bananas in a form that even banana haters will love, thanks to the chocolate and coconut.

4 teaspoons cocoa powder

¼ cup (112 g) unsweetened shredded coconut, toasted

2 bananas, sliced in half on the diagonal

Spread the cocoa and coconut on separate plates. Roll each banana slice in the cocoa, shake off the excess, then dip in the coconut.

Yield: 4 servings

Per serving: 118 calories (35% from fat, 5% from protein, 60% from carbohydrate); 2 g protein; 5 g total fat; 4 g saturated fat; 0 g monounsaturated fat; 0 g polyunsaturated fat; 20 g carbohydrate; 4 g fiber; 10 g sugar; 44 mg phosphorus; 8 mg calcium; 4 mg sodium; 334 mg potassium; 48 IU vitamin A; 0 mg ATE vitamin E; 7 mg vitamin C; 0 mg cholesterol

Grilled Chocolate-Filled Bananas

These chocolate-filled bananas are sure to be a hot dessert. To make a hot banana split, top the bananas with ice cream and a cherry.

4 bananas, unpeeled

2 tablespoons (28 g) unsalted butter, melted

2 tablespoons (25 g) sugar

4 ounces (112 g) chocolate chips

Cut a small piece off the curved side of each banana so they'll sit level, then make a deep slit down the center of each through the peel; place on separate sheets of foil. Open the slits and brush the inside of each banana with the melted butter, sprinkle with ½ tablespoon (6 g) of the sugar, and place 1 ounce (28 g) of the chocolate chips inside; fold up the foil. Grill the packets in a skillet over high heat until the chocolate melts, 6 to 8 minutes. Open the foil, peel the bananas, and serve.

Yield: 4 servings

Per serving: 360 calories (35% from fat, 4% from protein, 61% from carbohydrate); 4 g protein; 15 g total fat; 8 g saturated fat; 5 g monounsaturated fat; 1 g polyunsaturated fat; 57 g carbohydrate; 5 g fiber; 39 g sugar; 94 mg phosphorus; 63 mg calcium; 25 mg sodium; 644 mg potassium; 323 IU vitamin A; 61 mg ATE vitamin E; 13 mg vitamin C; 22 mg cholesterol

Fruit Dip

Orange marmalade adds a nice level of sweetness to yogurt in the dip. Full of nutrition and taste, but fast to put together, it also makes a great party or snack plate.

8 ounces (225 g) low-fat vanilla yogurt

3 tablespoons (60 g) orange marmalade

1 tablespoon (8 g) confectioners' sugar

1 apple, cored and sliced ¼ inch (6 mm) thick

½ cup (85 g) sliced strawberries

1 cup (150 g) sliced seedless green grapes

In a small bowl, combine the yogurt, marmalade, and sugar. Arrange the fruit on a serving platter and serve with the dip.

Yield: 6 servings

Per serving: 89 calories (5% from fat, 9% from protein, 85% from carbohydrate); 2 g protein; 1 g total fat; 0 g saturated fat; 0 g monounsaturated fat; 0 g polyunsaturated fat; 20 g carbohydrate; 1 g fiber; 18 g sugar; 58 mg phosphorus; 75 mg calcium; 31 mg sodium; 162 mg potassium; 54 IU vitamin A; 5 mg ATE vitamin E; 10 mg vitamin C; 2 mg cholesterol

Layered Fall Dessert Dip

This pretty apple dip is perfect for a Halloween party or a fall get-together. It's also great for family nibbling. Layered like the traditional Mexican dips, it lets everyone get the most of the part they like best.

8 ounces (225 g) cream cheese, softened

4 ounces (112 g) caramel topping

1 cup (145 g) crushed unsalted peanuts

4 apples, peeled, cored, and sliced

Spread the cream cheese in the center of a serving platter with a spatula or spoon. Pour the caramel sauce over the cream cheese, then cover with the crushed peanuts. Place the apple slices around the edge of the platter to be used for dipping.

Yield: 16 servings

Per serving: 95 calories (53% from fat, 7% from protein, 40% from carbohydrate); 2 g protein; 6 g total fat; 3 g saturated fat; 2 g monounsaturated fat; 0 g polyunsaturated fat; 10 g carbohydrate; 1 g fiber; 3 g sugar; 29 mg phosphorus; 19 mg calcium; 96 mg sodium; 59 mg potassium; 209 IU vitamin A; 53 mg ATE vitamin E; 1 mg vitamin C; 16 mg cholesterol

Baking Mix Cookies

These are simple cookies with a taste similar to snickerdoodles. Because you use baking mix, dessert doesn't get any easier or tastier than this.

¾ cup (170 g) Buttermilk Baking Mix (page 27)

2 ounces (56 g) instant vanilla pudding mix

¼ cup (60 ml) canola oil

½ cup (125 g) egg substitute, or 2 eggs, beaten

Preheat the oven to 350°F (180°C, or gas mark 4). Grease 2 or 3 cookie sheets or line with parchment paper. Combine the baking mix and pudding mix in a bowl. Stir in the oil and eggs, and mix thoroughly. Form into thirty-six small balls and flatten on the baking sheets with your fingers. Bake for 12 minutes, or until lightly browned. Transfer to cooling racks to cool.

Yield: 36 cookies

Per cookie: 32 calories (52% from fat, 8% from protein, 40% from carbohydrate); 1 g protein; 2 g total fat; 0 g saturated fat; 1 g monounsaturated fat; 1 g polyunsaturated fat; 3 g carbohydrate; 0 g fiber; 2 g sugar; 29 mg phosphorus; 6 mg calcium; 30 mg sodium; 16 mg potassium; 13 IU vitamin A; 0 mg ATE vitamin E; 0 mg vitamin C; 0 mg cholesterol

Tip: This will work with any flavor of pudding, so let your imagination run wild.

No-Bake Tea Cookies

These cookies are slightly sweet with orange and coconut flavors. Okay, you may have to hurry to make 60 of these in 15 minutes. But unless you're having a BIG party, you could cut the recipe in half and finish with time to spare.

1 pound (454 g) vanilla wafers, crushed

½ cup (112 g) unsalted butter

1 pound (454 g) confectioners' sugar, sifted

12 ounces (340 g) condensed frozen orange juice, thawed

1 cup (80 g) shredded coconut

Combine the vanilla wafers, butter, sugar, and orange juice in a bowl and mix well. Form into 60 small balls. Roll each in the coconut to coat.

Yield: 60 cookies

Per cookie: 84 calories (32% from fat, 2% from protein, 65% from carbohydrate); 0 g protein; 3 g total fat; 2 g saturated fat; 1 g monounsaturated fat; 0 g polyunsaturated fat; 14 g carbohydrate; 0 g fiber; 10 g sugar; 10 mg phosphorus; 5 mg calcium; 24 mg sodium; 23 mg potassium; 54 IU vitamin A; 13 mg ATE vitamin E; 2 mg vitamin C; 8 mg cholesterol

Chocolate Cookies

Nothing fancy here, just a full flavored chocolate cookie that goes perfectly with a glass of milk. Mix them up, bake for 8 minutes, and you'll have enough for the whole family, even if you have a *really* big family.

2 cups (240 g) all-purpose flour

1½ cups (300 g) sugar

1 teaspoon sodium-free baking soda

1 teaspoon sodium-free baking powder

3 tablespoons (23 g) nonfat dry milk

1 cup (225 g) unsalted butter, melted

⅓ cup (40 g) cocoa powder

½ cup (125 g) egg substitute, or 2 eggs, beaten

Preheat the oven to 350°F (180°C, or gas mark 4). Grease 4 cookie sheets or line with parchment paper. Mix all the ingredients together in a bowl. Form into 48 cookies and place on the cookie sheets. Bake for 8 to 10 minutes, or until lightly browned around edges. Transfer to cooling racks to cool. The cookies will not appear done when removed from the oven, but they will rise like cake, then fall when cool.

Yield: 48 cookies

Per cookie: 82 calories (43% from fat, 5% from protein, 51% from carbohydrate); 1 g protein; 4 g total fat; 3 g saturated fat; 1 g monounsaturated fat; 0 g polyunsaturated fat; 11 g carbohydrate; 0 g fiber; 6 g sugar; 24 mg phosphorus; 12 mg calcium; 7 mg sodium; 40 mg potassium; 134 IU vitamin A; 34 mg ATE vitamin E; 0 mg vitamin C; 10 mg cholesterol

Boiled Chocolate Peanut Butter Cookies

Yes, that's what it says: boiled cookies. Don't laugh until you've tried them, especially because they can be made start to finish in less than 15 minutes. Also because they contain chocolate and peanut butter, which is always a good combination.

2 cups (400 g) sugar

½ cup (112 g) unsalted butter

½ cup (120 ml) skim milk

½ cup (60 g) cocoa powder

½ cup (40 g) shredded coconut

½ cup (130 g) no-salt-added peanut butter

1 tablespoon (15 ml) vanilla extract

3 cups (240 g) quick-cooking oats

Combine the sugar, butter, milk, cocoa, coconut, peanut butter, and vanilla in a saucepot. Bring to a boil over high heat, boil for 1 minute, then add the oatmeal and stir to combine. Remove from the heat and spoon 48 balls onto waxed paper to cool.

Yield: 48 cookies

Per cookie: 76 calories (30% from fat, 6% from protein, 65% from carbohydrate); 1 g protein; 3 g total fat; 2 g saturated fat; 1 g monounsaturated fat; 0 g polyunsaturated fat; 13 g carbohydrate; 1 g fiber; 9 g sugar; 35 mg phosphorus; 8 mg calcium; 2 mg sodium; 40 mg potassium; 64 IU vitamin A; 17 mg ATE vitamin E; 0 mg vitamin C; 5 mg cholesterol

Peanut Butter and Honey Balls

These sweet little treats are a cross between a candy and a cookie, but whatever you call them they are sure to please. They only contain 4 ingredients, but they have a lot of flavor.

½ cup (130 g) no-salt-added peanut butter
½ cup (160 g) honey
1 cup (120 g) nonfat dry milk
1 cup (80 g) quick-cooking oats

Combine the peanut butter and honey in a bowl. Slowly add the dry milk and oatmeal and stir to combine. Form into 32 small balls and place on waxed paper to set.

Yield: 32 cookies

Per cookie: 57 calories (33% from fat, 14% from protein, 53% from carbohydrate); 2 g protein; 2 g total fat; 0 g saturated fat; 1 g monounsaturated fat; 1 g polyunsaturated fat; 8 g carbohydrate; 1 g fiber; 6 g sugar; 46 mg phosphorus; 29 mg calcium; 13 mg sodium; 78 mg potassium; 50 IU vitamin A; 15 mg ATE vitamin E; 0 mg vitamin C; 0 mg cholesterol

Tip: Roll in confectioners' sugar and/or coconut, if desired.

Cinnamon Tostada

This is a sweet little snack with a brown sugar and cinnamon flavor similar to Mexican churros, but a lot quicker to make.

2 8 inch (20 cm) whole wheat tortillas
1 tablespoon (15 g) packed brown sugar
¼ teaspoon ground cinnamon
1½ teaspoons unsalted butter, softened

Preheat the broiler and set the oven rack 4 inches (10 cm) from the heat source. Place the tortillas on a baking sheet. In a small bowl, combine the sugar and cinnamon. Spread the butter on one side of each tortilla and sprinkle with the cinnamon sugar. Broil until the sugar is golden brown and the butter has melted, 1 to 2 minutes. Cut each tortilla into 8 wedges.

Yield: 4 servings

Per serving: 78 calories (30% from fat, 7% from protein, 63% from carbohydrate); 1 g protein; 3 g total fat; 1 g saturated fat; 1 g monounsaturated fat; 0 g polyunsaturated fat; 12 g carbohydrate; 1 g fiber; 3 g sugar; 21 mg phosphorus; 11 mg calcium; 78 mg sodium; 34 mg potassium; 45 IU vitamin A; 12 mg ATE vitamin E; 0 mg vitamin C; 4 mg cholesterol

Chocolate Pudding Cake

This is similar to the pudding or lava cake mixes you can buy at the supermarket but with a lot less sodium. It goes together quickly and cooks in the microwave, giving you an impressive dessert.

½ cup (120 ml) water
1 cup (200 g) plus 3 tablespoons (38 g) sugar, divided

(continued on page 222)

⅔ cup (80 g) all-purpose flour

⅔ cup (80 g) cocoa powder

1 teaspoon sodium-free baking powder

¾ cup (188 g) egg substitute, or 3 eggs, beaten

2 tablespoons (28 g) unsalted butter, melted

1 teaspoon vanilla extract

Bring the water and 3 tablespoons (38 g) of the sugar to a boil in a small pan and set aside. Combine the remaining 1 cup (200 g) sugar, flour, cocoa, and baking powder in a bowl, and then add the eggs, melted butter, and vanilla and stir until well blended; the mixture will be thick. Butter a 9-inch (23-cm) microwave-safe baking dish. Spread the mixture evenly into the buttered pan. Very slowly pour the sugar water into the center of the mixture and do not stir. Cover well with plastic wrap or a lid. Microwave on regular power for 5 minutes, or until set.

Yield: 8 servings

Per serving: 218 calories (18% from fat, 9% from protein, 73% from carbohydrate); 5 g protein; 5 g total fat; 3 g saturated fat; 1 g monounsaturated fat; 1 g polyunsaturated fat; 42 g carbohydrate; 3 g fiber; 30 g sugar; 136 mg phosphorus; 52 mg calcium; 41 mg sodium; 263 mg potassium; 173 IU vitamin A; 24 mg ATE vitamin E; 0 mg vitamin C; 8 mg cholesterol

Tip: Sprinkle with confectioners' sugar or serve with your favorite toppings.

The World's Quickest Chocolate Cake

If you need a dessert in a hurry this microwave-cooked chocolate cake may be just what you are looking for. Each serving takes only two minutes to cook, but you'll be surprised at the outcome. It's actually more moist and flavorful than many oven-baked cakes.

¼ cup (30 g) all-purpose flour

5 tablespoons (63 g) sugar

2 tablespoons (16 g) cocoa powder

¼ cup (63 g) egg substitute, or 1 egg, beaten

3 tablespoons (45 ml) skim milk

3 tablespoons (45 ml) canola oil

Dash of vanilla extract

Whisk all the ingredients together in a large mug until smooth. Microwave until puffed, about 2 minutes.

Yield: 2 servings

Per serving: 408 calories (48% from fat, 7% from protein, 45% from carbohydrate); 7 g protein; 22 g total fat; 2 g saturated fat; 13 g monounsaturated fat; 7 g polyunsaturated fat; 48 g carbohydrate; 2 g fiber; 32 g sugar; 120 mg phosphorus; 59 mg calcium; 65 mg sodium; 245 mg potassium; 160 IU vitamin A; 14 mg ATE vitamin E; 0 mg vitamin C; 1 mg cholesterol

Tip: You can save yourself even more time by measuring and mixing the dry ingredients ahead of time and sealing each portion in a resealable bag. They'll keep at least a year on your pantry shelf.

Instant Rice Pudding

Vanilla ice cream melts in hot rice, giving it a sweet, creamy texture and flavor.

2 cups (390 g) instant rice, such as Minute Rice
½ cup (70 g) vanilla ice cream
½ teaspoon ground cinnamon

Prepare the rice according to the package directions. Uncover, add the ice cream and cinnamon, and stir. Divide the pudding among 4 bowls and top with additional cinnamon, if desired. Serve warm or at room temperature.

Yield: 4 servings

Per serving: 151 calories (18% from fat, 8% from protein, 74% from carbohydrate); 3 g protein; 3 g total fat; 2 g saturated fat; 1 g monounsaturated fat; 0 g polyunsaturated fat; 27 g carbohydrate; 1 g fiber; 5 g sugar; 59 mg phosphorus; 40 mg calcium; 14 mg sodium; 67 mg potassium; 127 IU vitamin A; 34 mg ATE vitamin E; 0 mg vitamin C; 20 mg cholesterol

Cider Punch

This is a nice party drink, but it also works well as a tasty, easy, healthy alternative to soft drinks. The basic flavors are cranberry and apple, with a little lemon for tartness and ginger ale for sparkle. Make sure all the ingredients are well chilled for a refreshing beverage.

2 quarts (1.9 L) apple cider
2 cups (470 ml) cranberry juice
2 teaspoons lemon juice
4 cups (940 ml) ginger ale

In a large punch bowl combine the cider, cranberry juice, and lemon juice. Add the ginger ale and stir to combine just before serving.

Yield: 15 servings

Per serving: 103 calories (1% from fat, 0% from protein, 98% from carbohydrate); 0 g protein; 0 g total fat; 0 g saturated fat; 0 g monounsaturated fat; 0 g polyunsaturated fat; 26 g carbohydrate; 0 g fiber; 20 g sugar; 10 mg phosphorus; 13 mg calcium; 10 mg sodium; 164 mg potassium; 5 IU vitamin A; 0 mg ATE vitamin E; 5 mg vitamin C; 0 mg cholesterol

Tip: This is good without the ginger ale too; simply keep in a jug in the refrigerator.

How Would You Like a Punch?

This is a great-tasting hot punch, starting with cider and cranberry juice and then adding other fruit and spice accents. It's perfect for Halloween, football parties, or just for the family.

5 cups (1175 ml) apple cider
5 cups (1175 ml) cranberry juice
1½ cups (55 ml) mango nectar
¼ cup (60 ml) lime juice

(continued on page 224)

1 teaspoon ground ginger

½ teaspoon ground cinnamon

½ teaspoon ground allspice

Honey, to taste (optional)

In a 4-quart (4-L) Dutch oven, combine the apple cider, cranberry juice, mango juice, lime juice, ginger, cinnamon, and allspice. Bring to a boil over high heat, and then reduce the heat to a simmer. Simmer, uncovered, for 5 minutes, stirring occasionally. If desired, sweeten to taste with honey.

Yield: 10 servings

Per serving: 130 calories (1% from fat, 0% from protein, 98% from carbohydrate); 0 g protein; 0 g total fat; 0 g saturated fat; 0 g monounsaturated fat; 0 g polyunsaturated fat; 33 g carbohydrate; 0 g fiber; 14 g sugar; 11 mg phosphorus; 18 mg calcium; 8 mg sodium; 176 mg potassium; 18 IU vitamin A; 0 mg ATE vitamin E; 15 mg vitamin C; 0 mg cholesterol

Pink Punch

This punch is perfect for a birthday party, bridal shower, or any other occasion. And it takes almost no time to make. Pineapple juice and Kool-Aid form the base. The recipe calls for strawberry, but you can vary the flavor (and the color) to suit any occasion or taste.

3 cups (600 g) sugar

2 cups (470 ml) boiling water

4 cups (940 ml) pineapple juice

2 envelopes strawberry-flavored Kool-Aid

10 ounces (280 g) frozen strawberries

1 cup (235 ml) lemon juice

3 quarts (2.8 L) cold water

In a punch bowl, combine the sugar and boiling water and stir until dissolved. Add the juice, Kool-Aid, strawberries, lemon juice, and cold water, stir to combine, and chill in the refrigerator.

Yield: 40 servings

Per serving: 75 calories (0% from fat, 1% from protein, 99% from carbohydrate); 0 g protein; 0 g total fat; 0 g saturated fat; 0 g monounsaturated fat; 0 g polyunsaturated fat; 19 g carbohydrate; 0 g fiber; 19 g sugar; 3 mg phosphorus; 8 mg calcium; 3 mg sodium; 49 mg potassium; 5 IU vitamin A; 0 mg ATE vitamin E; 8 mg vitamin C; 0 mg cholesterol

Sangria for Everyone

Sangria without the wine. But just as good and suitable for the entire family. White grape juice gets the citrus and fruit sparkle in this version, which is just as appropriate for a party punch or a family dinner.

3 cups (705 ml) white grape juice

1 cup (235 ml) orange juice

1 cup (150 g) sliced seedless green grapes

1 cup (170 g) sliced strawberries

1 cup (125 g) raspberries

3 oranges, peeled and sliced

Combine all the ingredients in a pitcher and stir to mix.

Yield: 6 servings

Per serving: 164 calories (3% from fat, 5% from protein, 92% from carbohydrate); 2 g protein; 1 g total fat; 0 g saturated fat; 0 g monounsaturated fat; 0 g polyunsaturated fat; 40 g carbohydrate; 5 g fiber; 31 g sugar; 42 mg phosphorus; 64 mg calcium; 5 mg sodium; 510 mg potassium; 287 IU vitamin A; 0 mg ATE vitamin E; 84 mg vitamin C; 0 mg cholesterol

Tip: Nibbling the fruit after you drink the punch is at least half the fun.

Part II

Fix-It-in-15 and Let-It-Cook Meals

14

Fix-It-in-15 Make-Aheads

In chapter 3 we created a number of quick-to-fix ingredients that could be stored on your shelf or in the refrigerator and used in place of the similar products with high-sodium levels available commercially. But there are some things that would be handy to have that just don't cook within 15 minutes. For example, one of the tricks that many 15-minute recipe websites and cookbooks use is to base a lot of dishes on deli chicken or beef. We know how much sodium they typically contain, but it's not hard to cook your own roast beef or rotisserie-style chicken; it just can't be finished in 15 minutes. That's where "Fix It in 15" recipes come in. This chapter contains recipes that can be prepared in 15 minutes and then left to cook on their own, with the result being ingredients you can then use as a springboard to other quick meals. Here you'll find rotisserie chicken, roast beef, and roast turkey breast as well as condiments used in a number of recipes in this book, including salsa, chili sauce, and chicken and beef stock, which can provide an even more flavorful, lower-sodium alternative to their commercial counterparts. And just for good measure, I've added a couple of good long-cooked pasta sauces.

"Instant" Rice

This is a little trick I invented to solve the problem that I didn't like the taste and (especially) texture of Minute Rice, but I didn't want to pay the price for the little two-serving microwave pouches. So now I buy big bags of rice and steam a couple of cups at a time to freeze until the night I want to prepare a quick side dish.

2 cups (390 g) long-cooking rice

Prepare the rice according to package directions, either on the stove top or using a steamer or rice cooker. Cool. Pack 1½ cups (250 g) rice into 1-quart (1-L) resealable freezer bags. To use, remove the bag from the freezer, puncture near the top with a knife, and microwave on high for 2 to 3 minutes, until heated through.

Yield: 10 servings

Per serving: 135 calories (2% from fat, 8% from protein, 90% from carbohydrate); 3 g protein; 0 g total fat; 0 g saturated fat; 0 g monounsaturated fat; 0 g polyunsaturated fat; 30 g carbohydrate; 0 g fiber; 0 g sugar; 43 mg phosphorus; 10 mg calcium; 2 mg sodium; 43 mg potassium; 0 IU vitamin A; 0 mg ATE vitamin E; 0 mg vitamin C; 0 mg cholesterol

Tip: This same idea also works just as well with brown rice.

Rotisserie-Style Chicken

Many of the 15- and 30-minute recipes you find online start with rotisserie chicken. There are even whole cookbooks based on it. But commercial rotisserie chicken contains a lot of sodium. So I make my own, which is just as tasty and convenient, but a lot healthier. The chicken may be stored in the refrigerator for up to a week. For longer storage remove the meat from the bones, separate into meal-size portions, pack in covered airtight containers or resealable freezer bags, and freeze. The flavor will be best if used within 4 months. The bones can be used for the Chicken Stock on page 232 or frozen in resealable freezer bags for up to four months.

¼ cup (80 g) honey

1 teaspoon paprika

1 teaspoon onion powder

½ teaspoon freshly ground black pepper

½ teaspoon dried thyme

¼ teaspoon garlic powder

6½ pounds (3 kg) roasting chicken

Preheat the oven to 325°F (170°C, or gas mark 3). Stir the spices into the honey in a small bowl. Brush onto the chicken. Place in a roasting pan and cook, uncovered, basting occasionally with the pan juices, for 1½ to 2 hours, or until a meat thermometer inserted in the thickest part of the thigh reads 165° F (74°C).

Yield: 8 servings

Per serving: 71 calories (18% from fat, 30% from protein, 51% from carbohydrate); 5 g protein; 1 g total fat; 0 g saturated fat; 1 g monounsaturated fat; 0 g polyunsaturated fat; 9 g carbohydrate; 0 g fiber; 9 g sugar; 7 mg calcium; 0 mg Iron; 37 mg sodium; 67 mg potassium; 163 IU vitamin A; 0 mg vitamin C; 16 mg cholesterol

Tip: You can also cook this on a rotisserie if you have one or, as I often do, split it in half and grill it over an indirect fire.

Roast Beef

It really doesn't get any easier than this. This is the perfect roast for slicing for sandwiches or using in other recipes that call for leftover roast beef. The meat may be stored in the refrigerator for up to a week. For longer storage separate into meal-size portions, pack in covered airtight containers or resealable freezer bags, and freeze. The flavor will be best if used within 4 months.

3½ pounds (1590 g) beef round roast
½ teaspoon freshly ground black pepper
1 cup (160 g) sliced onion

Preheat the oven to 350°F (180°C, or gas mark 4). Place the beef, fat side up, on a rack in a roasting pan. Season with the pepper, then top with the onion slices. Add enough water to cover the bottom of the pan. Bake, uncovered, for about 3½ hours, or until a meat thermometer registers 165°F (74°C) when inserted into the thickest part for well done. Let stand for 10 minutes before carving.

Yield: 10 servings

Per serving: 210 calories (26% from fat, 71% from protein, 3% from carbohydrate); 35 g protein; 6 g total fat; 2 g saturated fat; 2 g monounsaturated fat; 0 g polyunsaturated fat; 2 g carbohydrate; 0 g fiber; 1 g sugar; 349 mg phosphorus; 37 mg calcium; 99 mg sodium; 598 mg potassium; 1 IU vitamin A; 0 mg ATE vitamin E; 1 mg vitamin C; 79 mg cholesterol

Tip: Skim the fat off the pan juices and save to dilute with water and use in place of canned beef broth. The 3½ hour cooking time will give you a roast that is well done, but that is a good thing with a round roast, which is much more tender when cooked for a longer time.

Roast Turkey Breast

There are a huge number of recipes that call for leftover deli turkey or chicken. Save the money and the sodium by buying turkey breasts when they are on sale and roasting them yourself. Not only do they make a good meal at the time, but you'll also have plenty of leftovers that you can freeze and pull out for other quick meals. The turkey may be stored in the refrigerator for up to a week. For longer storage remove the meat from the bones, separate into meal-size portions, pack in covered airtight containers or resealable freezer bags, and freeze. The flavor will be best if used within 4 months. The bones can be used to make stock or frozen in resealable freezer bags for up to 4 months.

1 turkey breast, about 8½ pounds (3860 g)
3 tablespoons (45 ml) lemon juice, divided
2 tablespoons (30 ml) olive oil, divided

½ teaspoon minced garlic

1 teaspoon lemon zest

1 teaspoon dried thyme

¾ teaspoon freshly ground black pepper

½ teaspoon crumbled sage

Preheat the oven to 350°F (180°C, or gas mark 4). Loosen the skin from the turkey with your fingers, leaving the skin attached along the bottom edges. In a small bowl, combine 1 tablespoon (15 ml) of the lemon juice, 1 tablespoon (15 ml) of the oil, the garlic, and the seasonings. Spread under the turkey skin. In a small bowl, combine the remaining 2 tablespoons (30 ml) lemon juice and 1 tablespoon (15 ml) oil; set aside. Place the turkey on a rack in a shallow roasting pan. Bake, uncovered, for 2½ to 3 hours, or until a meat thermometer registers 170°F (77°C) when inserted into the thickest part, basting occasionally with the lemon juice mixture. Let stand for 10 minutes. Discard the skin before carving.

Yield: 16 servings

Per serving: 124 calories (24% from fat, 75% from protein, 1% from carbohydrate); 22 g protein; 3 g total fat; 1 g saturated fat; 2 g monounsaturated fat; 1 g polyunsaturated fat; 0 g carbohydrate; 0 g fiber; 0 g sugar; 192 mg phosphorus; 14 mg calcium; 59 mg sodium; 292 mg potassium; 5 IU vitamin A; 0 mg ATE vitamin E; 2 mg vitamin C; 56 mg cholesterol

Carnitas

Make this ahead of time and freeze it in meal-size portions to make great Mexican meals super quick. It's perfect for fajitas, in taco salad, or in place of the more typical beef in any Mexican recipe. The meat may be stored in the refrigerator for up to a week. For longer storage separate into meal-size portions, pack in covered airtight containers or resealable freezer bags, and freeze. The flavor will be best if used within four months.

3 pounds (1362 g) boneless pork loin roast, cut into 3-inch (7.5-cm) cubes

½ cup (120 ml) lime juice

½ teaspoon freshly ground black pepper

½ teaspoon red pepper flakes

Coat the inside of a 3-quart (3-L) slow cooker with cooking spray. Combine the pork, lime juice, pepper, and red pepper flakes in the slow cooker. Cover and cook on high for 1 hour; stir. Reduce the heat to low and cook for 8 to 10 hours longer, or until the meat is tender. Let stand for 10 minutes, then shred the pork with two forks.

Yield: 10 servings

Per serving: 211 calories (39% from fat, 58% from protein, 2% from carbohydrate); 30 g protein; 9 g total fat; 3 g saturated fat; 4 g monounsaturated fat; 1 g polyunsaturated fat; 1 g carbohydrate; 0 g fiber; 0 g sugar; 283 mg phosphorus; 9 mg calcium; 61 mg sodium; 589 mg potassium; 53 IU vitamin A; 3 mg ATE vitamin E; 4 mg vitamin C; 75 mg cholesterol

Low-Sodium Beef Stock

The main difference between broth and stock is that broth is usually just meat simmered with water and vegetables, while stock is made by browning meaty bones, and then simmering them. This produces a richer, more flavorful liquid. This recipe produces stock that can be diluted before using. It cooks easily in the slow cooker and gives you a good size quantity of stock. Freeze stock that is not going to be used within a week by packing one cup portions in covered airtight containers or resealable freezer bags and freezing. The flavor will be best if used within 6 months.

1½ pounds (680 g) beef chuck with bones

1 cup (160 g) sliced onion

1 cup (130 g) sliced carrot

1 cup (100 g) chopped celery

1½ cups (355 ml) water

½ teaspoon freshly ground black pepper

1 teaspoon dried thyme

Preheat the oven to 350°F (180°C, or gas mark 4). Place the beef and vegetables in a single layer in a roasting pan and roast, uncovered, until browned, about 1 hour. Transfer to a 4-quart (4-L) slow cooker. Pour the water over, add the pepper and thyme, and cook on low for 8 to 9 hours. Remove the meat from the pot and let rest until cool enough to handle. Remove the meat from the bones and save for another use. Strain the veggies from the stock and discard. Cool the stock in the refrigerator and remove the fat from the top. Both the beef and the stock may be frozen until needed.

To make beef broth: Mix the stock with an equal amount of water and use in any recipe calling for beef broth.

Yield: You should have about 4 cups (950 ml) of stock, or 8 ½-cup (120-ml) servings

Per serving: 70 calories (66% from fat, 27% from protein, 7% from carbohydrate); 4 g protein; 3 g total fat; 2 g saturated fat; 1 g monounsaturated fat; 1 g polyunsaturated fat; 4 g carbohydrate; 1 g fiber; 2 g sugar; 153 mg phosphorus; 28 mg calcium; 2 mg Iron; 81 mg sodium; 347 mg potassium; 2752 IU vitamin A; 0 mg ATE vitamin E; 3 mg vitamin C; 60 mg cholesterol

Tip: For more convenient storage and thawing, pour stock into ice cube trays and freeze. Once stock is frozen, transfer cubes to a resealable freezer bag. Each cube will hold ¼ cup of stock, enough for ½ cup (120 ml) of prepared broth.

Low-Sodium Chicken Stock

The main difference between broth and stock is that broth is usually just meat simmered with water and vegetables, while stock is made by browning meaty bones, and then simmering them. This produces a richer, more flavorful stock. This recipe produces stock that can be diluted before using. It cooks easily in the slow cooker and gives you a good size quantity of stock. You can use any chicken bones that have most of the meat removed. I often buy chicken breasts, remove most of the meat to make a much cheaper boneless, skinless

(continued on page 232)

breast piece, then use the bones to make stock. You can also use the bones from a roasted chicken. Freeze stock that is not going to be used within a week by packing one cup portions in covered airtight containers or resealable freezer bags and freezing. The flavor will be best if used within 6 months.

1½ pounds (680 g) meaty chicken bones

1 cup (160 g) sliced onion

1 cup (130 g) sliced carrot

1 cup (100 g) chopped celery

½ cup (120 ml) water

½ teaspoon freshly ground black pepper

1 teaspoon thyme

Preheat the oven to 350°F (180°C, or gas mark 4). Place the bones and vegetables in a single layer in a roasting pan and roast, uncovered, until browned, about 1 hour. Transfer to a 4-quart (4-L) slow cooker. Pour the water over, add the pepper and thyme, and cook on low for 8 to 9 hours. Remove the bones from pot and let stand until cool enough to handle. Remove the meat from the bones and save for another use. Strain the veggies from the stock and discard. Cool the stock in the refrigerator and remove the fat from the top. Both the chicken and the stock may be frozen until needed.

To make chicken broth: Mix the stock with an equal amount of water and use in any recipe calling for chicken broth.

Yield: You should have about 4 cups (950 ml) of stock, or 8 ½-cup (120 ml) servings

Per serving: 134 calories (35% from fat, 53% from protein, 12% from carbohydrate); 17 g protein; 5 g total fat; 1 g saturated fat; 2 g monounsaturated fat; 1 g polyunsaturated fat; 4 g carbohydrate; 1 g fiber; 2 g sugar; 143 mg phosphorus; 33 mg calcium; 1 mg Iron; 92 mg sodium; 290 mg potassium; 2836 IU vitamin A; 26 mg ATE vitamin E; 3 mg vitamin C; 69 mg cholesterol

Tip: For more convenient storage and thawing, pour stock into ice cube trays and freeze. Once stock is frozen, transfer cubes to a resealable freezer bag. Each cube will hold ¼ cup of stock, enough for ½ cup of prepared broth.

The World's Best Low-Sodium Salsa

Okay, I can't really prove it's the best. It took me a lot of experimenting, but I finally came up with a recipe for salsa that satisfies me and that I actually wrote down the ingredients for. It's been popular with our kids and their friends, so that's probably a good recommendation. This makes a mild version. You could add another chile pepper or two depending on how hot you like it.

3 pounds (1362 g) plum tomatoes, peeled and chopped

½ cup (125 g) cooked black beans

½ cup (65 g) frozen corn kernels

1 can (8 ounces, or 225 g) no-salt-added tomato sauce

1 chile pepper, seeded and minced

¼ cup (60 ml) red wine vinegar

½ cup (80 g) chopped onion

1 teaspoon minced garlic

1½ teaspoons chopped fresh cilantro

½ teaspoon dried oregano

1½ teaspoons ground cumin

Combine all the ingredients in a large pot over medium-low heat. Simmer until thickened, about 15 minutes. Pack into jars and store in the refrigerator. Salsa will keep in the refrigerator for up to a month or may be frozen. If freezing in jars be sure to leave 1½ inches (3.8 cm) of headspace for expansion and do not tighten the lid until after it is frozen. Frozen salsa will be best if used with 3 months.

Yield: 3 pints (1425 g), or 48 servings (2 tablespoons, or 28 g, per serving)

Per serving: 18 calories (7% from fat, 19% from protein, 74% from carbohydrate); 1 g protein; 0 g total fat; 0 g saturated fat; 0 g monounsaturated fat; 0 g polyunsaturated fat; 4 g carbohydrate; 1 g fiber; 1 g sugar; 21 mg phosphorus; 8 mg calcium; 0 mg Iron; 25 mg sodium; 132 mg potassium; 305 IU vitamin A; 0 mg ATE vitamin E; 7 mg vitamin C; 0 mg cholesterol

Tip: To peel tomatoes, slip them into boiling water for about 30 seconds; then, transfer to an ice bath. The skins will come right off.

Chili Sauce

I've got to admit, I've never been a really big fan of bottled chili sauce. The kids used it on hot dogs for a while, but I've always been a mustard and relish type of guy. Anyway, I much prefer the flavor of this chili sauce, which was adapted from a recipe from the American Heart Association, to the kind found in stores. There are enough veggies in it to give it something more than a glorified ketchup taste.

1 can (14.5 ounces, or 411 g) no-salt-added tomatoes

1 can (8 ounces, or 225 g) no-salt-added tomato sauce

½ cup (80 g) chopped onion

½ cup (100 g) sugar

½ cup (50 g) chopped celery

½ cup (75 g) chopped green bell pepper

1 tablespoon (15 ml) lemon juice

1 tablespoon (15 g) packed brown sugar

1 tablespoon (20 g) molasses

¼ teaspoon hot pepper sauce

⅛ teaspoon ground cloves

⅛ teaspoon ground cinnamon

⅛ teaspoon freshly ground black pepper

⅛ teaspoon dried basil

⅛ teaspoon dried tarragon

½ cup (120 ml) cider vinegar

Combine all the ingredients in a large saucepan. Bring to a boil over high heat, reduce the heat to a simmer, and cook, uncovered, for 1½ hours, or until the mixture is reduced by half. Pack into jars and store in the refrigerator for up to 4 weeks or freeze for up to 6 months.

Yield: 3 pints (1425 g), or 48 servings (2 tablespoons, or 28 g, per serving)

(continued on page 234)

Per serving: 15 calories (2% from fat, 4% from protein, 94% from carbohydrate); 0 g protein; 0 g total fat; 0 g saturated fat; 0 g monounsaturated fat; 0 g polyunsaturated fat; 4 g carbohydrate; 0 g fiber; 3 g sugar; 4 mg phosphorus; 6 mg calcium; 27 mg sodium; 53 mg potassium; 39 IU vitamin A; 0 mg ATE vitamin E; 3 mg vitamin C; 0 mg cholesterol

Tip: If freezing allow 1½ inches (3.8 cm) headspace and do not put the lid on tight until after the mixture has frozen.

Low-Sodium Spaghetti Sauce

This recipe makes a fairly large quantity, but you can freeze the extra in meal-size portions so it can be easily thawed and heated in the microwave when needed.

4 pounds (1.8 kg) Roma tomatoes, roughly chopped

1 pound (454 g) extra-lean ground beef

1 cup (160 g) chopped onion

2 tablespoons (20 g) minced garlic, divided

¼ cup (38 g) chopped green bell pepper

2 tablespoons (30 ml) extra-virgin olive oil

1 teaspoon dried basil

1 teaspoon white pepper

¼ teaspoon dried oregano

¼ teaspoon dried thyme

2 tablespoons (25 g) sugar

Coat the inside of a 4-quart (4-L) slow cooker with cooking spray. Place the tomatoes in a

food processor and process until puréed. In a skillet or wok over medium-high heat, brown the ground beef, breaking it up with a spatula. Add the onion and 1 tablespoon (10 g) of the minced garlic. When the meat is no longer pink, remove from the heat and add the green pepper. Add to the slow cooker, along with the remaining 1 tablespoon (10 g) garlic, oil, spices, and sugar. Cook on low for 2 to 4 hours. Sauce will keep in the refrigerator for up to a week or may be frozen in meal-size portions in an airtight container or resealable freezer bag. The flavor will be best if used within 6 months.

Yield: About 6 cups (1470 g), or 12 ½-cup (125 g) servings

Per serving: 101 calories (63% from fat, 23% from protein, 14% from carbohydrate); 7 g protein; 9 g total fat; 3 g saturated fat; 4 g monounsaturated fat; 1 g polyunsaturated fat; 4 g carbohydrate; 0 g fiber; 3 g sugar; 60 mg phosphorus; 11 mg calcium; 26 mg sodium; 140 mg potassium; 19 IU vitamin A; 0 mg ATE vitamin E; 4 mg vitamin C; 26 mg cholesterol

Roasted Red Pepper Sauce

This makes a big batch of a great-tasting sauce that you can freeze in meal-size portions. It has a bit more sodium than most of the recipes here because of the canned red peppers. If you roast or freeze your own while they are plentiful in the summer, you can get the same great taste with a fraction of the sodium.

4 pounds (1816 g) plum tomatoes, coarsely chopped

1 cup (160 g) chopped sweet onion

2 cans (14.5 ounces, or 190 g, each) no-salt-added puréed tomatoes

21 ounces (588 g) roasted red peppers, drained and chopped

8 ounces (225 g) mushrooms, quartered

¼ cup (50 g) sugar

¼ cup (60 ml) balsamic vinegar

¼ cup (60 ml) olive oil

1 teaspoon minced garlic

1 tablespoon (2 g) basil

1 tablespoon (3 g) oregano

Coat the inside of a 5-quart (5-L) slow cooker with cooking spray. Combine all the ingredients in the slow cooker. Cover and cook on high for 4 hours, or until the flavors are blended. The sauce will keep in the refrigerator for up to a week or may be frozen in meal-size portions in an airtight container or resealable freezer bag. The flavor will be best if used within 6 months.

Yield: About 15 cups, or 30 servings (½ cup, or 125 g, per serving)

Per serving: 49 calories (36% from fat, 9% from protein, 55% from carbohydrate); 1 g protein; 2 g total fat; 0 g saturated fat; 1 g monounsaturated fat; 0 g polyunsaturated fat; 7 g carbohydrate; 1 g fiber; 3 g sugar; 32 mg phosphorus; 24 mg calcium; 280 mg sodium; 263 mg potassium; 529 IU vitamin A; 0 mg ATE vitamin E; 29 mg vitamin C; 0 mg cholesterol

15

Fix-It-in-15 Breakfasts

Do you ever run into a situation where you need a breakfast for a number of people, either family or perhaps holiday guests, but don't want to spend a lot of time fixing it? This chapter contains recipes that will solve that problem. They all are assembled quickly, then cooked in either the slow cooker or the oven while you sleep late or do other things. There are some great egg dishes here as well as things such as potatoes, french toast, and cereal.

Creamy Egg and Veggie Casserole

Throw it in the slow cooker and forget it. If you have a timer on your cooker, it can even start it up in the middle of the night and have breakfast waiting when you get up. Unlike many breakfast casseroles containing high sodium meats such as sausage or ham, this one gets a rich flavor and added nutrition from vegetables and cottage cheese.

24 ounces (672 g) no-salt-added cottage cheese

10 ounces (280 g) frozen chopped broccoli, thawed and drained

1 cup (160 g) chopped onion

½ cup (75 g) shredded red bell pepper

8 ounces (225 g) Swiss cheese, shredded

1½ cups (375 g) egg substitute, or 6 eggs, lightly beaten

⅓ cup (40 g) all-purpose flour

¼ cup (112 g) unsalted butter, melted

Coat a 3-quart (3-L) slow cooker with cooking spray. Combine all the ingredients in a large bowl. Transfer to the slow cooker. Cover and cook on low for 4 to 5 hours, or egg are set in the center.

Yield: 6 servings

Per serving: 432 calories (53% from fat, 32% from protein, 15% from carbohydrate); 35 g protein; 25 g total fat; 15 g saturated fat; 7 g monounsaturated fat; 2 g polyunsaturated fat; 16 g carbohydrate; 2 g fiber; 4 g sugar; 498 mg phosphorus; 490 mg calcium; 193 mg sodium; 486 mg potassium; 1874 IU vitamin A; 192 mg ATE vitamin E; 44 mg vitamin C; 73 mg cholesterol

Hash Brown Egg Bake

Toss this breakfast casserole into the oven and go about the rest of your life for the next 50 minutes or so. Then come back for a tasty, hot breakfast. The generous amount of Swiss cheese will ensure that no one complains about the lack of meat.

32 ounces (896 g) frozen hash brown potatoes, thawed

1 cup (110 g) shredded Swiss cheese, divided

2 cups (500 g) egg substitute, or 8 eggs

2 cups (470 ml) skim milk

Pinch of paprika

Preheat the oven to 350°F (180°C, or gas mark 4). Grease a 13 × 9-inch (33 × 23-cm) baking dish. In a large bowl, combine the hash browns and ½ cup (55 g) of the cheese. Spoon into in the prepared baking dish. In another large bowl, whisk together the eggs and milk until smooth; pour over the hash brown mixture. Sprinkle with the paprika. Bake, uncovered, for 45 to 50 minutes, until a knife inserted near the center comes out clean. Sprinkle with the remaining ½ cup (55 g) cheese and serve.

Yield: 8 servings

Per serving: 224 calories (27% from fat, 29% from protein, 44% from carbohydrate); 16 g protein;

7 g total fat; 3 g saturated fat; 2 g monounsaturated fat; 1 g polyunsaturated fat; 24 g carbohydrate; 2 g fiber; 1 g sugar; 284 mg phosphorus; 269 mg calcium; 163 mg sodium; 658 mg potassium; 467 IU vitamin A; 67 mg ATE vitamin E; 10 mg vitamin C; 15 mg cholesterol

Slow-Cooked Mexican Egg Scramble

Mexican-accented eggs cook overnight while you sleep. These are great topped with sour cream or fresh salsa for an extra little bit of flavor.

1 cup (160 g) chopped onion

1 cup (150 g) chopped green bell pepper

4 ounces (112 g) chopped green chiles, drained

2 cups (220 g) grated Swiss cheese

4 cups (1000 g) egg substitute, or 16 eggs, beaten

Coat the inside of a 3- to 4-quart (3- to 4-L) slow cooker with cooking spray. Layer the onion, pepper, chiles, and cheese in the slow cooker, repeating the layering process until all the ingredients are used. Pour the eggs over the mixture, cover, and cook on low for 7 to 8 hours, until eggs are set.

Yield: 12 servings

Per serving: 163 calories (50% from fat, 41% from protein, 9% from carbohydrate); 17 g protein; 9 g total fat; 4 g saturated fat; 2 g monounsaturated fat; 2 g polyunsaturated fat; 4 g

carbohydrate; 1 g fiber; 2 g sugar; 241 mg phosphorus; 263 mg calcium; 189 mg sodium; 352 mg potassium; 539 IU vitamin A; 46 mg ATE vitamin E; 14 mg vitamin C; 21 mg cholesterol

Tip: Make this a grab and go breakfast by providing warmed corn tortillas to place the mixture in taco-style.

Overnight Omelet

This makes a big batch of breakfast. It's great if you have a number of people staying over because you can put it in the night before and have a nice hot breakfast with no work in the morning.

32 ounces (896 g) frozen hash brown potatoes, thawed

¾ cup (120 g) chopped onion

½ cup (75 g) chopped green bell pepper

3 cups (750 g) egg substitute, or 12 eggs

1 cup (235 ml) skim milk

Coat the inside of a 3- to 4-quart (3- to 4-L) slow cooker with cooking spray. Layer half the potatoes and half the vegetables in the slow cooker, and then repeat to make another layer. Beat together the eggs and milk in a bowl, pour over the mixture in the slow cooker, cover, and cook on low for 8 to 10 hours, until eggs are set.

Yield: 10 servings

Per serving: 278 calories (41% from fat, 18% from protein, 41% from carbohydrate); 13 g protein; 13 g total fat; 5 g saturated fat; 5 g

monounsaturated fat; 2 g polyunsaturated fat; 29 g carbohydrate; 2 g fiber; 3 g sugar; 189 mg phosphorus; 92 mg calcium; 179 mg sodium; 719 mg potassium; 349 IU vitamin A; 15 mg ATE vitamin E; 13 mg vitamin C; 1 mg cholesterol

Broccoli Hash Brown Quiche

Here's another hot breakfast that you can get into the oven in a few minutes and then forget for an hour. If you're like me, there are a lot of things you could use that hour for on a weekend morning.

3 cups (330 g) frozen hash brown potatoes, thawed

1½ cups (105 g) frozen broccoli, thawed

1 cup (250 g) egg substitute, or 4 eggs

8 ounces (225 g) sour cream

4 ounces (112 g) Swiss cheese, shredded

Preheat the oven to 350°F (180°C, or gas mark 4). Grease a 9-inch (23-cm) pie plate. Press the hash browns onto the bottom and up the sides of the prepared pie plate, forming a shell. Layer the broccoli on top. In a bowl, beat together the eggs and sour cream, stir in the cheese, then pour over the broccoli. Bake for 55 to 65 minutes, or until a knife inserted near the center comes out clean. Let stand for 5 minutes before cutting.

Yield: 6 servings

Per serving: 256 calories (41% from fat, 23% from protein, 36% from carbohydrate); 15 g protein;

12 g total fat; 7 g saturated fat; 3 g monounsaturated fat; 1 g polyunsaturated fat; 24 g carbohydrate; 3 g fiber; 1 g sugar; 273 mg phosphorus; 269 mg calcium; 113 mg sodium; 572 mg potassium; 960 IU vitamin A; 78 mg ATE vitamin E; 27 mg vitamin C; 33 mg cholesterol

Ready When You Are Breakfast Potatoes

This is an easy, cheesy version of home-fried potatoes that cooks overnight. Not only does it go well with traditional breakfasts, it also is great as a side dish if cooked during the day.

4 large red potatoes

1 cup (160 g) coarsely chopped onion

4 ounces (112 g) Swiss cheese, shredded

1 tablespoon (14 g) unsalted butter

Coat the inside of a 4-quart (4-L) slow cooker with cooking spray. Thinly slice the potatoes. Layer half of the potatoes, onion, and cheese in the slow cooker, dot with half of the butter, then repeat to make a second layer. Cook on high for 8 to 10 hours, until potatoes are soft.

Yield: 6 servings

Per serving: 276 calories (24% from fat, 15% from protein, 61% from carbohydrate); 10 g protein; 7 g total fat; 5 g saturated fat; 2 g monounsaturated fat; 0 g polyunsaturated fat; 42 g carbohydrate; 5 g fiber; 4 g sugar; 272 mg phosphorus; 213 mg calcium; 18 mg sodium; 1179 mg potassium; 231 IU vitamin A; 56 mg ATE vitamin E; 50 mg vitamin C; 22 mg cholesterol

Baked French Toast

This is an easy make-ahead breakfast for a weekend or holiday. The whole wheat bread adds both flavor and fiber. The blueberries make it a special treat,

8 slices Low-Sodium Whole Wheat Bread (page 312), cubed

¾ cup (188 g) egg substitute, or 3 eggs, beaten

3 tablespoons (38 g) granulated sugar

1 teaspoon vanilla extract

2¼ cups (530 ml) skim milk

¼ cup (30 g) all-purpose flour

6 tablespoons (90 g) packed brown sugar

½ teaspoon ground cinnamon

2 tablespoons (28 g) unsalted butter

2 cups (290 g) fresh or frozen blueberries

Grease a 9 × 13-inch (23 × 33-cm) baking dish. Place the bread cubes in the prepared baking dish. In a medium bowl, lightly beat eggs, granulated sugar, and vanilla. Stir in the milk until well blended. Pour over the bread, turning the pieces to coat well. Cover and refrigerate overnight.

Preheat the oven to 375°F (190°C, or gas mark 5). In a small bowl, combine the flour, brown sugar, and cinnamon. Cut in the butter until the mixture resembles coarse crumbs. Turn the bread over in the baking dish. Cover with the blueberries and sprinkle evenly with the crumb mixture. Bake for about 40 minutes, until golden brown.

Yield: 6 servings

Per serving: 310 calories (19% from fat, 15% from protein, 66% from carbohydrate); 11 g protein; 7 g total fat; 3 g saturated fat; 2 g monounsaturated fat; 1 g polyunsaturated fat; 52 g carbohydrate; 3 g fiber; 26 g sugar; 207 mg phosphorus; 203 mg calcium; 128 mg sodium; 432 mg potassium; 445 IU vitamin A; 88 mg ATE vitamin E; 6 mg vitamin C; 12 mg cholesterol

Tip: You can substitute strawberries or raspberries, or use some combination, if you prefer.

Banana Nut Muesli

This breakfast "cooks" overnight in the refrigerator. What could be more convenient than that? The bananas, raisins, and nuts make it more than just plain oatmeal and the flavor is superior to any of those instant oatmeal packages.

1 cup (235 ml) water

⅔ cup (53 g) quick-cooking oats

1 banana, sliced

¼ cup (36 g) raisins

¼ cup (27 g) chopped almonds

¼ teaspoon ground cinnamon

Combine all of the ingredients in a bowl. Cover and refrigerate overnight. Serve chilled.

Yield: 2 servings

Per serving: 352 calories (31% from fat, 11% from protein, 59% from carbohydrate); 10 g protein; 13 g total fat; 1 g saturated fat; 7 g monounsaturated fat; 3 g polyunsaturated fat; 55 g carbohydrate; 8 g fiber; 23 g sugar; 257 mg phosphorus; 91 mg calcium; 7 mg sodium; 656 mg potassium; 49 IU vitamin A; 0 mg ATE vitamin E; 7 mg vitamin C; 0 mg cholesterol

Easy Overnight Apple Oatmeal

Full of fruit, this breakfast cereal is sure to please. Topped with yogurt and granola, it looks as good as it tastes. Even better, it cooks overnight and is ready to serve when you get up in the morning.

3 cups (705 ml) water

1¾ cups (410 ml) apple juice

1½ cups (120 g) rolled oats

7 ounces (196 g) dried mixed fruit

⅓ cup (75 g) packed brown sugar

½ teaspoon ground cinnamon

12 ounces (340 g) low-fat vanilla yogurt

1 cup (240 g) granola

Coat the inside of a 4-quart (4-L) slow cooker with cooking spray. Combine the water, juice, oats, mixed fruit, brown sugar, and cinnamon in the slow cooker. Cover and cook on low for 6 to 8 hours, until oats are cooked and fruit is soft. Top with the yogurt and granola and serve.

Yield: 8 servings

Per serving: 254 calories (7% from fat, 9% from protein, 84% from carbohydrate); 6 g protein; 2 g total fat; 1 g saturated fat; 1 g monounsaturated fat; 1 g polyunsaturated fat; 55 g carbohydrate; 4 g

fiber; 24 g sugar; 182 mg phosphorus; 108 mg calcium; 81 mg sodium; 471 mg potassium; 624 IU vitamin A; 5 mg ATE vitamin E; 2 mg vitamin C; 2 mg cholesterol

Muesli

Muesli is a traditional make-ahead breakfast. The oats soften in liquid overnight and the flavors blend for a morning taste treat. This version contains the added flavor of orange juice.

2 cups (160 g) quick-cooking oats

1¼ cups (295 ml) skim milk

¾ cup (109 g) raisins

½ cup (120 ml) orange juice

⅓ cup (37 g) wheat germ

2 tablespoons (40 g) honey

Combine all the ingredients in a bowl, mixing well. Cover and refrigerate overnight or for at least 8 hours. Mix well before serving.

Yield: 6 servings

Per serving: 241 calories (9% from fat, 14% from protein, 76% from carbohydrate); 9 g protein; 3 g total fat; 1 g saturated fat; 1 g monounsaturated fat; 1 g polyunsaturated fat; 48 g carbohydrate; 4 g fiber; 19 g sugar; 281 mg phosphorus; 103 mg calcium; 34 mg sodium; 445 mg potassium; 127 IU vitamin A; 31 mg ATE vitamin E; 8 mg vitamin C; 1 mg cholesterol

Tip: This is also good heated in the microwave for a hot breakfast.

16

Fix-It-in-15 Poultry Dishes

This chapter contains some recipes for chicken and turkey that fall into my easy fix-ahead scheme. Some will give you leftovers that you can use for future meals. Many make use of the slow cooker to give you a break from the kitchen and do other things while dinner fixes itself. All will give you the kind of homemade meals that are full of flavor while providing great nutrition.

Broth-Injected Turkey

If you're looking for a BIG batch of already cooked meat to add to quick meals, consider a turkey. You can get the same kind of extra juiciness that the pre-basted turkeys have while saving lots of sodium by injecting your own turkey. Using a low-sodium chicken broth adds almost no sodium per serving. Starting the cooking at a high temperature seals in the juices and gives you nice crispy skin.

12-pound (5448-g) turkey

1 cup (235 ml) Low-Sodium Chicken Broth (page 232) or turkey broth

Preheat the oven to 500°F (250°C, or gas mark 10). Place the turkey in a roasting pan. Using an injector, inject the broth into the turkey. Put the turkey in the oven and cook, uncovered, for 20 minutes, or until the exterior is crisp, but not golden brown. Reduce the temperature to 375°F (190°C, or gas mark 5). Roast until meat thermometer inserted in thickest part of thigh reads 165°F (74°C), about 2 hours. The turkey may be stored in the refrigerator for up to a week. For longer storage remove the meat from the bones, separate into meal-size portions, pack in covered airtight containers or resealable freezer bags, and freeze. The flavor will be best if used within 4 months. The bones can be used to make stock or frozen in resealable freezer bags for up to 4 months.

Yield: 36 servings

Per serving: 177 calories (22% from fat, 78% from protein, 0% from carbohydrate); 33 g protein; 4 g total fat; 1 g saturated fat; 1 g monounsaturated fat; 1 g polyunsaturated fat; 0 g carbohydrate; 0 g fiber; 0 g sugar; 299 mg phosphorus; 21 mg calcium; 110 mg sodium; 457 mg potassium; 0 IU vitamin A; 0 mg ATE vitamin E; 0 mg vitamin C; 103 mg cholesterol

Tip: You can find injectors in the gadget aisle of many large supermarkets or any kitchen supply store or buy one online for only a few dollars.

Herbed Turkey Breast

Turkey breast is given incredible flavor by marinating, then cooking in fresh herbs. This gives you not only a meal that is sure to please but also meat that adds extra flavor to soups, salads, or sandwiches.

4 cups (940 ml) Low-Sodium Chicken Broth (page 232)

1 cup (235 ml) lemon juice

½ cup (120 g) packed brown sugar

½ cup (20 g) minced fresh sage

½ cup (20 g) minced fresh thyme

2 tablespoons (4 g) fresh marjoram

1 tablespoon (7 g) paprika

2 teaspoons garlic powder

2 teaspoons freshly ground black pepper

½ cup (120 ml) lime juice

½ cup (120 ml) cider vinegar

½ cup (120 ml) olive oil

¼ cup (30 g) Onion Soup Mix (page 34)

¼ cup (44 g) Dijon mustard

8-pound (3632-g) turkey breast

(continued on page 244)

In a blender, process the broth, lemon juice, sugar, spices, lime juice, vinegar, oil, soup mix, and mustard until blended. Pour 3½ cups (823 ml) of the marinade into a large resealable plastic bag; add the turkey. Seal the bag and turn to coat. Refrigerate for 8 hours or overnight. Cover and refrigerate the remaining marinade.

When ready to cook, coat the inside of a 4- to 5-quart (4- to 5-L) slow cooker with cooking spray. Drain the turkey and discard the marinade. Place the turkey in the slow cooker and add the reserved marinade. Cover and cook on high for 3½ to 4½ hours, or until a meat thermometer registers 170°F (77°C) when inserted into the thickest part. The turkey may be stored in the refrigerator for up to a week. For longer storage remove the meat from the bones, separate into meal-size portions, pack in covered airtight containers or resealable freezer bags, and freeze. The flavor will be best if used within four months. The bones can be used to make stock or frozen in resealable freezer bags for up to four months.

Yield: 16 servings

Per serving: 288 calories (31% from fat, 52% from protein, 17% from carbohydrate); 37 g protein; 10 g total fat; 2 g saturated fat; 6 g monounsaturated fat; 1 g polyunsaturated fat; 12 g carbohydrate; 1 g fiber; 8 g sugar; 339 mg phosphorus; 82 mg calcium; 161 mg sodium; 615 mg potassium; 385 IU vitamin A; 0 mg ATE vitamin E; 12 mg vitamin C; 90 mg cholesterol

Basic Turkey Meatballs

These meatballs are not only lower in sodium and fat than commercial ones, they also have great flavor and are easier to make that they sound. Make them ahead of time and freeze them in meal-size batches to add to soups or pasta sauce. But plan on at least one meal while they are fresh.

2 pounds (908 g) ground turkey
½ cup (125 g) egg substitute, or 2 eggs
¾ cup (86 g) Italian-Style Bread Crumbs (page 33)
½ cup (80 g) finely chopped onion
1 teaspoon dried parsley
¼ teaspoon freshly ground black pepper
¼ teaspoon garlic powder

Preheat the oven to 325°F (170°C, or gas mark 3). Grease 1 or 2 cookie sheets or line with parchment paper. Combine all the ingredients in a large bowl. Shape into 48 walnut-size balls. Place on the cookie sheets. Bake for 30 minutes, or until no longer pink in the middle. Let cool, and then place in a plastic bag and store in the freezer until needed. They will keep indefinitely, but the flavor will be best if used within four months.

Yield: 8 servings, 6 meatballs per serving

Per serving: 251 calories (25% from fat, 61% from protein, 14% from carbohydrate); 37 g protein; 7 g total fat; 2 g saturated fat; 1 g monounsaturated fat; 2 g polyunsaturated fat; 9 g carbohydrate; 1 g fiber; 1 g sugar; 281 mg phosphorus; 58 mg calcium; 108 mg sodium;

427 mg potassium; 70 IU vitamin A; 0 mg ATE vitamin E; 1 mg vitamin C; 86 mg cholesterol

Tips: For even easier thawing of just the right amount, freeze them individually on a clean baking sheet before packing them into bags. For a more distinct Italian flavor, add a teaspoon of Italian seasoning.

Classic Chicken Stew

Chicken stew like Grandma used to make, only easier because she didn't have a slow cooker to do all the work. This is the kind of classic comfort food that many people think they have to give up on a low sodium diet, but the easy preparation and great nutrition will make it a favorite.

2 pounds (908 g) boneless skinless chicken breasts, cut into 1-inch (2.5-cm) cubes

4 cups (940 ml) Low-Sodium Chicken Broth (page 232)

3 red potatoes, peeled and cubed

1 cup (160 g) chopped onion

1 cup (100 g) sliced celery

1 cup (130 g) thinly sliced carrots

1 teaspoon paprika

½ teaspoon freshly ground black pepper

½ teaspoon crumbled sage

½ teaspoon thyme

1 can (6 ounces, or 170 g) no-salt-added tomato paste

Coat the inside of a 4- to 5-quart (4- to 5-L) slow cooker with cooking spray. Add all the ingredients to the slow cooker, stir to combine, cover, and cook on high for 4 to 5 hours, until the chicken is no longer pink in the center and the vegetables are tender.

Yield: 6 servings

Per serving: 384 calories (8% from fat, 46% from protein, 47% from carbohydrate); 44 g protein; 3 g total fat; 1 g saturated fat; 1 g monounsaturated fat; 1 g polyunsaturated fat; 45 g carbohydrate; 6 g fiber; 5 g sugar; 495 mg phosphorus; 84 mg calcium; 218 mg sodium; 1802 mg potassium; 3352 IU vitamin A; 9 mg ATE vitamin E; 32 mg vitamin C; 88 mg cholesterol

Creamy Italian Chicken

Creamy chicken is made easy with the make-aheads from chapter 3. Load it into the slow cooker and forget it. But be prepared for a dish that tastes like it took a long time to cook and contains all the things you aren't supposed to eat. This recipe works well served over either pasta or rice. Use whole grain pasta or brown rice for an additional nutrient boost.

4 boneless skinless chicken breasts

1½ cups (355 ml) Condensed Cream of Mushroom Soup (page 31)

1 cup (235 ml) skim milk

2 tablespoons (16 g) Italian Dressing Mix (page 35)

1 teaspoon thyme

1 teaspoon parsley flakes

(continued on page 246)

Coat the inside of a 4- to 5-quart (4- to 5-L) slow cooker with cooking spray. Place the chicken in the slow cooker. Combine the soup, milk, dressing mix, thyme, and parsley in a bowl; pour over the chicken. Cover and cook on low for 4 to 5 hours, or until the chicken is tender and no longer pink in the center.

Yield: 4 servings

Per serving: 132 calories (15% from fat, 66% from protein, 19% from carbohydrate); 21 g protein; 2 g total fat; 1 g saturated fat; 1 g monounsaturated fat; 0 g polyunsaturated fat; 6 g carbohydrate; 0 g fiber; 0 g sugar; 222 mg phosphorus; 104 mg calcium; 94 mg sodium; 357 mg potassium; 160 IU vitamin A; 42 mg ATE vitamin E; 4 mg vitamin C; 45 mg cholesterol

Curried Chicken with Tomatoes

I usually use mild curry powder, so this isn't as hot as you might think from the quantity. But that doesn't mean it doesn't have a depth of flavor, because the long slow cooking ensures that it does. You can vary the amount and heat of the spices to suit your own taste. This would traditionally be served over rice, but it's also good over small pasta such as orzo or couscous.

2 cans (14.5 ounces, or 411 g each) no-salt-added tomatoes

4 boneless skinless chicken breasts, cut in half

1 cup (160 g) coarsely chopped onion

½ cup (75 g) chopped green bell pepper

½ cup (65 g) chopped carrot

½ cup (50 g) chopped celery

2 tablespoons (12.5 g) curry powder

1 teaspoon turmeric

¼ teaspoon freshly ground black pepper

1 tablespoon (12 g) sugar

Coat the inside of a 4- to 5-quart (4- to 5-L) slow cooker with cooking spray. Combine all the ingredients in the slow cooker. Cover and cook on high for 2 to 3 hours, or on low for 5 to 6 hours, until the chicken is tender and no longer pink in the center.

Yield: 6 servings

Per serving: 113 calories (9% from fat, 44% from protein, 47% from carbohydrate); 13 g protein; 1 g total fat; 0 g saturated fat; 0 g monounsaturated fat; 0 g polyunsaturated fat; 14 g carbohydrate; 3 g fiber; 8 g sugar; 142 mg phosphorus; 71 mg calcium; 62 mg sodium; 584 mg potassium; 1579 IU vitamin A; 3 mg ATE vitamin E; 32 mg vitamin C; 27 mg cholesterol

Long and Slow Chicken Jambalaya

I'm a big fan of jambalaya and similar rice dishes. This is an way to make it simple in preparation. And there's something very nice about coming home to a house that smells of Cajun cooking. Add a salad for a complete meal.

1 pound (454 g) boneless chicken breast, cut into 1-inch (2.5-cm) cubes

2 cans (14.5 ounces, or 411 g each) no-salt-added tomatoes

½ cup (75 g) chopped green bell pepper

1 cup (235 ml) Low-Sodium Chicken Broth (page 232)

½ cup (120 ml) white wine

2 teaspoons dried oregano

2 teaspoons dried parsley

2 teaspoons Salt-Free Cajun Seasoning (page 29)

1 teaspoon cayenne pepper

2 cups (330 g) cooked rice

Coat the inside of a 4- to 5-quart (4- to 5-L) slow cooker with cooking spray. Combine the chicken, tomatoes, bell pepper, broth, wine, and seasonings in the slow cooker. Cover and cook on low for 6 to 8 hours, until the chicken is tender and no longer pink in the center. About 30 minutes before the end of the cooking, add the cooked rice and heat through.

Yield: 6 servings

Per serving: 204 calories (8% from fat, 44% from protein, 48% from carbohydrate); 21 g protein; 2 g total fat; 0 g saturated fat; 0 g monounsaturated fat; 0 g polyunsaturated fat; 23 g carbohydrate; 2 g fiber; 5 g sugar; 222 mg phosphorus; 78 mg calcium; 81 mg sodium; 663 mg potassium; 451 IU vitamin A; 5 mg ATE vitamin E; 35 mg vitamin C; 44 mg cholesterol

Full-Flavored Teriyaki Chicken

Overnight marinating gives these chicken legs great deep-down flavor, and then they can bake in the oven while you are busy with other things. Our low-sodium teriyaki sauce and generous amounts of garlic and ginger provide flavor without sodium. Steamed vegetables make a great accompaniment.

¾ cup (180 ml) Low-Sodium Teriyaki Sauce (page 30)

¼ cup (60 ml) canola oil

3 tablespoons (45 g) packed brown sugar

2 tablespoons (30 ml) sherry (optional)

½ teaspoon ground ginger

½ teaspoon garlic powder

12 chicken drumsticks

In a large resealable plastic bag, combine the teriyaki sauce, oil, brown sugar, sherry, ginger, and garlic powder; shake to combine. Add the drumsticks, seal the bag, and turn to coat; refrigerate overnight, turning occasionally.

When ready to cook, preheat the oven to 375°F (190°C, or gas mark 5). Drain the chicken and discard the marinade. Place the chicken in a single layer on a foil-lined baking sheet. Bake, uncovered, for 35 to 45 minutes, or until a meat thermometer registers 180°F (82°C) when inserted into the thickest part away from the bone and the juices run clear when pricked with a fork.

Yield: 6 servings

(continued on page 248)

Per serving: 222 calories (50% from fat, 30% from protein, 19% from carbohydrate); 16 g protein; 12 g total fat; 1 g saturated fat; 6 g monounsaturated fat; 3 g polyunsaturated fat; 10 g carbohydrate; 0 g fiber; 8 g sugar; 134 mg phosphorus; 18 mg calcium; 133 mg sodium; 218 mg potassium; 31 IU vitamin A; 9 mg ATE vitamin E; 0 mg vitamin C; 48 mg cholesterol

Just Like You Remember Orange Chicken

Do you sometimes long for the days when you could go to the Asian takeout in the food court and order the orange chicken? This dish will take you back. All the flavor is there, enhanced by the long cooking time in the slow cooker, but without the sodium. To complete the food-court picture, serve over brown rice with stir-fried cabbage, broccoli, and carrots.

2 oranges, cut into wedges

1 cup (150 g) chopped green bell pepper

1 chicken, 3 to 4 pounds (1362 to 1816 g), cut up and skin removed

1 cup (235 ml) orange juice

½ cup (125 g) Chili Sauce (page 233)

2 tablespoons (30 ml) Low-Sodium Soy Sauce (page 29)

1 tablespoon (20 g) molasses

1 teaspoon dry mustard powder

1 teaspoon minced garlic

¼ teaspoon freshly ground black pepper

Coat the inside of a 4- to 5-quart (4- to 5-L) slow cooker with cooking spray. Place the oranges and green pepper in the slow cooker and top with the chicken. Combine the juice, chili sauce, soy sauce, molasses, mustard powder, garlic, and black pepper in a bowl; pour over the chicken. Cover and cook on low for 4 to 5 hours, or until the chicken is tender and the juices run clear when pricked with a fork.

Yield: 4 servings

Per serving: 172 calories (11% from fat, 30% from protein, 60% from carbohydrate); 13 g protein; 2 g total fat; 0 g saturated fat; 1 g monounsaturated fat; 0 g polyunsaturated fat; 26 g carbohydrate; 3 g fiber; 15 g sugar; 124 mg phosphorus; 74 mg calcium; 102 mg sodium; 561 mg potassium; 923 IU vitamin A; 8 mg ATE vitamin E; 106 mg vitamin C; 34 mg cholesterol

Spanish Style Chicken and Rice

This is a slow cooker version of the classic Spanish arroz con pollo, but without the classic time spent in preparation. Serve with a green salad for a complete meal.

1 tablespoon (15 ml) olive oil

3 pounds (1362 g) chicken pieces

1 cup (160 g) finely chopped onion

1 teaspoon minced garlic

¼ teaspoon freshly ground black pepper

1½ cups (285 g) long-grain rice

1 can (14.5 ounces, or 411 g) no-salt-added tomatoes

1½ cups (355 ml) Low-Sodium Chicken Broth (page 232)

½ cup (120 ml) white wine

¾ cup (112 g) finely chopped green bell pepper

1 cup (130 g) no-salt-added frozen peas, thawed

Coat the inside of a 4- to 5-quart (4- to 5-L) slow cooker with cooking spray. In a nonstick skillet, heat the oil over medium-high heat. Add the chicken and brown lightly on all sides, about 4 to 5 minutes per side. Transfer the chicken to the slow cooker. Reduce the heat to medium, add the onion to the skillet, and cook, stirring, until softened, 5 minutes. Add the garlic and pepper and cook, stirring, for 1 minute. Add the rice and stir until the grains are well coated with the mixture. Stir in the tomatoes, chicken broth, and wine. Transfer to the slow cooker and stir to combine with the chicken. Cover and cook on low for 6 to 8 hours, until the chicken is tender and the juices run clear when pricked with a fork. Stir in the green pepper and peas, cover, increase the heat to high, and cook for 20 minutes, until the vegetables are heated through.

Yield: 6 servings

Per serving: 598 calories (41% from fat, 25% from protein, 34% from carbohydrate); 36 g protein; 26 g total fat; 7 g saturated fat; 11 g monounsaturated fat; 5 g polyunsaturated fat; 49 g carbohydrate; 4 g fiber; 5 g sugar; 121 mg phosphorus; 74 mg calcium; 160 mg sodium; 702 mg potassium; 1944 IU vitamin A; 0 mg ATE vitamin E; 35 mg vitamin C; 141 mg cholesterol

Slow Cooker Moroccan Chicken Stew

Dried apricots and cinnamon add a hard-to-define sweetness to this easy-to-prepare stew. The flavors are typical of North African cooking. Serve the traditional way over couscous.

6 boneless chicken thighs, skin removed

1 cup (160 g) chopped onion

1 cup (130 g) sliced carrots

¾ cup (180 ml) apple juice

½ teaspoon minced garlic

½ teaspoon ground cinnamon

½ teaspoon freshly ground black pepper

1 cup (130 g) chopped dried apricots

Coat the inside of a 4- to 5-quart (4- to 5-L) slow cooker with cooking spray. Place the chicken, onion, and carrots in the slow cooker. In a small bowl, combine the apple juice, garlic, cinnamon, and pepper; pour over the chicken and vegetables. Cover and cook on low for 6 to 8 hours, or until the chicken is tender and the juices run clear when pricked with a fork. Remove the chicken from the slow cooker and shred the meat with two forks. Skim the fat from the cooking juices and stir in the apricots. Return the shredded chicken to the slow cooker and heat though.

Yield: 6 servings

Per serving: 103 calories (15% from fat, 34% from protein, 51% from carbohydrate); 9 g protein; 2 g total fat; 0 g saturated fat; 1 g

(continued on page 250)

monounsaturated fat; 0 g polyunsaturated fat; 13 g carbohydrate; 2 g fiber; 10 g sugar; 94 mg phosphorus; 26 mg calcium; 55 mg sodium; 309 mg potassium; 3291 IU vitamin A; 8 mg ATE vitamin E; 6 mg vitamin C; 34 mg cholesterol

South Pacific Chicken

It doesn't get much better than this tender, sweet chicken. The taste and ingredients are typical sweet and sour chicken. However, the fat is less than 10% and the sodium is only about 20% of that found in a typical carryout sweet and sour.

8 boneless skinless chicken breasts

2 cups (500 g) Barbecue Sauce (page 30)

20 ounces (560 g) pineapple chunks, undrained

1 cup (150 g) chopped green bell pepper

1 cup (160 g) chopped onion

½ teaspoon minced garlic

Coat the inside of a 5-quart (5-L) slow cooker with cooking spray. Place 4 of the chicken breasts in the slow cooker. Combine the barbecue sauce, pineapple, green pepper, onion, and garlic in a bowl; pour half over the chicken. Top with the remaining 4 chicken breasts and the remaining sauce. Cover and cook on low for 8 to 9 hours, or until the chicken is tender and the juices run clear when pricked with a fork.

Yield: 8 servings

Per serving: 239 calories (4% from fat, 30% from protein, 66% from carbohydrate); 18 g protein; 1 g

total fat; 0 g saturated fat; 0 g monounsaturated fat; 0 g polyunsaturated fat; 39 g carbohydrate; 1 g fiber; 30 g sugar; 151 mg phosphorus; 25 mg calcium; 68 mg sodium; 333 mg potassium; 110 IU vitamin A; 4 mg ATE vitamin E; 23 mg vitamin C; 41 mg cholesterol

Tip: Serve both the chicken and the sauce over rice.

Tex-Mex Chicken Breasts

Zippy chicken cooks while you work. This is great as is with rice or noodles, but it can also be shredded for tacos, fajitas, or other Mexican meals.

6 boneless skinless chicken breasts

1 can (14.5 ounces, or 411 g) no-salt-added tomatoes, undrained

1 cup (160 g) chopped onion

1 cup (150 g) chopped green bell pepper

1 teaspoon minced garlic

2 tablespoons (30 ml) lime juice

1 teaspoon hot pepper sauce

¼ teaspoon freshly ground black pepper

1 tablespoon (7.5 g) chili powder

Coat the inside of a 4- to 5-quart (4- to 5-L) slow cooker with cooking spray. Place the chicken in the slow cooker. In a large bowl, combine the tomatoes, onion, green pepper, garlic, lime juice, hot pepper sauce, pepper, and chili powder. Pour over the chicken, cover, and cook on low for 3 to 4 hours, or until the chicken is tender and the juices run clear when pricked with a fork.

Yield: 6 servings

Per serving: 109 calories (9% from fat, 64% from protein, 27% from carbohydrate); 18 g protein; 1 g total fat; 0 g saturated fat; 0 g monounsaturated fat; 0 g polyunsaturated fat; 7 g carbohydrate; 1 g fiber; 4 g sugar; 165 mg phosphorus; 37 mg calcium; 59 mg sodium; 422 mg potassium; 213 IU vitamin A; 4 mg ATE vitamin E; 34 mg vitamin C; 41 mg cholesterol

Tip: Use more or less hot pepper sauce depending on how spicy you like your food.

Turkey Chili

Mild, low-fat chili that's perfect for a family. This recipe, which cooks more quickly than some slow cooker recipes, is great for a weekend, when you can start it in the middle of the day and have it ready for dinner.

1 pound (454 g) ground turkey

1 cup (150 g) finely chopped green bell pepper

1 cup (160 g) finely chopped red onion

½ teaspoon minced garlic

2 cans (14.5 ounces, or 411 g, each) no-salt-added tomatoes, undrained

2 cups (500 g) kidney beans, cooked or canned, drained

2 cups (500 g) black beans, cooked or canned, drained

2 cups (470 ml) Low-Sodium Chicken Broth (page 232)

12 ounces (336 g) frozen corn kernels, thawed

1 can (6 ounces, or 170 g) no-salt-added tomato paste

1 tablespoon (7.5 g) chili powder

½ teaspoon freshly ground black pepper

¼ teaspoon ground cumin

¼ teaspoon garlic powder

Coat the inside of a 4-quart (4-L) slow cooker with cooking spray. In a large nonstick skillet, cook the turkey, green pepper, and onion over medium heat until the meat is no longer pink. Add the garlic; cook 1 minute longer. Drain. Transfer to the slow cooker. Stir in the tomatoes, kidney beans, black beans, broth, corn, tomato paste, chili powder, pepper, cumin, and garlic powder. Cover and cook on low for 4 to 5 hours, or until cooked through.

Yield: 6 servings

Per serving: 362 calories (8% from fat, 36% from protein, 56% from carbohydrate); 35 g protein; 3 g total fat; 1 g saturated fat; 1 g monounsaturated fat; 1 g polyunsaturated fat; 53 g carbohydrate; 16 g fiber; 10 g sugar; 451 mg phosphorus; 131 mg calcium; 138 mg sodium; 1587 mg potassium; 1190 IU vitamin A; 0 mg ATE vitamin E; 52 mg vitamin C; 46 mg cholesterol

Turkey Stew

This stew would be a great use for leftover Thanksgiving turkey or one of the turkey breast recipes in this chapter or on page 229.

(continued on page 252)

It contains a generous portion of vegetables to make it a meal in a bowl.

¼ cup (112 g) unsalted butter

1 cup (130 g) 1-inch (2.5-cm) chunks carrot

½ cup (50 g) 1-inch (2.5-cm) chunks celery

1 cup (160 g) chopped onion

4 cups (940 ml) Low-Sodium Chicken Broth (page 232)

3 cups (705 ml) water

¼ teaspoon freshly ground black pepper

3 cups (420 g) cubed cooked turkey

20 ounces (560 g) frozen green beans, thawed

2 teaspoons Worcestershire sauce

Coat the inside of a 4- to 5-quart (4- to 5-L) slow cooker with cooking spray. In a Dutch oven, melt the butter and sauté the carrot, celery, and onion until softened, about 5 minutes. Transfer to the slow cooker. Add the broth, water, pepper, turkey, green beans, and Worcestershire sauce, stirring to combine. Cover and cook on low for 2½ to 3 hours, until cooked through.

Yield: 8 servings

Per serving: 188 calories (37% from fat, 41% from protein, 22% from carbohydrate); 20 g protein; 8 g total fat; 4 g saturated fat; 2 g monounsaturated fat; 1 g polyunsaturated fat; 11 g carbohydrate; 3 g fiber; 3 g sugar; 187 mg phosphorus; 58 mg calcium; 108 mg sodium; 501 mg potassium; 2631 IU vitamin A; 48 mg ATE vitamin E; 16 mg vitamin C; 67 mg cholesterol

17

Fix-It-in-15 Beef Dishes

Like the poultry recipes in the previous chapter, this chapter contains mostly recipes that cook all day in the slow cooker. For beef this has multiple benefits. Not only does it get you away from the kitchen, but it also allows you to use cheaper cuts of beef like round roast and get falling-apart-tender results. And the slow cooking tends to make the meat more flavorful than marinating would. I also include a couple of meatball recipes that can be used as is or frozen and used as great meal starters in the future.

Traditional Pot Roast

Tender and flavorful, this is sure to become a family favorite. The use of make-ahead dressing mixtures saves time and adds an Italian flavor enhanced further by the herbs in the ranch dressing,

2 tablespoons (30 ml) olive oil

3 pounds (1362 g) beef chuck roast

1½ tablespoons (12 g) Italian Dressing Mix (page 35)

2 tablespoons (16 g) Ranch Dressing Mix (page 34)

2 cups (470 ml) Low-Sodium Beef Broth (page 231)

1 large onion, diced

Coat the inside of a 4- to 5-quart (4- to 5-L) slow cooker with cooking spray. Heat oil in a large skillet over medium-high heat, add the roast, and brown on all sides, about 5 minutes per side. Place the roast in the slow cooker. In a small cup or bowl, mix together the Italian dressing mix, ranch dressing mix, and broth. Pour over the roast. Add the chopped onion. Cover and cook on low for 8 to 10 hours, or until the meat is tender.

Yield: 9 servings

Per serving: 350 calories (39% from fat, 60% from protein, 2% from carbohydrate); 50 g protein; 15 g total fat; 5 g saturated fat; 6 g monounsaturated fat; 2 g polyunsaturated fat; 1 g carbohydrate; 0 g fiber; 1 g sugar; 409 mg phosphorus; 17 mg calcium; 100 mg sodium; 456 mg potassium; 0 IU vitamin A; 0 mg ATE vitamin E; 1 mg vitamin C; 153 mg cholesterol

Roast Beef with Gravy

Use your make-ahead items and your slow cooker to produce a great comfort food meal with almost no time spent. The mushroom and onion soups not only flavor the meat but also produce a gravy that can be served over noodles or mashed potatoes.

3 pounds (1362 g) beef round roast

3 cups (705 ml) Condensed Cream of Mushroom Soup (page 31)

⅓ cup (80 ml) Low-Sodium Beef Broth (page 231)

2 tablespoons (16 g) Onion Soup Mix (page 34)

Coat the inside of a 4- to 5-quart (4- to 5-L) slow cooker with cooking spray. Cut the roast in half; place in the slow cooker. In a large bowl, combine the soup, broth, and soup mix; pour over the roast. Cover and cook on low for 8 to 10 hours, or until the meat is tender.

Yield: 9 servings

Per serving: 219 calories (28% from fat, 68% from protein, 4% from carbohydrate); 36 g protein; 7 g total fat; 2 g saturated fat; 3 g monounsaturated fat; 0 g polyunsaturated fat; 2 g carbohydrate; 0 g fiber; 0 g sugar; 342 mg phosphorus; 35 mg calcium; 116 mg sodium; 609 mg potassium; 0 IU vitamin A; 0 mg ATE vitamin E; 2 mg vitamin C; 78 mg cholesterol

Southwestern Pot Roast with Beans

Great flavor abounds in this pot roast, thanks to the tomatoes, chiles, onion, and spices. It can be served with mashed potatoes or as part of a Mexican meal but is hearty enough to be a meal in itself.

2 cans (14.5 ounces, or 411 g each) no-salt-added tomatoes

4 ounces (112 g) chopped green chiles

1 onion, cut into 8 wedges

1 tablespoon (7.5 g) chili powder

2 tablespoons (30 ml) olive oil

3 pounds (1362 g) beef round roast, trimmed of fat

4 cups (1024 g) pinto beans, drained, divided

Coat the inside of a 4- to 5-quart (4- to 5-L) slow cooker with cooking spray. Combine the tomatoes, chiles, onion, and chili powder in a medium bowl. Heat the oil in a large Dutch oven over medium-high heat, add the roast, and brown for 2 to 3 minutes on each side, or until browned all over. Transfer to the slow cooker. Pour the tomato mixture over the roast. Cover and cook on low for 8 to 10 hours, or until the meat shreds easily with a fork. Remove the roast from the slow cooker and cut into large chunks, removing any large pieces of fat; keep warm. Mash 2 cups (512 g) of the pinto beans; add to the slow cooker, and stir to combine with the tomato sauce. Stir in the remaining 2 cups (512 g) beans. Add the roast pieces back to the slow cooker; cover and cook on high for 20 to 25 minutes, until the beans are heated through.

Yield: 10 servings

Per serving: 527 calories (46% from fat, 36% from protein, 18% from carbohydrate); 48 g protein; 27 g total fat; 9 g saturated fat; 12 g monounsaturated fat; 1 g polyunsaturated fat; 22 g carbohydrate; 7 g fiber; 3 g sugar; 440 mg phosphorus; 76 mg calcium; 153 mg sodium; 786 mg potassium; 356 IU vitamin A; 0 mg ATE vitamin E; 18 mg vitamin C; 136 mg cholesterol

Italian Pot Roast

You can make this ahead of time and freeze in meal-size portions to add to pasta sauce and other Italian dishes. But when you walk in the door and smell it you'll have to eat some that night. It also makes great sandwiches.

8 ounces (225 g) mushrooms, sliced

1 cup (160 g) sliced onion

3 pounds (1362 g) beef round roast, trimmed of fat

1 teaspoon freshly ground black pepper

2 tablespoons (30 ml) olive oil

2 tablespoons (16 g) Onion Soup Mix (page 34)

2 cups (470 ml) Low-Sodium Beef Broth (page 231)

1 can (8 ounces, or 225 g) no-salt-added tomato sauce

(continued on page 256)

3 tablespoons (48 g) no-salt-added tomato paste

1 teaspoon Italian seasoning

2 tablespoons (16 g) cornstarch

Coat the inside of a 5- to 6-quart (5- to 6-L) slow cooker with cooking spray. Place the mushrooms and onion in the slow cooker. Sprinkle the roast with the pepper. Heat the oil in a large skillet over medium-high heat, add the roast, and brown for 2 to 3 minutes on each side, or until browned all over. Place the roast on top of the mushrooms and onion in the slow cooker. Sprinkle the onion soup mix over the roast, then pour the beef broth and tomato sauce over. Cover and cook on low for 8 to 10 hours, or until the meat shreds easily with a fork. Transfer the roast to a cutting board; cut into large chunks, removing any large pieces of fat. Keep the roast warm. Skim the fat from the juices in the slow cooker, and then stir in the tomato paste, Italian seasoning, and cornstarch. Increase the heat to high and stir in the roast pieces. Cover and cook for 20 minutes, or until thickened.

Yield: 9 servings

Per serving: 448 calories (55% from fat, 39% from protein, 6% from carbohydrate); 47 g protein; 29 g total fat; 11 g saturated fat; 13 g monounsaturated fat; 1 g polyunsaturated fat; 7 g carbohydrate; 1 g fiber; 3 g sugar; 408 mg phosphorus; 30 mg calcium; 135 mg sodium; 683 mg potassium; 190 IU vitamin A; 0 mg ATE vitamin E; 7 mg vitamin C; 151 mg cholesterol

Basic Beef Meatballs

Like the turkey meatballs from the last chapter, these meatballs can be used for a number of different recipes. They are a fairly traditional meatball, with both cracker crumbs and oatmeal to hold them together and simple flavoring from onions and garlic, so they go well with just about anything from tomato sauce to stroganoff.

3 pounds (1362 g) extra-lean ground beef

5 ounces (140 g) nonfat evaporated milk

1 cup (80 g) rolled or quick-cooking oats

1 cup (80 g) cracker crumbs

½ cup (125 g) egg substitute, or 2 eggs, beaten

½ cup (80 g) chopped onion

½ teaspoon garlic powder

½ teaspoon freshly ground black pepper

Preheat the oven to 325°F (170°C, or gas mark 3). Grease 2 or 3 cookie sheets or line with parchment paper. Combine all the ingredients in a large bowl. Shape into 72 walnut-size balls. Place on the cookie sheets. Bake for 30 minutes, or until no longer pink in the middle. Let cool, and then place in a plastic bag and store in the freezer until needed. They will keep indefinitely, but the flavor will be best if used within 4 months.

Yield: 12 servings, 6 meatballs per serving

Per serving: 249 calories (58% from fat, 31% from protein, 11% from carbohydrate); 25 g protein; 20 g total fat; 8 g saturated fat; 9 g

monounsaturated fat; 1 g polyunsaturated fat; 9 g carbohydrate; 1 g fiber; 2 g sugar; 213 mg phosphorus; 66 mg calcium; 107 mg sodium; 425 mg potassium; 85 IU vitamin A; 14 mg ATE vitamin E; 1 mg vitamin C; 79 mg cholesterol

Mama's Italian Meatballs

I discovered this recipe years ago. I was looking for a recipe to take to some get-together, and it has served that purpose many times over the years. The meatballs are good by themselves with an Italian flavor from the seasoning and Parmesan cheese that goes well in any tomato sauce. But are even better if allowed to simmer in this sauce in a slow cooker for a few hours. It has a kind of sweet and sour flavor that makes them prefect for appetizers as well as in a meal over rice or pasta. Don't be afraid of the amount of onion in the sauce. It may not have been the inspiration for our old family phrase "you can never have too many onions," but it certainly exemplifies that.

1½ pounds (680 g) extra-lean ground beef

¾ cup (188 g) egg substitute, or 3 eggs, beaten

¼ cup (25 g) grated Parmesan cheese

½ teaspoon garlic powder

1 tablespoon (2 g) chopped fresh parsley

1½ teaspoons dried oregano

4 slices Low-Sodium Bread (pages 312 to 324), crumbled

3 onions, chopped

1 can (6 ounces, or 170 g) no-salt-added tomato paste

1½ cups (355 ml) water

½ cup (120 ml) red wine vinegar

3 tablespoons (45 g) packed brown sugar

Preheat the oven to 375°F (190°C, or gas mark 5). Grease 1 or 2 cookie sheets or line with parchment paper. Combine the beef, eggs, cheese, seasonings, and bread in a large bowl. Form into 36 balls, 1-inch, or 2.5-cm, and place on the cookie sheets. Bake for 30 to 40 minutes, turning once. Scoop up a few tablespoons (15 ml) of the meat drippings and pour into a skillet. Add the onions and sauté for 3 to 4 minutes, until softened. Coat the inside of a slow cooker with cooking spray. Combine the sautéed onions, tomato paste, water, vinegar, and brown sugar in the slow cooker. Add the meatballs, stir to coat with the sauce, and cook on low for 5 hours, until 142.

Yield: 6 servings, 6 meatballs per serving

Per serving: 359 calories (47% from fat, 28% from protein, 26% from carbohydrate); 30 g protein; 22 g total fat; 9 g saturated fat; 9 g monounsaturated fat; 2 g polyunsaturated fat; 28 g carbohydrate; 3 g fiber; 15 g sugar; 298 mg phosphorus; 125 mg calcium; 234 mg sodium; 894 mg potassium; 635 IU vitamin A; 5 mg ATE vitamin E; 11 mg vitamin C; 83 mg cholesterol

Tip: Baking the meatballs is much easier than frying them, and they don't fall apart from the handling.

Multi-Cultural Meatball Stew

This stew is a complete meal in a bowl. Using previously frozen meatballs makes preparation a snap. The herbs used are typical of Mediterranean cooking, but the vegetables are more the traditional American stew mixture.

6 medium red potatoes, cubed

1 cup (160 g) sliced onion

1½ cups (195 g) sliced carrots

2 pounds (908 g) Meatballs (page 256 or 257)

1 cup (240 g) no-salt-added ketchup

1 cup (235 ml) water

2 tablespoons (30 ml) vinegar

1 teaspoon dried basil

1 teaspoon dried oregano

¼ teaspoon freshly ground black pepper

Coat the inside of a 4- to 5-quart (4- to 5-L) slow cooker with cooking spray. Place the potatoes, onion, and carrots in the slow cooker, then place the meatballs on top. Combine the ketchup, water, vinegar, basil, oregano, and pepper in a bowl. Pour over the meatballs, cover, and cook on high for 4 to 5 hours, or until the vegetables are tender.

Yield: 8 servings

Per serving: 485 calories (29% from fat, 20% from protein, 51% from carbohydrate); 25 g protein; 16 g total fat; 6 g saturated fat; 7 g monounsaturated fat; 1 g polyunsaturated fat; 63 g carbohydrate; 7 g fiber; 13 g sugar; 355 mg phosphorus; 96 mg calcium; 5 mg Iron; 122 mg sodium; 1807 mg potassium; 4418 IU vitamin A; 11 mg ATE vitamin E; 31 mg vitamin C; 60 mg cholesterol

Ready When You Are Mexican Steak

This is kind of like Swiss steak, but with a real Mexican flavor. It is good with rice or tucked into tortillas.

2 pounds (908 g) flank steak

¼ teaspoon garlic powder

2 cups (520 g) Low-Sodium Salsa (page 232)

1 can (8 ounces, or 225 g) no-salt-added tomato sauce

Dash of hot pepper sauce

Coat the inside of a 3- to 4-quart (3- to 4-L) slow cooker with cooking spray. Pound the meat on both sides with a meat mallet, and then sprinkle with the garlic powder. Place in the slow cooker. Combine the salsa, tomato sauce, and hot pepper sauce in a small bowl. Pour over the meat; cover and cook on low for 8 to 10 hours, until meat is very tender.

Yield: 6 servings

Per serving: 328 calories (36% from fat, 55% from protein, 9% from carbohydrate); 43 g protein; 13 g total fat; 5 g saturated fat; 5 g monounsaturated fat; 1 g polyunsaturated fat; 7 g carbohydrate; 2 g fiber; 5 g sugar; 350 mg phosphorus; 49 mg calcium; 159 mg sodium; 804 mg potassium; 606 IU vitamin A; 0 mg ATE vitamin E; 15 mg vitamin C; 83 mg cholesterol

Old-Time Flavor Braised Short Ribs

Okay, this may not be the healthiest recipe in the book. The sodium is low, but short ribs do tend to contain a lot of fat calories. But they do taste good. Just don't have them four days a week. The flavorings in this recipe are fairly traditional, headed by onions, but the allspice gives it that little hard-to-identify subplot.

1 cup (120 g) all-purpose flour

½ teaspoon freshly ground black pepper

3 pounds (1362 g) beef short ribs, cut up

2 tablespoons (30 ml) olive oil

1½ cups (240 g) sliced onion

1 bay leaf

½ teaspoon whole allspice

1 cup (235 ml) Low-Sodium Beef Broth (page 231)

Coat the inside of a 4- to 5-quart (4- to 5-L) slow cooker with cooking spray. Combine the flour and pepper on a plate; then, dredge the beef ribs in the mixture. Heat the oil in skillet over medium-high heat, add the meat, and brown well on all sides, 2 to 3 minutes perside. Place in the slow cooker, add the onion, bay leaf, allspice, and broth, cover, and cook on low for 8 to 10 hours or on high for 4 to 6 hours, until meat is very tender. Before serving, remove the bay leaf and allspice.

Yield: 6 servings

Per serving: 528 calories (49% from fat, 36% from protein, 16% from carbohydrate); 46 g protein; 28 g total fat; 11 g saturated fat; 13 g monounsaturated fat; 1 g polyunsaturated fat; 20 g carbohydrate; 1 g fiber; 2 g sugar; 470 mg phosphorus; 34 mg calcium; 173 mg sodium; 913 mg potassium; 10 IU vitamin A; 0 mg ATE vitamin E; 3 mg vitamin C; 134 mg cholesterol

Tip: Since short ribs tend to be rather fatty, skim off the excess fat after cooking or refrigerate overnight and then do so.

Long and Slow Beer-Braised Short Ribs

These ribs are about the most tender and full flavored that you'll find. The simple seasonings enhance, rather than hide, the flavor of the meat. The beer helps to break down the meat so it is extremely tender. They are great served with mashed potatoes or noodles.

3 pounds (1.4 kg) beef short ribs, cut up

2 tablespoons (30 g) packed brown sugar

1 teaspoon minced garlic

¼ cup (30 g) all-purpose flour

1 cup (160 g) chopped onion

1 cup (235 ml) Low-Sodium Beef Broth (page 231)

12 ounces (355 ml) beer, ale or dark beer preferred

Coat the inside of a 4- to 5-quart (4- to 5-L) slow cooker with cooking spray. Place the beef in the slow cooker. Add the brown sugar, garlic, and flour and toss to coat. Place the onion on top. Stir the broth and beer together

(continued on page 260)

in a small bowl, and then pour over the beef. Cover and cook on low for 8 to 9 hours, or until the beef is fork-tender.

Yield: 6 servings

Per serving: 440 calories (47% from fat, 41% from protein, 12% from carbohydrate);44 g protein; 23 g total fat; 10 g saturated fat; 10 g monounsaturated fat; 1 g polyunsaturated fat; 11 g carbohydrate; 1 g fiber; 6 g sugar; 451 mg phosphorus; 32 mg calcium; 174 mg sodium; 693 mg potassium; 1 IU vitamin A; 0 mg ATE vitamin E; 2 mg vitamin C; 134 mg cholesterol

Come Home from the Fields Shepherd's Pie

This is a shepherd's pie in the slow cooker. The flavor and ingredients are traditional, but the use of the slow cooker to make it easy to fix is new.

1 pound (454 g) extra-lean ground beef

1 cup (160 g) chopped onion

1 can (8 ounces, or 225 g) no-salt added tomato sauce

12 ounces (340 g) frozen corn kernels, thawed

1½ cups (140 g) potato flakes

1½ cups (345 g) sour cream

⅓ cup (80 ml) water

1½ cups (165 g) grated Swiss cheese

Coat the inside of a 3- to 4-quart (3- to 4-L) slow cooker with cooking spray. Add the beef and onion to a skillet and brown over medium heat until no longer pink, about 5 minutes.

Drain well. Place in the slow cooker, add the tomato sauce, and corn, and mix well. In a bowl, combine the potato flakes, sour cream, and water. Spread the mixture over the beef and top with the grated cheese. Cover and cook on low for 7 to 10 hours.

Yield: 4 servings

Per serving: 649 calories (55% from fat, 23% from protein, 22% from carbohydrate); 42 g protein; 44 g total fat; 23 g saturated fat; 15 g monounsaturated fat; 2 g polyunsaturated fat; 41 g carbohydrate; 4 g fiber; 6 g sugar; 633 mg phosphorus; 595 mg calcium; 144 mg sodium; 872 mg potassium; 748 IU vitamin A; 195 mg ATE vitamin E; 21 mg vitamin C; 159 mg cholesterol

Not Your Usual Beef and Beans

Here's an updated version of beef and beans. The addition of corn and Swiss cheese adds new flavor elements that the cowboy cooks never knew about. Use either no-salt-added canned beans or precooked dried beans.

1 pound (454 g) extra-lean ground beef

12 ounces (420 g) frozen corn kernels, thawed

2 cups (512 g) no-salt-added kidney beans

1 can (8 ounces, or 225 g) no-salt-added tomato sauce

1 cup (110 g) shredded Swiss cheese

¼ cup (60 ml) skim milk

1 teaspoon onion flakes

½ teaspoon chili powder

Coat the inside of a 3- to 4-quart (3- to 4-L) slow cooker with cooking spray. Add the beef to a skillet and brown over medium heat until no longer pink, about 5 minutes. Drain well. Place in the slow cooker, add the corn, beans, tomato sauce, cheese, milk, onion flakes, and chili powder, cover, and cook on low for 3 to 4 hours.

Yield: 5 servings
(With the addition of the beans, it has less meat per serving.)

Per serving: 442 calories (43% from fat, 27% from protein, 30% from carbohydrate); 34 g protein; 24 g total fat; 11 g saturated fat; 9 g monounsaturated fat; 1 g polyunsaturated fat; 39 g carbohydrate; 10 g fiber; 6 g sugar; 483 mg phosphorus; 288 mg calcium; 140 mg sodium; 1044 mg potassium; 694 IU vitamin A; 64 mg ATE vitamin E; 14 mg vitamin C; 87 mg cholesterol

Sweet-and-Sour Beef Stew

Beef is not a traditional meat for sweet-and-sour dishes, but this easy slow cooker recipe changed that. The rest of the ingredients are a fairly standard combination of the usual components of both stew and sweet-and-sour. It can be served over rice or just by itself.

¼ cup (30 g) all-purpose flour

⅛ teaspoon freshly ground black pepper

2 pounds (908 g) beef round steak, cut into 1½-inch (3.8-cm) cubes

2 tablespoons (30 ml) olive oil

1½ cups (195 g) ¾-inch (2-cm) pieces carrot

1 cup (160 g) chopped onion

¼ cup (60 g) packed brown sugar

½ cup (120 ml) cider vinegar

1 tablespoon (15 ml) Worcestershire sauce

Coat the inside of a 3- to 4-quart (3- to 4-L) slow cooker with cooking spray. Combine the flour and pepper on a plate; then, dredge the beef in the mixture. Heat the oil in a skillet over medium-high heat and brown the meat well on all sides, about 5 minutes per side. Place the carrots in the bottom of the slow cooker. Add the meat and onion. Combine the sugar, vinegar, and Worcestershire sauce in a bowl, and then add to the slow cooker, stirring to combine. Cover and cook on low for 7 to 8 hours, until meat is tender and vegetables are done.

Yield: 6 servings

Per serving: 317 calories (28% from fat, 46% from protein, 26% from carbohydrate); 36 g protein; 10 g total fat; 2 g saturated fat; 5 g monounsaturated fat; 1 g polyunsaturated fat; 20 g carbohydrate; 1 g fiber; 13 g sugar; 369 mg phosphorus; 60 mg calcium; 148 mg sodium; 782 mg potassium; 3857 IU vitamin A; 0 mg ATE vitamin E; 8 mg vitamin C; 70 mg cholesterol

Down Home Beef Barley Soup

This has been a family favorite for quite a while. I've made it on the stove also, but the slow cooker recipe is even more convenient.

(continued on page 262)

And the depth of flavor achieved by the long slow cooking enhances the overall impression.

1 pound (454 g) extra-lean ground beef

1 large onion, chopped

8 ounces (225 g) mushrooms, chopped

2 cups (470 ml) Low-Sodium Chicken Broth (page 232)

4 cups (940 ml) Low-Sodium Beef Broth (page 231)

1 cup (184 g) barley

½ teaspoon garlic powder

2 teaspoons Worcestershire sauce

½ teaspoon dried thyme

1 cup (110 g) shredded carrot

½ teaspoon freshly ground black pepper

Coat the inside of a 3- to 4-quart (3- to 4-L) slow cooker with cooking spray. Add the ground beef and onion to a large skillet and brown over medium heat until no longer pink, about 5 minutes. When the beef is almost done, add the mushrooms and cook a few minutes more, until they begin to release their water. Transfer to the slow cooker, add the broths, barley, garlic powder, Worcestershire sauce, thyme, carrot, and pepper, cover, and cook on low for 6 to 8 hours, until meat is tender and barley is done.

Yield: 6 servings

Per serving: 291 calories (36% from fat, 26% from protein, 38% from carbohydrate); 22 g protein; 14 g total fat; 5 g saturated fat; 6 g monounsaturated fat; 1 g polyunsaturated fat; 32 g carbohydrate; 7 g fiber; 3 g sugar; 264 mg

phosphorus; 46 mg calcium; 225 mg sodium; 697 mg potassium; 2581 IU vitamin A; 0 mg ATE vitamin E; 7 mg vitamin C; 52 mg cholesterol

Tex-Mex Chili

This makes a moderately spicy chili, great with cornbread or just by itself. The flavors are traditional Tex-Mex, developed over the long cooking period with a number of herbs and spices playing into the final product.

1 tablespoon (15 ml) olive oil

3 pounds (1.4 kg) beef round steak, cut into ½ inch (1.3 cm) cubes

1 teaspoon minced garlic

6 cups (1.5 kg) kidney beans, cooked or canned, drained

3 cans (8 ounces, or 225 g, each) no-salt-added tomato sauce

1 can (14.5 ounces, or 411 g) no-salt-added tomatoes, undrained

1 can (6 ounces, or 170 g) no-salt-added tomato paste

1 cup (235 ml) water

¾ cup (195 g) Low-Sodium Salsa (page 232)

2 tablespoons (16 g) Salt-Free Taco Seasoning (page 28)

2 teaspoons minced onion

1 teaspoon chili powder

½ teaspoon ground cumin

½ teaspoon cayenne pepper

¾ cup shredded Cheddar cheese

¼ cup (4 g) chopped fresh cilantro

Coat the inside of a 6-quart (6-L) slow cooker with cooking spray. Heat the oil in a large skillet over medium-high heat, add the beef in batches, and brown on all sides, about 5 minutes. Add the garlic to the pan; cook and stir for 1 minute longer. Transfer to the slow cooker. Stir in the beans, tomato sauce, tomatoes, tomato paste, water, salsa, taco seasoning, onion, chili powder, cumin, and cayenne. Cover and cook on low for 6 to 8 hours, or until the meat is tender. Garnish each serving with some of the cheese and cilantro.

Yield: 12 servings

Per serving: 349 calories (21% from fat, 34% from protein,45% from carbohydrate); 39 g protein; 8 g total fat; 3 g saturated fat; 3 g monounsaturated fat; 1 g polyunsaturated fat; 31 g carbohydrate; 11 g fiber; 6 g sugar; 465 mg phosphorus; 176 mg calcium; 175 mg sodium; 1331 mg potassium; 874 IU vitamin A; 21 mg ATE vitamin E; 20 mg vitamin C; 61 mg cholesterol

Tip: If you prefer milder food, reduce or leave out the cayenne.

18

Fix-It-in-15 Pork Dishes

Same story here as with the beef, with pork being another meat that can be prepared using long, slow cooking to produce tender and flavorful results. There are a couple of roasts that make great leftovers. If you use the method I spoke about on page 121 and buy whole pork loins, you can cut part of it into roasts of the desired size. I usually aim for something that just fits inside my slow cooker. For those of you thinking that quick preparation means no ribs, I have a couple of recipes here to prove that idea wrong also.

Classic Pork Roast

I like to make this pork roast on the weekend so we have the leftovers (or sometimes we keep the whole thing) to use for other recipes during the week. Of course I also have to eat a little while it's hot and juicy. It works well leftover for everything from Asian dishes to barbecued pork sandwiches.

3 pounds (1.4 kg) boneless pork loin roast

1 teaspoon sliced garlic

⅔ cup (160 ml) Low-Sodium Chicken Broth (page 232)

⅔ cup (160 ml) lemon juice

¼ cup (60 ml) olive oil

1½ cups (240 g) chopped onion

2 bay leaves

1 tablespoon (2 g) minced fresh thyme

½ teaspoon freshly ground black pepper

Cut tiny slits in the roast and insert the garlic slices. Place the roast in a large resealable plastic bag or shallow glass bowl. Combine the broth, lemon juice, oil, onion, bay leaves, thyme, and pepper in a bowl; pour over the roast and turn to coat. Seal the bag or cover the dish and refrigerate overnight, turning occasionally.

When ready to cook, preheat the oven to 350°F (180°C, or gas mark 4). Remove the roast from the marinade and place it, fat side up, in a shallow roasting pan; pour the marinade over. Bake, uncovered, for 2 to 2½ hours, or until a meat thermometer registers 160 to 170°F (71 to 77°C) when inserted into the thickest part. Let rest for 10 minutes before carving.

Yield: 10 servings

Per serving: 240 calories (43% from fat, 50% from protein, 7% from carbohydrate); 29 g protein; 11 g total fat; 3 g saturated fat; 7 g monounsaturated fat; 1 g polyunsaturated fat; 4 g carbohydrate; 1 g fiber; 1 g sugar; 310 mg phosphorus; 31 mg calcium; 76 mg sodium; 577 mg potassium; 25 IU vitamin A; 3 mg ATE vitamin E; 11 mg vitamin C; 86 mg cholesterol

Cranberry Pork Roast

A real company kind of meal, this roast is made in the slow cooker with almost no preparation time. In addition to the cranberry flavor, mustard and cloves contribute to the overall goodness. This goes well with potatoes. If I'm home on a weekend cooking it I'll roast some in the oven. If it's a weeknight it's more likely to be mashed.

3 pounds (1362 g) boneless pork loin roast

14 ounces (392 g) jellied cranberry sauce

½ cup (100 g) sugar

½ cup (120 ml) cranberry juice

1 teaspoon dry mustard powder

¼ teaspoon ground cloves

Coat the inside of a 5-quart (5-L) slow cooker with cooking spray. Place the pork roast in the cooker. In a small bowl, mash the cranberry sauce; stir in the sugar, cranberry juice, mustard, and cloves. Pour over the roast.

(continued on page 266)

Cover and cook on low for 6 to 8 hours, or until the meat is tender.

Yield: 10 servings

Per serving: 313 calories (26% from fat, 39% from protein, 35% from carbohydrate); 30 g protein; 9 g total fat; 3 g saturated fat; 4 g monounsaturated fat; 1 g polyunsaturated fat; 27 g carbohydrate; 0 g fiber; 24 g sugar; 284 mg phosphorus; 10 mg calcium; 73 mg sodium; 587 mg potassium; 28 IU vitamin A; 3 mg ATE vitamin E; 2 mg vitamin C; 75 mg cholesterol

Tip: The juices can be thickened with cornstarch and used as a sauce.

Southwestern Pork Roast

The chili powder gives this a Southwestern flavor, but the other herbs, such as the rosemary, add some different highlights. Serve this with the Instant Mexican Rice on page 210. The leftovers make great tacos or fajitas.

1 tablespoon (15 ml) olive oil

5 teaspoons (12.5 g) chili powder

½ teaspoon ground cloves

1 teaspoon oregano

¾ teaspoon ground cumin

½ teaspoon crushed rosemary

3 pounds (1362 g) boneless pork loin roast

Combine the oil and the spices in a small bowl. Place the pork roast, fat side up, in a shallow baking dish and rub the spice mixture over the roast. Cover and refrigerate overnight.

When ready to cook, preheat the oven to 350°F (180°C, or gas mark 4). Bake the roast, uncovered, for 1¼ to 1½ hours, or until meat thermometer registers 160°F (71°C) when inserted into the thickest part. Let rest for 10 minutes before carving.

Yield: 10 servings

Per serving: 224 calories (43% from fat, 55% from protein, 2% from carbohydrate); 30 g protein; 10 g total fat; 3 g saturated fat; 5 g monounsaturated fat; 1 g polyunsaturated fat; 1 g carbohydrate; 1 g fiber; 0 g sugar; 287 mg phosphorus; 14 mg calcium; 74 mg sodium; 603 mg potassium; 390 IU vitamin A; 3 mg ATE vitamin E; 1 mg vitamin C; 75 mg cholesterol

Hawaiian Pork Roast

Pork loin roast cooks to tender perfection with island flavors, highlighted especially with pineapple and ginger. This is good served with rice and steamed vegetables.

1½ pounds (680 g) pork loin roast

1 cup (235 ml) pineapple juice

¼ cup (60 ml) sherry

2 tablespoons (30 ml) Low-Sodium Soy Sauce (page 29)

1 teaspoon ground ginger

1 tablespoon (12 g) sugar

Coat the inside of a 4-quart (4-L) slow cooker with cooking spray. Place the pork in the slow cooker. Combine the juice, sherry, soy sauce, ginger, and sugar in a small bowl and pour over the pork. Cover and cook on low for 4 to 5 hours, until a meat thermometer registers 160 to 170°F (71 to 77°C) when inserted into the thickest part.

Yield: 4 servings

Per serving: 294 calories (24% from fat, 54% from protein, 22% from carbohydrate); 37 g protein; 7 g total fat; 2 g saturated fat; 3 g monounsaturated fat; 1 g polyunsaturated fat; 15 g carbohydrate; 0 g fiber; 13 g sugar; 387 mg phosphorus; 36 mg calcium; 109 mg sodium; 747 mg potassium; 16 IU vitamin A; 3 mg ATE vitamin E; 8 mg vitamin C; 107 mg cholesterol

Multi-Purpose Mexican Pork with Beans

This Mexican pork and bean mixture is very versatile. Serve it spooned over cornbread or rolled up burrito style in tortillas. It can be used in nachos, quesadillas, or tacos, too. It can even be used as a meaty addition to Mexican egg dishes for breakfast.

1 pound (454 g) dried pinto beans

3½ pounds (1590 g) pork loin roast

4 ounces (112 g) chopped green chiles

½ teaspoon chopped garlic

1 tablespoon (7.5 g) chili powder

1 teaspoon dried oregano

1 teaspoon ground cumin

4 cups (940 ml) Low-Sodium Chicken Broth (page 232)

1 can (14.5 ounces, or 411 g) no-salt-added diced tomatoes

2 tablespoons (30 ml) lime juice

¼ cup (4 g) chopped fresh cilantro

Coat the inside of a 6-quart (6-L) slow cooker with cooking spray. Rinse and sort the beans. Place the beans in the slow cooker; add the roast, chiles, garlic, chili powder, oregano, and cumin and stir to combine. Pour the chicken broth evenly over the top of the roast. Cover and cook on low for 9 hours, until a meat thermometer registers 160 to 170°F (71 to 77°C) when inserted into the thickest part. Remove the fat from the roast and shred into large pieces with two forks. Stir in the diced tomatoes. Cook, uncovered, on high for 1 more hour, or until the liquid is slightly thickened. Stir in the lime juice and cilantro.

Yield: 10 servings

Per serving: 233 calories (30% from fat, 63% from protein, 8% from carbohydrate); 36 g protein; 8 g total fat; 3 g saturated fat; 3 g monounsaturated fat; 1 g polyunsaturated fat; 4 g carbohydrate; 1 g fiber; 1 g sugar; 388 mg phosphorus; 47 mg calcium; 167 mg sodium; 802 mg potassium; 381 IU vitamin A; 3 mg ATE vitamin E; 13 mg vitamin C; 100 mg cholesterol

Almost Traditional Sweet-and-Sour Pork

This is exactly what you'd expect, with the tender pork simmered in the sweet-and-sour sauce along with onions, green pepper and

(continued on page 268)

pineapple. What is not traditional is the preparation. Throw this together in the slow cooker in the morning and you'll have not only a great dinner waiting for you when you get home but also a house that smells marvelous.

1½ pounds (680 g) boneless pork loin, cut into 2-inch (5-cm) strips

1 teaspoon paprika

2 tablespoons (30 ml) olive oil

½ cup (80 g) thinly sliced onion

½ cup (75 g) sliced green bell pepper

3 tablespoons (45 g) packed brown sugar

¼ cup (30 g) instant nonfat dry milk

2 tablespoons (16 g) cornstarch

15 ounces (420 g) pineapple tidbits, drained (reserve the syrup)

⅓ cup (80 ml) vinegar

1 tablespoon (15 ml) Low-Sodium Soy Sauce (page 29)

1 tablespoon (15 ml) Worcestershire sauce

Coat the inside of a 4-quart (4-L) slow cooker with cooking spray. Sprinkle the pork pieces with the paprika. Heat the oil in skillet over medium heat. Add the pork and sauté until browned on all sides, about 5 minutes. Drain well. Place the meat in the slow cooker. Add the onion and pepper. Combine the sugar, dry milk, cornstarch, and pineapple tidbits in a bowl, then add the vinegar, soy sauce, Worcestershire sauce, and ⅔ cup (160 ml) of the pineapple liquid (if the juice does not make this much, add water to make up the difference). Pour the mixture into the slow cooker, cover, and cook on low for 8 to 9

hours or on high for 4 to 5 hours, until meat is tender and vegetables are soft.

Yield: 6 servings

Per serving: 348 calories (49% from fat, 28% from protein, 23% from carbohydrate); 24 g protein; 19 g total fat; 6 g saturated fat; 10 g monounsaturated fat; 2 g polyunsaturated fat; 20 g carbohydrate; 1 g fiber; 15 g sugar; 270 mg phosphorus; 78 mg calcium; 108 mg sodium; 654 mg potassium; 353 IU vitamin A; 22 mg ATE vitamin E; 22 mg vitamin C; 72 mg cholesterol

Cook All Day Pork and Sweet Potatoes

This is one of those meals that you might like to have more often, but it just takes too long to fix when you get home from work. I've transformed it into an easy slow cooker creation. The pork cooks to a delicious tenderness along with the sweet potatoes, flavored by brown sugar and just enough spices to make you take notice.

4 sweet potatoes, peeled and sliced

2 pounds (908 g) pork loin roast

½ cup (120 g) packed brown sugar

¼ teaspoon cayenne pepper

¼ teaspoon freshly ground black pepper

¼ teaspoon garlic powder

½ teaspoon onion powder

Coat the inside of a 4- to 5-quart (4- to 5-L) slow cooker with cooking spray. Place the potatoes in the bottom of the slow cooker, and then place the pork on top. Combine the sugar, cayenne pepper, black pepper, garlic powder, and onion powder in a small bowl and sprinkle over the pork and potatoes. Cover and cook on low for 8 to 10 hours, until a meat thermometer registers 160 to 170°F (71 to 77°C) when inserted into the thickest part. Remove the pork from the slow cooker, let rest for 10 minutes, and slice. Serve the juices over the pork and potatoes.

Yield: 8 servings

Per serving: 256 calories (18% from fat, 40% from protein, 43% from carbohydrate); 25 g protein; 5 g total fat; 2 g saturated fat; 2 g monounsaturated fat; 1 g polyunsaturated fat; 27 g carbohydrate; 2 g fiber; 18 g sugar; 276 mg phosphorus; 48 mg calcium; 84 mg sodium; 645 mg potassium; 11937 IU vitamin A; 2 mg ATE vitamin E; 11 mg vitamin C; 71 mg cholesterol

Super Flavorful Slow Cooker Spareribs

If you want perfectly sauced, falling-off-the-bone spareribs, but don't want the amount of effort that usually goes into them, let the slow cooker do the work for you. Then all you have to do is enjoy. This recipe couldn't be easier, with only 4 ingredients going into the slow cooker along with the ribs, but the flavor is excellent and you won't find more tender meat.

3 pounds (1362 g) pork spareribs, cut into serving-size pieces

2 cans (14.5 ounces, or 411 g each) no-salt-added tomatoes, undrained

2 cups (500 g) Barbecue Sauce (page 30)

¼ cup (60 g) packed brown sugar

¼ cup (60 ml) white wine vinegar

Coat the inside of a 5-quart (5-L) slow cooker. Place the ribs on the bottom of the slow cooker. Combine the tomatoes, barbecue sauce, sugar, and vinegar in a bowl; pour over the ribs. Cover and cook on low for 6 to 7 hours, or until the meat is tender. Serve with the sauce spooned over the top.

Yield: 9 servings

Per serving: 589 calories (55% from fat, 19% from protein, 26% from carbohydrate); 28 g protein; 36 g total fat; 14 g saturated fat; 15 g monounsaturated fat; 3 g polyunsaturated fat; 38 g carbohydrate; 1 g fiber; 30 g sugar; 383 mg phosphorus; 84 mg calcium; 146 mg sodium; 656 mg potassium; 155 IU vitamin A; 5 mg ATE vitamin E; 15 mg vitamin C; 118 mg cholesterol

Asian Ribs

Country-style ribs cook in the slow cooker all day in an Asian sauce, for marvelous flavor and tenderness. They may not be as crispy as the little appetizer ribs served in Asian restaurants, but they are a lot more tender and every bit as flavorful.

¼ cup (60 g) packed brown sugar

1 cup (235 ml) Low-Sodium Soy Sauce (page 29)

(continued on page 270)

¼ cup (60 ml) sesame oil

2 tablespoons (30 ml) olive oil

2 tablespoons (30 ml) rice vinegar

2 tablespoons (30 ml) lime juice

2 tablespoon (10 g) minced garlic

2 tablespoons (12 g) minced fresh ginger

½ teaspoon hot pepper sauce

3 pounds (1362 g) country-style pork ribs

Coat the inside of a 4- to 5-quart (4- to 5-L) slow cooker with cooking spray. Stir together the brown sugar, soy sauce, sesame oil, olive oil, rice vinegar, lime juice, garlic, ginger, and hot pepper sauce. Place the ribs in the slow cooker and pour the sauce over. Cover and cook on low for 8 to 10 hours, until meat is falling off the bones.

Yield: 9 servings

Per serving: 341 calories (58% from fat, 37% from protein, 5% from carbohydrate); 31 g protein; 22 g total fat; 6 g saturated fat; 10 g monounsaturated fat; 4 g polyunsaturated fat; 4 g carbohydrate; 0 g fiber; 1 g sugar; 325 mg phosphorus; 45 mg calcium; 175 mg sodium; 596 mg potassium; 18 IU vitamin A; 3 mg ATE vitamin E; 3 mg vitamin C; 97 mg cholesterol

Barbecued Pork Chops

Trust me on this. I know it's not *normal* to cook potatoes and carrots in barbecue sauce. But just because you've never tried does not mean it isn't good. In this case it's one of those things that you wonder why you didn't think of before. This is a barbecue-flavored meal all in one pot. All you need to do is load it in the slow cooker in the morning and dinner is taken care of.

6 red potatoes, cut into quarters

1½ cups (195 g) 1-inch (2.5-cm) pieces carrot

8 boneless pork loin chops

¼ teaspoon freshly ground black pepper

1½ cups (375 g) Barbecue Sauce (page 30)

1 cup (240 g) no-salt-added ketchup

1 cup (235 ml) cola

2 tablespoons (30 ml) Worcestershire sauce

Coat the inside of a 5-quart (5-L) slow cooker with cooking spray. Place the potatoes and carrots in the bottom of the slow cooker. Top with the pork chops. Sprinkle with the pepper. In a small bowl, combine the barbecue sauce, ketchup, cola, and Worcestershire sauce; pour over the chops. Cover and cook on low for 8 to 9 hours, or until the meat and vegetables are tender.

Yield: 8 servings

Per serving: 480 calories (9% from fat, 23% from protein, 68% from carbohydrate); 28 g protein; 5 g total fat; 2 g saturated fat; 2 g monounsaturated fat; 1 g polyunsaturated fat; 81 g carbohydrate; 6 g fiber; 31 g sugar; 417 mg phosphorus; 56 mg calcium; 144 mg sodium; 1885 mg potassium; 3232 IU vitamin A; 2 mg ATE vitamin E; 68 mg vitamin C; 64 mg cholesterol

Slow Cooker Asian Pork Chops

Tender, slow-cooked chops are paired with an Asian-flavored sauce. The slow cooking allows the flavor to permeate the meat. Serve with rice and stir-fried vegetables and spoon the cooking juices over everything.

6 boneless pork loin chops

¾ cup (120 g) finely chopped onion

⅓ cup (160 g) no-salt-added ketchup

3 tablespoons (45 g) packed brown sugar

3 tablespoons (45 ml) water

3 tablespoons (45 ml) Low-Sodium Soy Sauce (page 29)

½ teaspoon minced garlic

1 teaspoon ground ginger

Coat the inside of a 4- to 5-quart (4- to 5-L) slow cooker with cooking spray. Place the chops in the slow cooker. In a small bowl, combine the onion, ketchup, brown sugar, water, soy sauce, garlic, and ginger. Pour over the chops. Cover and cook on low for 8 to 10 hours, or until the meat is tender.

Yield: 6 servings

Per serving: 183 calories (22% from fat, 49% from protein, 29% from carbohydrate); 22 g protein; 4 g total fat; 1 g saturated fat; 2 g monounsaturated fat; 0 g polyunsaturated fat; 13 g carbohydrate; 1 g fiber; 11 g sugar; 242 mg phosphorus; 28 mg calcium; 78 mg sodium; 510 mg potassium; 147 IU vitamin A; 2 mg ATE vitamin E; 4 mg vitamin C; 64 mg cholesterol

Slow Cooker Barbecued Pork Chops

Feel like some barbecue, but don't want to fire up the grill? These chops are a perfect alternative, cooked with minimum effort in the slow cooker. They will be so tender that you can shred them like you would a smoked pork shoulder and the sauce is already part of the dish.

4 pork loin chops

1 cup (160 g) sliced onion

1 tablespoon (15 ml) packed brown sugar

¼ cup (60 g) no-salt-added ketchup

1 tablespoon (15 ml) lemon juice

¼ cup (60 ml) water

Coat the inside of a 3- to 4-quart (3- to 4-L) slow cooker with cooking spray. Layer the chops and onion in the slow cooker. In a small bowl, combine the brown sugar, ketchup, lemon juice, and water. Pour over the chops. Cook on low for 8 to 10 hours, until meat is tender.

Yield: 4 servings

Per serving: 176 calories (23% from fat, 50% from protein, 27% from carbohydrate); 22 g protein; 4 g total fat; 1 g saturated fat; 2 g monounsaturated fat; 1 g polyunsaturated fat; 12 g carbohydrate; 1 g fiber; 9 g sugar; 238 mg phosphorus; 28 mg calcium; 57 mg sodium; 520 mg potassium; 165 IU vitamin A; 2 mg ATE vitamin E; 7 mg vitamin C; 64 mg cholesterol

Brunswick Stew

Brunswick stew is a traditional dish in the southern United States. There are many versions, often using game such as squirrel or rabbit. This one uses a pork loin roast, holding down the fat and providing great flavor.

3 pounds (1362 g) boneless pork loin roast

2 medium red potatoes, peeled and chopped

1 cup (160 g) chopped onion

10 ounces (280 g) frozen lima beans, thawed

12 ounces (280 g) frozen corn kernels, thawed

2 cans (14.5 ounces, or 411 g each) no-salt-added tomatoes

1 cup (250 g) Barbecue Sauce (page 30)

2 cups (470 ml) Low-Sodium Chicken Broth (page 232)

2 tablespoons (30 g) packed brown sugar

Coat the inside of a 6-quart (6-L) slow cooker with cooking spray. Trim the fat off the roast and cut into 2-inch (5-cm) pieces. Layer the roast, potatoes, onion, lima beans, and corn in the slow cooker. In a bowl, combine the tomatoes, barbecue sauce, broth, and brown sugar. Pour over the pork and vegetables. Cover and cook on low for 10 to 12 hours, or until the meat and potatoes are tender. Remove the pork with a slotted spoon and shred with two forks. Return the shredded pork to the slow cooker and stir well.

Yield: 8 servings

Per serving: 599 calories (34% from fat, 28% from protein, 38% from carbohydrate); 42 g protein; 23 g total fat; 8 g saturated fat; 10 g monounsaturated fat; 3 g polyunsaturated fat; 57 g carbohydrate; 6 g fiber; 20 g sugar; 500 mg phosphorus; 97 mg calcium; 155 mg sodium; 1590 mg potassium; 290 IU vitamin A; 3 mg ATE vitamin E; 31 mg vitamin C; 107 mg cholesterol

Tip: If you like the flavor of okra you could add 10 ounces of fresh or frozen okra along with the other vegetables.

Taste of Fall Stew

What could say cooler temperatures and falling leaves better than the flavors of apples, cider, pork, and root vegetables? This version cooks in the slow cooker while you're at work. It's a great full meal, especially if you also put one of the bread recipes on pages 312 to 324 in the bread maker in the morning so you have a slice of warm bread to go with it.

2 pounds (908 g) boneless pork loin roast, cut into 1-inch (2.5-cm) cubes

2 cups (220 g) sliced parsnips

1 cup (130 g) ½-inch (1.3-cm) pieces carrot

1 cup (160 g) sliced onion

1 apple, cored and coarsely chopped

½ cup (50 g) chopped celery

1 cup (235 ml) water

1 cup (235 ml) apple cider

1 teaspoon freshly ground black pepper

Coat the inside of a 3- to 4-quart (3- to 4-L) slow cooker with cooking spray. Layer the pork, parsnips, carrot, onion, apple, and celery in the slow cooker. Combine the water, cider, and pepper in a bowl, then pour over the meat and vegetables. Cover and cook on low for 10 to 12 hours, until the meat is tender.

Yield: 6 servings

Per serving: 279 calories (22% from fat, 48% from protein, 30% from carbohydrate); 33 g protein; 7 g total fat; 2 g saturated fat; 3 g monounsaturated fat; 1 g polyunsaturated fat; 21 g carbohydrate; 4 g fiber; 11 g sugar; 384 mg phosphorus; 59 mg calcium; 107 mg sodium; 931 mg potassium; 2633 IU vitamin A; 3 mg ATE vitamin E; 13 mg vitamin C; 95 mg cholesterol

Pork and Black Bean Chili

This makes a moderately spicy, traditional flavored pork and black bean chili. Prepared in the slow cooker while you work or sleep, it provides a flavorful meal that is ready when you are.

1 tablespoon (15 ml) olive oil

2 pounds (908 g) boneless pork loin roast, cut into ½-inch (1.3-cm) cubes

2 cans (14.5 ounces, or 411 g each) no-salt-added tomatoes

12 ounces (336 g) frozen corn kernels, thawed

2 cups (512 g) black beans, cooked or canned, drained

1 cup (160 g) sliced onion

1 cup (235 ml) Low-Sodium Beef Broth (page 231)

4 ounces (112 g) chopped green chiles

1 tablespoon (7.5 g) chili powder

1 teaspoon minced garlic

¼ teaspoon cayenne pepper

½ teaspoon freshly ground black pepper

¼ cup (4 g) minced fresh cilantro

Coat the inside of a 5-quart (5-L) slow cooker with cooking spray. Heat the oil in a large skillet over medium-high heat, add the pork, and cook for 5 to 6 minutes, or until browned all over. Transfer the pork to the slow cooker. Stir in the tomatoes, corn, beans, onion, broth, chiles, chili powder, garlic, cayenne, and black pepper. Cover and cook on low for 6 to 7 hours, or until the pork is tender. Stir in the cilantro just before serving.

Yield: 6 servings

Per serving: 488 calories (41% from fat, 31% from protein, 27% from carbohydrate); 39 g protein; 23 g total fat; 7 g saturated fat; 10 g monounsaturated fat; 3 g polyunsaturated fat; 34 g carbohydrate; 9 g fiber; 7 g sugar; 469 mg phosphorus; 104 mg calcium; 210 mg sodium; 1300 mg potassium; 739 IU vitamin A; 3 mg ATE vitamin E; 34 mg vitamin C; 95 mg cholesterol

19

Fix-It-in-15 Fish and Seafood Dishes

Fish and seafood don't normally benefit from long cooking times, so the recipes here are a little different than those in the chapters before. Many of them still make use of the slow cooker, but they don't require all day cooking. But that doesn't mean they still can't be useful. I find they make perfect weekend recipes. You can put them in the slow cooker, go off to do all the things you need to do on the weekend, and come home several hours later to find dinner ready.

Spanish Halibut

This fish has a Mediterranean style, highlighted by the pimentos and onions, as well as the unique combination of herbs and spices. It doesn't need long cooking like most of the other make-ahead recipes, but it will get you out of the kitchen for 45 minutes to run an errand or take care of other things.

1 tablespoon (15 ml) olive oil

1 cup (160 g) thinly sliced onion

2 tablespoons (12.5 g) chopped pimento

1½ pounds boned halibut fillets

¼ teaspoon ground mace

¼ teaspoon cayenne pepper

¼ teaspoon freshly ground black pepper

6 thick slices tomato

8 ounces (225 g) mushrooms, thinly sliced

3 tablespoons (18 g) chopped scallion

¼ cup (60 ml) Dry White Wine or Low-Sodium Chicken Broth (page 232)

4 teaspoons unsalted butter

½ cup (60 g) Italian-Style Bread Crumbs (page 33)

Preheat the oven to 350°F (180°C, or gas mark 4). Brush the oil onto the bottom of a 9 × 13-inch (23 × 33-cm) baking dish; layer with the onion and pimento. Pat the fish dry. Combine the mace, cayenne, and black pepper in a small bowl; sprinkle over both sides of the fish. Arrange the fish over the onion and pimento layer. Top each fillet with a tomato slice; sprinkle with the mushrooms and scallion. Pour the wine over the fish and vegetables. In a nonstick skillet over medium heat, melt the butter; add the bread crumbs and cook, stirring, until lightly browned, 1 to 2 minutes. Sprinkle over the fish. Bake for 40 to 45 minutes, or until the fish flakes easily with a fork.

Yield: 6 servings

Per serving: 560 calories (25% from fat, 66% from protein, 9% from carbohydrate); 88 g protein; 15 g total fat; 3 g saturated fat; 6 g monounsaturated fat; 4 g polyunsaturated fat; 12 g carbohydrate; 2 g fiber; 3 g sugar; 970 mg phosphorus; 222 mg calcium; 226 mg sodium; 2096 mg potassium; 1095 IU vitamin A; 213 mg ATE vitamin E; 10 mg vitamin C; 137 mg cholesterol

Slow-Cooked Poached Catfish

This is a simple preparation, using only onion, parsley, and lemon to subtlely flavor the catfish. It is a great meal for weekends or that evening when you have some errands to run, because it doesn't need to cook all day like many slow cooker recipes. You can substitute any firm-fleshed white fish. Serve garnished with lemon slices and sprigs of fresh parsley.

1½ pounds (680 g) catfish fillets

½ cup (80 g) chopped onion

1 tablespoon (4 g) chopped fresh parsley

4 teaspoons (7 g) lemon zest

Coat the inside of a 3- to 4-quart (3- to 4-L) slow cooker with cooking spray. Place the fish

(continued on page 276)

in the slow cooker. Sprinkle the onion, parsley, and lemon zest over the fish. Cover and cook on low for 1½ hours, until the fish flakes easily with a fork.

Yield: 6 servings

Per serving: 160 calories (50% from fat, 46% from protein, 4% from carbohydrate); 18 g protein; 9 g total fat; 2 g saturated fat; 4 g monounsaturated fat; 2 g polyunsaturated fat; 2 g carbohydrate; 0 g fiber; 1 g sugar; 233 mg phosphorus; 16 mg calcium; 61 mg sodium; 364 mg potassium; 110 IU vitamin A; 17 mg ATE vitamin E; 4 mg vitamin C; 53 mg cholesterol

Slow-Cooked Italian Fish and Vegetables

Slow cooked in an Italian-oriented sauce with added vegetables, this fish really absorbs the multiple flavors. You won't believe how intense the flavor can be until you try it. Great served with pasta.

1 pound (454 g) flounder, cut into 2-inch (5-cm) pieces

1 cup (160 g) sliced onion

½ cup (75 g) 1-inch (2.5-cm) pieces green bell pepper

1½ cups (180 g) sliced zucchini

2 tablespoons (30 ml) olive oil

½ teaspoon minced garlic

1 can (14.5 ounces, or 411 g) no-salt-added tomatoes

½ teaspoon dried basil

½ teaspoon dried oregano

⅛ teaspoon freshly ground black pepper

¼ cup (60 ml) dry white wine

Coat the inside of a 3- to 4-quart (3- to 4-L) slow cooker with cooking spray. Place the fish in the slow cooker and cover with the onion, bell pepper, and zucchini. In a bowl, combine the oil, garlic, tomatoes, basil, oregano, black pepper, and wine; pour over the fish in the slow cooker. Cover and cook on low for 6 to 8 hours, until the fish flakes easily with a fork.

Yield: 4 servings

Per serving: 221 calories (35% from fat, 44% from protein, 21% from carbohydrate); 23 g protein; 8 g total fat; 1 g saturated fat; 5 g monounsaturated fat; 1 g polyunsaturated fat; 11 g carbohydrate; 2 g fiber; 6 g sugar; 263 mg phosphorus; 74 mg calcium; 109 mg sodium; 866 mg potassium; 347 IU vitamin A; 11 mg ATE vitamin E; 42 mg vitamin C; 54 mg cholesterol

Italian Salmon Loaf

Salmon loaf is one of those old-fashioned comfort foods I remember from my childhood. This version, which has Italian flavors from the bread crumbs and Parmesan cheese, cooks in the slow cooker, freeing you for other things.

½ cup (125 g) egg substitute, or 2 eggs, lightly beaten

2 cups (230 g) Italian-Style Bread Crumbs (page 33)

1 cup (235 ml) Low-Sodium Chicken Broth (page 232)

⅓ cup (33 g) grated Parmesan cheese

¼ teaspoon dry mustard powder

1 can (14 ounces, or 392 g) salmon, drained, bones and skin removed

Coat the inside of a 3-quart (3-L) slow cooker with cooking spray. Cut three 3 × 20-inch (7.5 × 50-cm) strips of heavy-duty foil; lay in a crisscross so they resemble spokes of a wheel. Place the strips on the bottom and up the sides of the slow cooker. In a large bowl, combine the eggs, bread crumbs, broth, cheese, and mustard. Add the salmon and mix well. Gently shape the mixture into a round loaf. Place in the center of the strips. Cover and cook on low for 4 to 6 hours, or until a meat thermometer inserted into the center registers 160°F (71°C). Using the foil strips as handles, transfer the loaf to a platter.

Yield: 6 servings

Per serving: 288 calories (23% from fat, 36% from protein, 41% from carbohydrate); 25 g protein; 7 g total fat, 2 g saturated fat; 2 g monounsaturated fat; 2 g polyunsaturated fat; 29 g carbohydrate; 2 g fiber; 0 g sugar; 365 mg phosphorus; 279 mg calcium; 197 mg sodium; 417 mg potassium; 146 IU vitamin A; 20 mg ATE vitamin E; 0 mg vitamin C; 31 mg cholesterol

Tuna Noodle Casserole

This is classic American comfort food. There's no need to describe the taste because it will be just the way you remember it. It will definitely remind you of the good old days, but is healthier and way easier to fix.

10 ounces (300 ml) Condensed Cream of Mushroom Soup (page 31)

⅓ cup (80 ml) Low-Sodium Chicken Broth (page 232)

⅔ cup (160 ml) skim milk

2 tablespoons (8 g) chopped fresh parsley

10 ounces (280 g) frozen no-salt-added peas, thawed

14 ounces (392 g) tuna packed in water, well drained

10 ounces (280 g) egg noodles, cooked according to package directions until just tender

3 tablespoons (21 g) Italian-Style Bread Crumbs (page 33)

Coat the inside of a 3- to 4-quart (3- to 4-L) slow cooker with cooking spray. In a large bowl, combine the soup, chicken broth, milk, parsley, peas, and tuna. Fold in the cooked noodles. Pour the mixture into the prepared slow cooker. Top with the bread crumbs. Cover and cook on low for 5 to 6 hours.

Yield: 6 servings

Per serving: 231 calories (14% from fat, 38% from protein, 49% from carbohydrate); 21 g protein; 3 g total fat; 1 g saturated fat; 1 g monounsaturated fat; 1 g polyunsaturated fat; 28 g carbohydrate; 5 g fiber; 3 g sugar; 277 mg phosphorus; 74 mg calcium; 265 mg sodium; 463 mg potassium; 1196 IU vitamin A; 22 mg ATE vitamin E; 7 mg vitamin C; 30 mg cholesterol

Marinated Shrimp

These shrimp are marinated in a vinaigrette similar to Italian dressing. They can sit in the marinate in the refrigerator for a day or more, allowing you to fix them when you have a few minutes and have them ready when you need them. Serve over a salad to make it a meal or use as appetizers.

2 pounds (908 g) medium shrimp, cooked, peeled, and deveined

1 cup (160 g) sliced red onion, separated into rings

2 lemons, sliced

½ cup (120 ml) olive oil

3 tablespoons (45 ml) lemon juice

3 tablespoons (45 ml) red wine vinegar

⅓ cup (20 g) minced fresh parsley

½ teaspoon minced garlic

1 bay leaf

1 teaspoon dried basil

1 teaspoon dry mustard powder

¼ teaspoon freshly ground black pepper

In a 3-quart (3-L) glass serving bowl, combine the shrimp, onion, and lemons. In a jar with a tight-fitting lid, combine the oil, lemon juice, vinegar, and seasonings; shake well. Pour over the shrimp mixture and stir gently to coat. Cover and refrigerate for 24 hours, stirring occasionally. Discard the bay leaf before serving.

Yield: 8 servings

Per serving: 258 calories (53% from fat, 36% from protein, 11% from carbohydrate); 24 g protein; 16 g total fat; 2 g saturated fat; 10 g monounsaturated fat; 2 g polyunsaturated fat; 7 g carbohydrate; 2 g fiber; 1 g sugar; 245 mg phosphorus; 87 mg calcium; 171 mg sodium; 310 mg potassium; 433 IU vitamin A; 61 mg ATE vitamin E; 30 mg vitamin C; 172 mg cholesterol

Shrimp Pasta Sauce

Pasta sauce is a perfect dish for the slow cooker because the long cooking gives you that depth of flavor that long simmering on the stove does, without needing to keep an eye on it. This is a fairly traditional Italian sauce, with shrimp added near the end so they don't get overcooked.

1 can (14.5 ounces, or 411 g) no-salt-added tomatoes, undrained

1 can (6 ounces, or 170 g) no-salt-added tomato paste

½ cup (120 ml) water

½ teaspoon minced garlic

2 tablespoons (8 g) minced fresh parsley

1 teaspoon dried oregano

½ teaspoon dried basil

¼ teaspoon freshly ground black pepper

1 pound (454 g) raw shrimp, peeled and deveined

Coat the inside of a 3- to 4-quart (3- to 4-L) slow cooker with cooking spray. Add the tomatoes, tomato paste, water, garlic, parsley, oregano, basil, and black pepper to the slow cooker. Cover and cook on low for 3 to 4 hours. Add the shrimp in the last 20 minutes.

Yield: 6 servings

Per serving: 118 calories (12% from fat, 57% from protein, 31% from carbohydrate); 17 g protein; 2 g total fat; 0 g saturated fat; 0 g monounsaturated fat; 1 g polyunsaturated fat; 9 g carbohydrate; 2 g fiber; 5 g sugar; 193 mg phosphorus; 76 mg calcium; 148 mg sodium; 591 mg potassium; 778 IU vitamin A; 41 mg ATE vitamin E; 19 mg vitamin C; 115 mg cholesterol

Tip: Need to be gone longer than 4 hours? No problem—the sauce can cook all day if needed.

Thai Shrimp

No one will even notice that this dish, filled with the flavors of Thailand, does not contain any salt. You can use more or less cayenne and ginger, depending on how spicy you like your food.

4 cups (910 ml) Low-Sodium Chicken Broth (page 232)

2 cups (380 g) raw rice

1 cup (110 g) shredded carrot

1 cup (160 g) chopped onion

½ cup (75 g) chopped red bell pepper

½ cup (75 g) chopped green bell pepper

½ cup (120 ml) water

½ cup (120 ml) coconut milk

⅓ cup (80 ml) lime juice

¼ cup (20 g) shredded coconut

½ cup (75 g) golden raisins

1½ teaspoons minced garlic

1 tablespoon (5 g) lime zest

1 tablespoon (6 g) minced fresh ginger

1 teaspoon ground coriander

1 teaspoon ground cumin

¼ teaspoon cayenne pepper

1 pound (454 g) raw shrimp, peeled and deveined

½ cup (38 g) snow peas, cut into thin strips

Coat the inside of a 4- to 5-quart (4- to 5-L) slow cooker with cooking spray. Combine the broth, rice, vegetables, water, coconut milk, lime juice, coconut, raisins, garlic, lime zest, ginger, and seasonings. Cover and cook on low for 3 to 4 hours, or until the rice is tender. Stir in the shrimp and snow peas. Cover and cook for 20 minutes longer, or until the shrimp just turn pink.

Yield: 8 servings

Per serving: 229 calories (22% from fat, 28% from protein, 50% from carbohydrate); 17 g protein; 6 g total fat; 4 g saturated fat; 1 g monounsaturated fat; 1 g polyunsaturated fat; 29 g carbohydrate; 2 g fiber; 9 g sugar; 220 mg phosphorus; 67 mg calcium; 138 mg sodium; 497 mg potassium; 2457 IU vitamin A; 31 mg ATE vitamin E; 36 mg vitamin C; 86 mg cholesterol

Cheesy Fish Chowder

Not cheesy like a bad comedian, but cheesy like full of the flavor of Swiss and Monterey Jack cheeses. With that as a starting point you don't need much else to produce full-flavored chowder, full of fish and broccoli, so I've kept the seasonings simple to allow the cheese to dominate.

1 tablespoon (14 g) unsalted butter

1 cup (160 g) chopped onion

2 cups (470 ml) skim milk

1 cup (235 ml) Ranch Dressing (page 34)

1 pound (454 g) cod fillets, skin and bones removed

10 ounces (280 g) frozen broccoli, thawed

1 cup (110 g) shredded Swiss cheese

½ cup (75 g) shredded Monterey Jack cheese

¼ teaspoon garlic powder

¼ teaspoon paprika

Coat the inside of a 3-quart (3-L) slow cooker with cooking spray. Melt the butter in a large skillet over medium heat, add the onion, and sauté until tender, about 5 minutes. Transfer to the slow cooker and add the milk, dressing, fish, broccoli, cheeses, and garlic powder. Cover and cook on high for 1½ to 2 hours, or until the soup is bubbly and the fish flakes easily with a fork. Sprinkle with the paprika before serving.

Yield: 6 servings

Per serving: 414 calories (54% from fat, 27% from protein, 19% from carbohydrate); 28 g protein; 25 g total fat; 9 g saturated fat; 7 g monounsaturated fat; 8 g polyunsaturated fat; 20 g carbohydrate; 2 g fiber; 5 g sugar; 469 mg phosphorus; 451 mg calcium; 178 mg sodium; 608 mg potassium; 1186 IU vitamin A; 147 mg ATE vitamin E; 22 mg vitamin C; 79 mg cholesterol

Italian Coast Seafood Stew

This is a great-tasting stew of scallops and shrimp based on spaghetti sauce. The flavor develops and permeates the vegetables during long cooking, with the shellfish added near the end so they don't get overcooked.

4 medium red potatoes, peeled and diced

1 cup (130 g) sliced carrot

3 cups (750 g) Low-Sodium Spaghetti Sauce (page 234)

8 ounces (225 g) mushrooms, sliced

1 teaspoon turmeric

1 teaspoon minced garlic

¼ teaspoon cayenne pepper

1½ cups (355 ml) water

1 pound (454 g) raw scallops

1 pound (454 g) raw shrimp, peeled and deveined

Coat the inside of a 3- to 4-quart (3- to 4-L) slow cooker with cooking spray. Add the potatoes, carrot, sauce, mushrooms, turmeric, garlic, and cayenne pepper to the slow cooker. Cover and cook on low for 4½ to 5 hours, or until the potatoes are fork-tender. Stir in the water, scallops, and shrimp. Cover and cook for 15 to 20 minutes longer, or until the scallops are opaque and the shrimp turn pink.

Yield: 9 servings

Per serving: 330 calories (15% from fat, 30% from protein, 55% from carbohydrate); 25 g protein; 6 g total fat; 1 g saturated fat; 3 g monounsaturated fat; 1 g polyunsaturated fat; 46 g carbohydrate; 6 g fiber; 11 g sugar; 366 mg phosphorus; 93 mg calcium; 203 mg sodium; 1439 mg potassium; 2373 IU vitamin A; 35 mg ATE vitamin E; 31 mg vitamin C; 93 mg cholesterol

20

Fix-It-in-15 Vegetarian Dishes

Here again you'll find mostly a collection of cook-all-day slow cooker recipes, many of them soups and stews. And that is just the ticket for these vegetarian meals. It allows you to cook meals with beans and other legumes without having to keep an eye on a simmering pot for several hours. And in the end they come out every bit as good as—and it seems to me in a lot of cases, better than—the same recipes cooked on the stove top.

Harvest Vegetable Soup

This may seem like an unusual combination when you first look at the ingredients, but it really works. Beans and butternut squash simmer in a tomato broth flavored with Southwestern herbs. The long cooking in the slow cooker allows all the different flavors to blend into one delicious whole.

1 cup (160 g) chopped onion

1 tablespoon (15 ml) olive oil

½ teaspoon ground cumin

¼ teaspoon ground cinnamon

½ teaspoon minced garlic

3 cups (450 g) 1-inch (2.5-cm) cubes butternut squash

1½ cups (355 ml) low-sodium vegetable broth

2 cups (512 g) Great Northern beans, rinsed and drained

1 can (14.5 ounces, or 411 g) no-salt-added tomatoes, undrained

1 tablespoon (1 g) chopped fresh cilantro

Combine all the ingredients in a 4- to 5-quart (4- to 5-L) slow cooker. Cover and cook on high for 1 hour. Reduce the heat to low and cook for 2 to 3 hours, until the vegetables are tender.

Yield: 6 servings

Per serving: 186 calories (15% from fat, 19% from protein, 67% from carbohydrate); 9 g protein; 3 g total fat; 1 g saturated fat; 2 g monounsaturated fat; 1 g polyunsaturated fat; 33 g carbohydrate; 7 g fiber; 5 g sugar; 181 mg phosphorus; 127 mg calcium; 82 mg sodium; 801 mg potassium; 7563 IU vitamin A; 1 mg ATE vitamin E; 27 mg vitamin C; 0 mg cholesterol

Irish Minestrone

Okay, I made up the Irish part. But with two of the main ingredients being beer and potatoes, it just came to me. Besides, a generous assortment of herbs provide flavor, beans add protein, and lots of vegetables produce a rather complex soup. But whatever you call it, it's full of both nutrition and flavor.

4 cups (940 ml) low-sodium vegetable broth

1 can (14.5 ounces, or 411 g) no-salt-added tomatoes

2 cups (512 g) kidney beans, rinsed and drained

2 cups (480 g) chickpeas, rinsed and drained

12 ounces (355 ml) dark beer

2 cups (220 g) frozen hash brown potatoes, thawed

1 tablespoon (10 g) minced onion

1 tablespoon (1 g) parsley flakes

1 teaspoon dried oregano

½ teaspoon garlic powder

½ teaspoon dried basil

½ teaspoon dried marjoram

10 ounces (280 g) frozen chopped spinach, thawed and drained

10 ounces (280 g) no-salt-added frozen peas and carrots, thawed

(continued on page 284)

In a 5-quart (5-L) slow cooker, combine the broth, tomatoes, beans, chickpeas, beer, hash browns, onion, parsley, oregano, garlic powder, basil, and marjoram. Cover and cook on low for 8 hours, until the beans and chickpeas are tender. Stir in the spinach and peas and carrots, cover, and cook until heated through, about 30 minutes.

Yield: 12 servings

Per serving: 164 calories (10% from fat, 24% from protein, 66% from carbohydrate); 10 g protein; 2 g total fat; 0 g saturated fat; 0 g monounsaturated fat; 1 g polyunsaturated fat; 26 g carbohydrate; 7 g fiber; 4 g sugar; 162 mg phosphorus; 118 mg calcium; 100 mg sodium; 571 mg potassium; 5138 IU vitamin A; 1 mg ATE vitamin E; 11 mg vitamin C; 0 mg cholesterol

Slow-Cooked Vegetable Chowder

This is a relatively simple vegetarian chowder, but don't let that fool you. The flavor is full and the soup is rich and warming. With the slow cooker doing most of the work while you're away all you have to do is stir in the milk at the end, and you're ready.

5 cups (1175 ml) low-sodium vegetable broth

8 medium red potatoes, cubed

1½ cups (240 g) chopped onion

1 cup (130 g) thinly sliced carrot

½ cup (50 g) thinly sliced celery

¼ cup (112 g) unsalted butter

¼ teaspoon freshly ground black pepper

12 ounces (355 ml) nonfat evaporated milk

1 tablespoon (4 g) minced fresh parsley

In a 5-quart (5-L) slow cooker, combine the broth, potatoes, onion, carrot, celery, butter, and black pepper. Cover and cook on high for 1 hour. Reduce the heat to low, cover, and cook for 5 to 6 hours, or until the vegetables are tender. Stir in the milk and parsley, cover, and cook until heated through, about 30 minutes.

Yield: 12 servings

Per serving: 295 calories (21% from fat, 13% from protein, 66% from carbohydrate); 10 g protein; 7 g total fat; 4 g saturated fat; 2 g monounsaturated fat; 0 g polyunsaturated fat; 49 g carbohydrate; 5 g fiber; 2 g sugar; 241 mg phosphorus; 152 mg calcium; 171 mg sodium; 1348 mg potassium; 1590 IU vitamin A; 64 mg ATE vitamin E; 29 mg vitamin C; 18 mg cholesterol

Tip: Serve with a thick slice of one of the whole grain breads in chapter 23.

Summer Vegetable Soup

Slow cooking adds a richness of flavor to this vegetarian soup chock-full of fresh summer veggies. Low sodium vegetable juice ensures that you will have a full flavored stock as the base. You couldn't ask for more nutrition for the amount of sodium and calories in this.

2 cans (14.5 ounces, or 411 g, each) no-salt-added chopped tomatoes

2 medium red potatoes, peeled and cubed

2 cups (200 g) fresh green beans

1 cup (120 g) cubed zucchini

1 cup (120 g) cubed yellow squash

¾ cup (98 g) thinly sliced carrot

½ cup (50 g) thinly sliced celery

1 cup (82 g) peeled and cubed eggplant

1 cup (70 g) sliced mushrooms

½ cup (75 g) chopped onion

1 tablespoon (4 g) minced fresh parsley

1 tablespoon (8 g) Salt-Free Seasoning
(page 27)

4 cups (940 ml) low-sodium vegetable juice

In a 5-quart (5-L) slow cooker, combine all the ingredients. Cover and cook on low for 7 to 8 hours, or until the vegetables are tender.

Yield: 12 servings

Per serving: 93 calories (4% from fat, 13% from protein, 83% from carbohydrate); 3 g protein; 0 g total fat; 0 g saturated fat; 0 g monounsaturated fat; 0 g polyunsaturated fat; 21 g carbohydrate; 4 g fiber; 4 g sugar; 88 mg phosphorus; 37 mg calcium; 66 mg sodium; 714 mg potassium; 2751 IU vitamin A; 0 mg ATE vitamin E; 50 mg vitamin C; 0 mg cholesterol

Tip: This soup is also good cold for a quick lunch the next day.

Vegetable Lentil Soup

People often seem to shy away from lentil dishes because they don't like the earthy flavor of this legume. But they will be hard pressed to find fault with this soup. Butternut squash and root vegetables play the main role here, with the lentil providing protein while playing in the background.

4 cups (940 ml) low-sodium vegetable broth

3 cups (450 g) peeled and cubed butternut squash

1 cup (192 g) lentils, rinsed

1 cup (130 g) chopped carrot

1 cup (160 g) chopped onion

2 teaspoons minced garlic

1 teaspoon dried oregano

1 teaspoon dried basil

1 can (14.5 ounces, or 411 g) no-salt-added tomatoes, undrained

9 ounces (252 g) frozen green beans

In a 5-quart (5-L) slow cooker, combine the broth, squash, lentils, carrot, onion, garlic, oregano, and basil. Cover and cook on low for 4 hours, or until the lentils are tender. Stir in the tomatoes and green beans. Cover and cook on high for 30 minutes, or until the beans are heated through.

Yield: 6 servings

Per serving: 144 calories (8% from fat, 23% from protein, 69% from carbohydrate); 9 g protein; 1 g total fat; 0 g saturated fat; 0 g monounsaturated fat; 0 g polyunsaturated fat; 27 g carbohydrate; 7 g fiber; 7 g sugar; 177 mg phosphorus; 144 mg calcium; 118 mg sodium; 864 mg potassium; 10421 IU vitamin A; 2 mg ATE vitamin E; 35 mg vitamin C; 0 mg cholesterol

Classic Potato Soup

This is a simple potato soup without a lot of frills and extras, making for great taste in a classic way. A creamy broth and the addition of onion, celery, and carrot provide just enough additional interest to make this a real winner.

6 medium red potatoes, peeled and diced

5 cups (1175 ml) low-sodium vegetable broth

2 cups (320 g) diced onion

½ cup (50 g) diced celery

½ cup (65 g) diced carrot

¼ teaspoon freshly ground black pepper

12 ounces (355 ml) nonfat evaporated milk

3 tablespoons (12 g) chopped fresh parsley

In a 5-quart (5-L) slow cooker, combine the potatoes, broth, onion, celery, carrot, and black pepper. Cover and cook on low for 7 to 8 hours, or until the vegetables are tender. Stir in the milk and parsley, cover, and cook until heated through, about 30 minutes.

Yield: 8 servings

Per serving: 278 calories (5% from fat, 17% from protein, 78% from carbohydrate); 12 g protein; 1 g total fat; 0 g saturated fat; 0 g monounsaturated fat; 0 g polyunsaturated fat; 55 g carbohydrate; 6 g fiber; 10 g sugar; 314 mg phosphorus; 213 mg calcium; 248 mg sodium; 1642 mg potassium; 1312 IU vitamin A; 52 mg ATE vitamin E; 60 mg vitamin C; 2 mg cholesterol

Mexican Bean Soup

No Mexican jumping beans (whatever they are) but a variety of other beans make this soup a filling meal in a bowl. Salsa and Mexican seasoning give it an easy flavor kick. For a little additional flavor top each bowl with a dollop of sour cream.

1 cup (160 g) chopped onion

1 can (14.5 ounces, or 411 g) no-salt-added tomatoes

2 cups (512 g) no-salt-added pinto beans, rinsed and drained

2 cups (512 g) no-salt-added black beans, rinsed and drained

2 cups (512 g) no-salt-added kidney beans, rinsed and drained

12 ounces (336 g) frozen corn kernels, thawed

12 ounces (340 g) Low-Sodium Salsa (page 232)

2 tablespoons (16 g) Salt-Free Mexican Seasoning (page 27)

Combine all the ingredients in a 4- to 5-quart (4- to 5-L) slow cooker. Cover and cook on low for 8 to 10 hours, until the beans are tender.

Yield: 8 servings

Per serving: 343 calories (5% from fat, 23% from protein, 72% from carbohydrate); 21 g protein; 2 g total fat; 0 g saturated fat; 0 g monounsaturated fat; 1 g polyunsaturated fat; 65 g carbohydrate; 18 g fiber; 7 g sugar; 393 mg phosphorus; 116 mg calcium; 67 mg sodium; 1387 mg potassium; 355 IU vitamin A; 0 mg ATE vitamin E; 22 mg vitamin C; 0 mg cholesterol

Bean and Bulgur Chili

The flavor is traditional chili, but the ingredient list may surprise you. This great-tasting meatless chili gets both a nutritional and a flavor bonus with the addition of bulgur. It might be fun to see whether anyone can guess what that secret ingredient is.

4 teaspoons (20 ml) olive oil

2 cups (320 g) chopped onion

1 cup (100 g) chopped celery

1 cup (150 g) chopped green bell pepper

1 teaspoon minced garlic

½ cup (55 g) shredded carrot

2 tablespoons (15 g) chili powder

1 teaspoon dried oregano

½ teaspoon freshly ground black pepper

½ teaspoon ground cumin

⅛ teaspoon ground cinnamon

⅛ teaspoon allspice

2 cans (14.5 ounces, or 411 g each) no-salt-added tomatoes, undrained

2 cups (512 g) no-salt-added kidney beans, rinsed and drained

2 cups (512 g) no-salt-added pinto beans, rinsed and drained

2 cups (512 g) black beans, rinsed and drained

2 cups (470 ml) vegetable broth

1 can (6 ounces, or 170 g) no-salt-added tomato paste

1 cup (184 g) bulgur

Heat the oil in a Dutch oven over medium heat, add the onion, celery, and green pepper, and sauté until tender, about 5 minutes. Add the garlic and cook, stirring, for 1 minute longer. Stir in the carrot and seasonings; cook, stirring, for 1 minute longer. Transfer to a 4- to 5-quart (4- to 5-L) slow cooker. Stir in the tomatoes, beans, broth, tomato paste, and bulgur. Cook on low for 8 to 10 hours, until the bulgur is tender.

Yield: 10 servings

Per serving: 278 calories (13% from fat, 19% from protein, 68% from carbohydrate); 14 g protein; 4 g total fat; 1 g saturated fat; 2 g monounsaturated fat; 1 g polyunsaturated fat; 50 g carbohydrate; 15 g fiber; 7 g sugar; 247 mg phosphorus; 112 mg calcium; 91 mg sodium; 958 mg potassium; 1702 IU vitamin A; 0 mg ATE vitamin E; 32 mg vitamin C; 0 mg cholesterol

Black Bean Chili

This tasty vegetarian chili contains an added bonus of vegetables that you don't typically think of when you think of chili. Celery and carrots join the more traditional ingredients to create a chili that has not only additional flavor nuances but also additional nutritional benefits.

1 cup (130 g) thinly sliced carrot

½ cup (50 g) thinly sliced celery

1 cup (160 g) chopped onion

1 teaspoon minced garlic

4 cups (1024 g) no-salt-added black beans, rinsed and drained

4 cups (940 ml) low-sodium vegetable broth

(continued on page 288)

1 can (14.5 ounces, or 411 g) no-salt-added
tomatoes

1½ teaspoons dried basil

½ teaspoon dried oregano

½ teaspoon ground cumin

½ teaspoon chili powder

½ teaspoon hot pepper sauce

In a 3-quart (3-L) slow cooker, combine all
the ingredients. Cover and cook on low for 9
to 11 hours, or until the vegetables and beans
are tender.

Yield: 8 servings

Per serving: 161 calories (8% from fat, 27% from
protein, 66% from carbohydrate); 11 g protein; 1 g
total fat; 0 g saturated fat; 0 g monounsaturated
fat; 0 g polyunsaturated fat; 27 g carbohydrate; 9 g
fiber; 3 g sugar; 182 mg phosphorus; 93 mg
calcium; 95 mg sodium; 635 mg potassium;
2104 IU vitamin A; 1 mg ATE vitamin E; 10 mg
vitamin C; 0 mg cholesterol

Tip: Serve over rice.

Many Vegetable Chili

Other than the beans, the ingredients aren't
what you'd expect for chili. But the taste
definitely is. And the amount of nutrition you
get for the amount of sodium and number of
calories is impressive.

1 cup (130 g) diced carrot

½ cup (50 g) diced celery

1 cup (160 g) diced onion

1 pound (454 g) mushrooms, sliced

1½ cups (180 g) diced zucchini

1 cup (120 g) chopped yellow squash

1 tablespoon (7.5 g) chili powder

1 teaspoon dried basil

1 teaspoon freshly ground black pepper

1 can (8 ounces, or 225 g) no-salt-added
tomato sauce

3 cups (705 ml) low-sodium tomato juice

2 cans (14.5 ounces, or 411 g, each) no-salt-
added diced tomatoes, undrained

2 cups (512 g) pinto beans, rinsed and
drained

1 cup (130 g) frozen corn kernels, thawed

Coat a large nonstick skillet with cooking
spray and sauté the carrot, celery, and onion
over medium-high heat 10 minutes, or until
the onion is translucent. Add the mushrooms,
zucchini, and squash; sauté for 3 more
minutes. Add the chili powder, basil, and black
pepper, and sauté for 5 more minutes. Stir
together the tomato sauce and tomato juice in
a 6-quart (6-L) slow cooker until blended. Stir
in the diced tomatoes, beans, corn, and carrot
mixture. Cover and cook on low for 8 hours.

Yield: 6 servings

Per serving: 213 calories (7% from fat, 21% from
protein, 73% from carbohydrate); 12 g protein; 2 g
total fat; 0 g saturated fat; 0 g monounsaturated
fat; 1 g polyunsaturated fat; 43 g carbohydrate;
11 g fiber; 16 g sugar; 264 mg phosphorus;
116 mg calcium; 82 mg sodium; 1486 mg
potassium; 4000 IU vitamin A; 0 mg ATE vitamin E;
63 mg vitamin C; 0 mg cholesterol

21

Fix-It-in-15 Side Dishes

Side dishes are an area where the fix-it-and-let-it-cook strategy can be very useful. This chapter is full of recipes that give you additional options for quick meals. There are vegetable casseroles and potato, rice, and barley dishes, all of which cook on their own in the slow cooker. There are also several versions of baked beans and some marinated vegetable recipes that just wait in the refrigerator until you are ready to pull them out and put them on the table.

Broccoli Rice Casserole

A hearty side dish of broccoli and rice in a creamy, cheesy sauce, this recipe only needs a piece of meat to make a complete meal. Cooking it in the slow cooker allows you to not worry about it at the last minute.

16 ounces (454 g) frozen broccoli, cooked and drained

10 ounces (300 ml) Condensed Cream of Mushroom Soup (page 31)

⅓ cup (53 g) chopped onion

½ cup (120 ml) skim milk

1½ cups (250 g) cooked rice

4 ounces (112 g) Swiss cheese, shredded

Coat the inside of a 3- to 4-quart (3- to 4-L) slow cooker with cooking spray. Combine all the ingredients in the slow cooker, reserving some cheese to sprinkle on top. Cook on low for 2 hours.

Yield: 4 servings

Per serving: 277 calories (31% from fat, 21% from protein, 48% from carbohydrate); 15 g protein; 10 g total fat; 6 g saturated fat; 2 g monounsaturated fat; 1 g polyunsaturated fat; 34 g carbohydrate; 4 g fiber; 4 g sugar; 346 mg phosphorus; 388 mg calcium; 75 mg sodium; 751 mg potassium; 1049 IU vitamin A; 80 mg ATE vitamin E; 102 mg vitamin C; 29 mg cholesterol

Vegetable Medley

These veggies make a great side dish, or you could freeze them and use them later in soups and other meals.

2 large Russet potatoes, peeled and diced

12 ounces (336 g) frozen corn kernels, thawed

1½ cups (270 g) seeded and diced tomato

1 cup (130 g) sliced carrot

½ cup (80 g) chopped onion

½ teaspoon sugar

½ teaspoon dillweed

⅛ teaspoon freshly ground black pepper

Coat the inside of a 3-quart (3-L) slow cooker with cooking spray. Combine all the ingredients in the slow cooker. Cover and cook on low for 5 to 6 hours, or until the vegetables are tender.

Yield: 6 servings

Per serving: 160 calories (4% from fat, 11% from protein, 84% from carbohydrate); 5 g protein; 1 g total fat; 0 g saturated fat; 0 g monounsaturated fat; 0 g polyunsaturated fat; 36 g carbohydrate; 5 g fiber; 4 g sugar; 133 mg phosphorus; 34 mg calcium; 32 mg sodium; 854 mg potassium; 2896 IU vitamin A; 0 mg ATE vitamin E; 23 mg vitamin C; 0 mg cholesterol

Slow Cooker Corn Soufflé

This creamy corn casserole is perfect with chicken or pork. Simple, comfort food, and taste that is the kind of thing that you can't get quickly, but that the slow cooker makes easy.

20 ounces (560 g) frozen corn kernels, thawed

8 ounces (225 g) fat-free cream cheese

¼ cup (112 g) unsalted butter

Coat the inside of a 2- to 3-quart (2- to 3-L) slow cooker with cooking spray. Combine all the ingredients in the slow cooker and cook on low until the cheese and butter are melted and the mixture is smooth, about 2 hours.

Yield: 6 servings

Per serving: 236 calories (56% from fat, 11% from protein, 33% from carbohydrate); 7 g protein; 15 g total fat; 9 g saturated fat; 4 g monounsaturated fat; 1 g polyunsaturated fat; 21 g carbohydrate; 3 g fiber; 3 g sugar; 142 mg phosphorus; 46 mg calcium; 127 mg sodium; 321 mg potassium; 690 IU vitamin A; 132 mg ATE vitamin E; 6 mg vitamin C; 42 mg cholesterol

Ratatouille

This is a fairly traditional version of this classic dish of Spain and southern France. The untraditional parts are the low-sodium level and the use of the slow cooker to get you out of the kitchen faster. This is the perfect eggplant dish for people who think they don't like eggplant because it has such rich flavor.

1 eggplant, peeled and cut into 1-inch (2.5-cm) cubes

3 cups (540 g) chopped tomatoes

3 cups (360 g) sliced zucchini

2 cups (320 g) chopped onion

1 cup (150 g) chopped green bell pepper

1 cup (150 g) chopped yellow bell pepper

1 can (6 ounces, or 170 g) no-salt-added tomato paste

½ cup (20 g) minced fresh basil

½ teaspoon minced garlic

½ teaspoon freshly ground black pepper

2 tablespoons (30 ml) olive oil

Coat the inside of a 5-quart (5-L) slow cooker with cooking spray. Combine all of the vegetables and seasonings in the slow cooker. Drizzle with the oil. Cover and cook on high for 3 to 4 hours, or until the vegetables are tender.

Yield: 10 servings

Per serving: 90 calories (29% from fat, 11% from protein, 60% from carbohydrate); 3 g protein; 3 g total fat; 0 g saturated fat; 2 g monounsaturated fat; 0 g polyunsaturated fat; 15 g carbohydrate; 5 g fiber; 5 g sugar; 75 mg phosphorus; 65 mg calcium; 28 mg sodium; 646 mg potassium; 875 IU vitamin A; 0 mg ATE vitamin E; 72 mg vitamin C; 0 mg cholesterol

Slow Cooker Acorn Squash

If you've never tried cooking acorn squash in the slow cooker you are doing it the hard way. It comes out soft and sweet and ready to eat. The version is sweetened even more with brown sugar, raisins, and spices that give it a flavor reminiscent of pumpkin pie.

¾ cup (170 g) packed brown sugar

1 teaspoon ground cinnamon

1 teaspoon nutmeg

2 acorn squash, halved and seeded

¾ cup (109 g) raisins

¼ cup (112 g) unsalted butter

½ cup (120 ml) water

In a small bowl, combine the brown sugar, cinnamon, and nutmeg; spoon into the squash halves. Sprinkle with the raisins. Top each with 1 tablespoon (14 g) of the butter. Wrap each squash half individually in heavy-duty foil; seal tightly. Pour water into a 5-quart (5-L) slow cooker. Place the squash, cut side up, in the slow cooker (packets may be stacked). Cover and cook on high for 4 hours, or until the squash is tender. Open the foil packets carefully to allow steam to escape.

Yield: 4 servings

Per serving: 440 calories (23% from fat, 2% from protein, 75% from carbohydrate); 3 g protein; 12 g total fat; 8 g saturated fat; 3 g monounsaturated fat; 1 g polyunsaturated fat; 88 g carbohydrate; 5 g fiber; 58 g sugar; 123 mg phosphorus; 134 mg calcium; 28 mg sodium; 1131 mg potassium; 1148 IU vitamin A; 95 mg ATE vitamin E; 25 mg vitamin C; 31 mg cholesterol

Italian Spaghetti Squash

I always used to cook spaghetti squash in the oven, watching it and turning it so it cooked evenly. Then I discovered how easy it is to cook in the slow cooker. Not only does it come out perfectly cooked, but this version also has Italian tomato sauce already cooked in, making it a perfect side dish with a simple piece of meat.

1 medium spaghetti squash

8 ounces (225 g) mushrooms, sliced

1 can (14.5 ounces, or 411 g) no-salt-added tomatoes, undrained

1 teaspoon dried oregano

¼ teaspoon freshly ground black pepper

¾ cup (90 g) shredded mozzarella cheese

Coat the inside of a 4- to 5-quart (4- to 5-L) slow cooker with cooking spray. Cut the squash in half lengthwise and scoop out and discard the seeds. Place the squash, cut side up, in the slow cooker. Layer on the mushrooms and tomatoes and sprinkle with the oregano and pepper. Cover and cook on low for 6 to 8 hours, or until the squash is tender. Sprinkle with the cheese. Cover and cook for 15 minutes longer, or until the cheese is melted. When the squash is cool enough to handle, separate into strands with two forks.

Yield: 4 servings

Per serving: 126 calories (37% from fat, 23% from protein, 40% from carbohydrate); 8 g protein; 6 g total fat; 3 g saturated fat; 1 g monounsaturated fat; 1 g polyunsaturated fat; 14 g carbohydrate; 2 g fiber; 4 g sugar; 154 mg phosphorus; 165 mg calcium; 161 mg sodium; 533 mg potassium; 346 IU vitamin A; 37 mg ATE vitamin E; 18 mg vitamin C; 17 mg cholesterol

Tip: Make sure the squash is on the small or medium side so that it fits into the slow cooker after being cut in half.

Baked Beans

This is a simple, but very good, baked bean recipe. There are only a few ingredients, but the long, slow cooking makes the most of them, cooking them up soft and sweet with just the hint of bacon flavor.

2½ cups (625 g) dried navy beans, rinsed and picked over

6 tablespoons (120 g) molasses

¼ cup (60 g) packed brown sugar

4 slices low-sodium bacon

¼ teaspoon freshly ground black pepper

Soak the beans in water to cover overnight to soften. Drain. Place the beans in a 4- to 5-quart (4- to 5-L) slow cooker and stir in the molasses, sugar, bacon, and pepper. Cook on low for 10 hours, or until the beans are tender.

Yield: 6 servings

Per serving: 232 calories (10% from fat, 14% from protein, 75% from carbohydrate); 9 g protein; 3 g total fat; 1 g saturated fat; 1 g monounsaturated fat; 0 g polyunsaturated fat; 45 g carbohydrate; 5 g fiber; 21 g sugar; 156 mg phosphorus; 105 mg calcium; 67 mg sodium; 650 mg potassium; 8 IU vitamin A; 1 mg ATE vitamin E; 1 mg vitamin C; 6 mg cholesterol

Boston Baked Beans

Sweet and delicious, these beans cook up perfectly in the slow cooker. The ingredients that make this a traditional New England recipe are the molasses and cloves, which not only add a unique flavor, but a darker color.

1 pound (454 g) dried navy beans, rinsed and picked over

6 cups (1.4 L) water, divided

1 cup (160 g) chopped onion

½ cup (115 g) packed brown sugar

½ cup (160 g) molasses

¼ cup (50 g) granulated sugar

1 teaspoon dry mustard powder

½ teaspoon ground cloves

½ teaspoon freshly ground black pepper

Coat the inside of a 4- to 5-quart (4- to 5-L) slow cooker with cooking spray. Place the beans in the slow cooker and add 4 cups (940 ml) of the water. Cover and let stand overnight. Drain and rinse the beans, discarding the liquid. Return the beans to the slow cooker. In a small bowl, combine the onion, brown sugar, molasses, granulated

(continued on page 294)

sugar, mustard, cloves, pepper, and remaining 2 cups (470 ml) water. Pour the mixture over the beans and stir to combine. Cover and cook on low for 10 to 12 hours, or until the beans are tender.

Yield: 10 servings

Per serving: 181 calories (2% from fat, 9% from protein, 90% from carbohydrate); 4 g protein; 0 g total fat; 0 g saturated fat; 0 g monounsaturated fat; 0 g polyunsaturated fat; 42 g carbohydrate; 3 g fiber; 26 g sugar; 83 mg phosphorus; 82 mg calcium; 14 mg sodium; 476 mg potassium; 6 IU vitamin A; 0 mg ATE vitamin E; 2 mg vitamin C; 0 mg cholesterol

Refried Beans

This makes a big batch of refried beans. The use of the slow cooker makes it easy to prepare. They freeze very nicely, so you can pack some away for future meals. The flavor is fairly traditional (despite the rather untraditional coffee in the ingredients) and not too spicy.

1 pound (454 g) dried pinto beans, rinsed and picked over

4 cups (940 ml) water

1 cup (235 ml) coffee

1 teaspoon minced garlic

1 cup (160 g) diced onion

1 tablespoon (7 g) ground cumin

2 teaspoons chili powder

1½ teaspoons dried oregano

Soak the beans in water to cover overnight to soften. Drain. Place the beans in a 4- to 5-quart (4- to 5-L) slow cooker and stir in the water, coffee, garlic, onion, cumin, chili powder, and oregano. Cover and cook on low for 8 to 10 hours, or until the beans are tender. Use a potato masher or large spoon to mash the beans to the desired consistency.

Yield: 12 servings

Per serving: 130 calories (5% from fat, 24% from protein, 71% from carbohydrate); 8 g protein; 1 g total fat; 0 g saturated fat; 0 g monounsaturated fat; 0 g polyunsaturated fat; 24 g carbohydrate; 6 g fiber; 1 g sugar; 160 mg phosphorus; 54 mg calcium; 14 mg sodium; 587 mg potassium; 139 IU vitamin A; 0 mg ATE vitamin E; 4 mg vitamin C; 0 mg cholesterol

Lemon Herb Potatoes

I have to admit that when I first saw this flavor combination, the thought of lemon and potatoes seemed a little strange. But I tried it and liked it. Now it's time for you to give it a try. These go particularly well with fish, but are also good with chicken or pork.

1½ pounds (680 g) red potatoes

¼ cup (60 ml) water

¼ cup (112 g) unsalted butter, melted

3 tablespoons (12 g) minced fresh parsley

1 tablespoon (15 ml) lemon juice

1 tablespoon (3 g) minced fresh chives

¼ teaspoon freshly ground black pepper

Coat the inside of a 3-quart (3-L) slow cooker with cooking spray. Peel a strip of skin from around the middle of each potato. Place the potatoes and the water in the slow cooker. Cover and cook on high for 2½ to 3 hours, or until tender (do not overcook); drain. In a small bowl, combine the butter, parsley, lemon juice, and chives. Pour over the potatoes and toss to coat. Season with the black pepper.

Yield: 6 servings

Per serving: 151 calories (46% from fat, 6% from protein, 48% from carbohydrate); 2 g protein; 8 g total fat; 5 g saturated fat; 2 g monounsaturated fat; 0 g polyunsaturated fat; 18 g carbohydrate; 2 g fiber; 1 g sugar; 73 mg phosphorus; 17 mg calcium; 9 mg sodium; 534 mg potassium; 426 IU vitamin A; 63 mg ATE vitamin E; 26 mg vitamin C; 20 mg cholesterol

Ranch Potatoes

A little of the make-ahead ranch dressing mix adds a lot of flavor to these slow-cooked potatoes, while cream cheese and mushroom soup give them their creamy sauce.

2 pounds (908 g) red potatoes, quartered

8 ounces (225 g) cream cheese, softened

1½ cups (355 ml) Condensed Cream of Mushroom Soup (page 31)

2 tablespoons (16 g) Ranch Dressing Mix (page 34)

Coat the inside of a 3-quart (3-L) slow cooker with cooking spray. Place the potatoes in the slow cooker. In a small bowl, beat the cream cheese, soup, and dressing mix until blended. Stir into the potatoes. Cover and cook on low for 8 hours, or until the potatoes are tender.

Yield: 6 servings

Per serving: 265 calories (54% from fat, 9% from protein, 38% from carbohydrate); 6 g protein; 16 g total fat; 9 g saturated fat; 4 g monounsaturated fat; 1 g polyunsaturated fat; 25 g carbohydrate; 3 g fiber; 2 g sugar; 136 mg phosphorus; 47 mg calcium; 169 mg sodium; 735 mg potassium; 521 IU vitamin A; 136 mg ATE vitamin E; 30 mg vitamin C; 43 mg cholesterol

Pineapple Sweet Potato Pudding

This would make a great pie or dessert, but it's also a perfect side dish for turkey or pork. The natural sweetness of the potatoes is enhanced by the pineapple and spices without reaching that overly sweet line that many sweet potato casseroles cross.

1 cup (250 g) egg substitute, or 4 eggs, beaten

1 cup (235 ml) skim milk

½ cup (225 g) unsalted butter, softened

6 cups (1350 g) mashed cooked sweet potato

1 teaspoon vanilla extract

1 teaspoon ground cinnamon

½ teaspoon nutmeg

½ teaspoon lemon extract

8 ounces (225 g) sliced pineapple, drained

¼ cup (28 g) chopped pecans

(continued on page 296)

Coat the inside of a 3-quart (3-L) slow cooker with cooking spray. In a large bowl, combine the eggs, milk, butter, sweet potato, vanilla, cinnamon, nutmeg, and lemon extract. Transfer to the slow cooker. Top with the pineapple slices and sprinkle with the pecans. Cover and cook on low for 4 to 5 hours, or until a knife inserted in the center comes out clean.

Yield: 12 servings

Per serving: 246 calories (37% from fat, 9% from protein, 53% from carbohydrate); 6 g protein; 10 g total fat; 5 g saturated fat; 3 g monounsaturated fat; 1 g polyunsaturated fat; 33 g carbohydrate; 5 g fiber; 12 g sugar; 111 mg phosphorus; 94 mg calcium; 91 mg sodium; 517 mg potassium; 26225 IU vitamin A; 76 mg ATE vitamin E; 23 mg vitamin C; 21 mg cholesterol

Beefy Rice Casserole

Similar to some of the packaged rice mixes, but with better taste and a LOT less sodium. You could make this on the stove if you had a half hour to wait or you can take this solution and turn it over to the slow cooker. The nice thing is that the rice is almost foolproof done this way.

1 cup (190 g) long-cooking rice

2 tablespoons (16 g) Onion Soup Mix (page 34)

4 ounces (112 g) mushrooms, sliced

3 cups (705 ml) Low-Sodium Beef Broth (page 231)

2 tablespoons (28 g) unsalted butter

Coat the inside of a 3-quart (3-L) slow cooker with cooking spray. Combine all the ingredients together in the slow cooker. Cover and cook on low for 3 hours, or until the rice is tender.

Yield: 4 servings

Per serving: 126 calories (45% from fat, 13% from protein, 42% from carbohydrate); 4 g protein; 6 g total fat; 4 g saturated fat; 2 g monounsaturated fat; 0 g polyunsaturated fat; 13 g carbohydrate; 1 g fiber; 1 g sugar; 66 mg phosphorus; 21 mg calcium; 111 mg sodium; 202 mg potassium; 177 IU vitamin A; 48 mg ATE vitamin E; 1 mg vitamin C; 15 mg cholesterol

Go Wild with Rice

Brown and wild rice rival the flavor of the high-sodium mixes on the grocery shelf. And they're even easier to fix using the slow cooker. This makes a lot of rice. Freeze the leftovers in meal-size portions in 1-quart (1-L) resealable plastic bags and all you need to do is pull one out, poke a little hole in it, and pop it in the microwave for a few minutes.

2¼ cups (530 ml) water

4 cups (940 ml) Low-Sodium Beef Broth (page 231)

2 tablespoons (16 g) Onion Soup Mix (page 34)

8 ounces (225 g) mushrooms, chopped

½ cup (225 g) unsalted butter, melted

1 cup (190 g) uncooked brown rice

1 cup (190 g) uncooked wild rice

Coat the inside of a 3-quart (3-L) slow cooker with cooking spray. Combine all the ingredients together in the slow cooker. Cover and cook on low for 3 hours, or until the rice is tender.

Yield: 12 servings

Per serving: 143 calories (50% from fat, 11% from protein, 39% from carbohydrate); 4 g protein; 8 g total fat; 5 g saturated fat; 2 g monounsaturated fat; 0 g polyunsaturated fat; 14 g carbohydrate; 1 g fiber; 1 g sugar; 99 mg phosphorus; 13 mg calcium; 50 mg sodium; 175 mg potassium; 239 IU vitamin A; 63 mg ATE vitamin E; 0 mg vitamin C; 20 mg cholesterol

Slow Cooker Creamy Rice

Creamy, cheesy rice cooks without any help from you. Swiss cheese, onion, and garlic provide the flavor base that makes this rice special.

3 cups (495 g) cooked rice

½ cup (125 g) egg substitute, or 2 eggs, lightly beaten

12 ounces (355 ml) nonfat evaporated milk

4 ounces (112 g) Swiss cheese, shredded

1 cup (160 g) chopped onion

½ cup (30 g) minced fresh parsley

6 tablespoons (90 ml) water

2 tablespoons (30 ml) canola oil

½ teaspoon minced garlic

¼ teaspoon freshly ground black pepper

Coat the inside of a 3-quart (3-L) slow cooker with cooking spray. Combine all the ingredients together in the slow cooker. Cover and cook on low for 2½ to 3 hours, or until a knife inserted in the center comes out clean.

Yield: 8 servings

Per serving: 241 calories (42% from fat, 18% from protein, 40% from carbohydrate); 11 g protein; 11 g total fat; 5 g saturated fat; 4 g monounsaturated fat; 2 g polyunsaturated fat; 24 g carbohydrate; 1 g fiber; 1 g sugar; 224 mg phosphorus; 272 mg calcium; 76 mg sodium; 268 mg potassium; 661 IU vitamin A; 77 mg ATE vitamin E; 7 mg vitamin C; 26 mg cholesterol

Tip: Have rice already frozen? Just break it up and put it in, checking the temperature to make sure everything has cooked properly.

Creamy Vegetable Salad

Broccoli, cauliflower, and peas form the basis for this salad. The creamy dressing is given an extra kick from horseradish, making it the perfect accompaniment to roast beef.

4 cups (280 g) broccoli florets

4 cups (400 g) cauliflower florets

10 ounces (280 g) no-salt-added frozen peas, thawed

¼ cup (25 g) sliced scallion

½ cup (115 g) sour cream

½ cup (112 g) mayonnaise

1 tablespoon (15 g) prepared horseradish

⅛ teaspoon freshly ground black pepper

(continued on page 298)

In a large bowl, combine the broccoli, cauliflower, peas, and scallion. In a small bowl, combine the sour cream, mayonnaise, horseradish, and pepper. Pour over the vegetables and toss to coat. Cover and refrigerate for several hours or overnight.

Yield: 9 servings

Per serving: 97 calories (38% from fat, 17% from protein, 46% from carbohydrate); 4 g protein; 4 g total fat; 1 g saturated fat; 1 g monounsaturated fat; 2 g polyunsaturated fat; 12 g carbohydrate; 4 g fiber; 3 g sugar; 79 mg phosphorus; 53 mg calcium; 70 mg sodium; 279 mg potassium; 1695 IU vitamin A; 13 mg ATE vitamin E; 59 mg vitamin C; 8 mg cholesterol

Make-Ahead Salad

Filled with vegetables that won't get soggy sitting in the dressing, this salad can be made well in advance and kept in the refrigerator until ready to serve. The dressing is a variation of a typical Italian vinaigrette.

2½ cups (250 g) cauliflower florets

2 cups (140 g) sliced mushrooms

1½ cups (105 g) broccoli florets

1½ cups (195 g) sliced carrot

1½ cups (180 g) sliced yellow squash

½ cup (120 ml) olive oil

½ cup (120 ml) cider vinegar

2 teaspoons sugar

1 teaspoon dillweed

½ teaspoon garlic powder

½ teaspoon freshly ground black pepper

In a large bowl, combine the vegetables; set aside. In a jar with a tight-fitting lid, combine the oil, vinegar, sugar, dillweed, garlic powder, and pepper and shake well. Pour over the vegetables and toss gently. Cover and refrigerate for 8 hours or overnight. Salad will keep in the refrigerator for at least a week.

Yield: 12 servings

Per serving: 105 calories (74% from fat, 6% from protein, 20% from carbohydrate); 2 g protein; 9 g total fat; 1 g saturated fat; 7 g monounsaturated fat; 1 g polyunsaturated fat; 6 g carbohydrate; 2 g fiber; 3 g sugar; 38 mg phosphorus; 21 mg calcium; 22 mg sodium; 220 mg potassium; 2233 IU vitamin A; 0 mg ATE vitamin E; 24 mg vitamin C; 0 mg cholesterol

Marinated Onions

These subtly flavored onions are great as a side dish or on salads and sandwiches. They keep for a nice long time in the refrigerator, and they don't require any preparation other than peeling and slicing the onions and putting them in the dressing.

¾ cup (150 g) sugar

¾ cup (180 ml) canola oil

¼ cup (60 ml) vinegar

⅛ teaspoon freshly ground black pepper

5 cups (800 g) sliced sweet onions, such as Vidalia

In a large bowl, combine the sugar, oil, vinegar, and pepper. Add the onions and toss to coat. Cover and refrigerate for 24 hours, stirring occasionally. Store in sealed jars in the refrigerator for up to 2 months.

Yield: 20 servings, ¼ cup (40 g) per serving

Per serving: 119 calories (60% from fat, 1% from protein, 38% from carbohydrate); 0 g protein; 8 g total fat; 1 g saturated fat; 5 g monounsaturated fat; 2 g polyunsaturated fat; 12 g carbohydrate; 1 g fiber; 9 g sugar; 11 mg phosphorus; 9 mg calcium; 1 mg sodium; 61 mg potassium; 1 IU vitamin A; 0 mg ATE vitamin E; 3 mg vitamin C; 0 mg cholesterol

Pickled Peppers

Try these and like Peter Piper you'll want a whole peck. And they are low enough in sodium that a peck wouldn't hurt you. I like them on salads to add a little extra crunch and flavor. They also work well on sandwiches.

1 cup (150 g) 1-inch (2.5-cm) pieces green bell pepper

1 cup (150 g) 1-inch (2.5-cm) pieces red bell pepper

1 cup (150 g) 1-inch (2.5-cm) pieces yellow bell pepper

1 cup (160 g) thinly sliced red onion

1 cup (235 ml) cider vinegar

1 cup (200 g) sugar

⅓ cup (80 ml) water

2 teaspoons mixed pickling spices

½ teaspoon celery seed

In a large glass bowl, combine the peppers and onion; set aside. In a saucepan, combine the vinegar, sugar, and water. Place the pickling spices and celery seed in a double thickness of cheesecloth; bring up the corners of cloth and tie with string to form a bag. Add to the saucepan. Bring to a boil over high heat; boil for 1 minute. Transfer the spice bag to the pepper mixture. Pour the vinegar mixture over all. Cover and refrigerate for 24 hours, stirring occasionally. Discard the spice bag. Store in sealed jars in the refrigerator for up to 1 month.

Yield: 16 servings, ¼ cup (40 g) per serving

Per serving: 63 calories (1% from fat, 2% from protein, 96% from carbohydrate); 0 g protein; 0 g total fat; 0 g saturated fat; 0 g monounsaturated fat; 0 g polyunsaturated fat; 16 g carbohydrate; 1 g fiber; 15 g sugar; 11 mg phosphorus; 7 mg calcium; 1 mg sodium; 91 mg potassium; 350 IU vitamin A; 0 mg ATE vitamin E; 47 mg vitamin C; 0 mg cholesterol

Stewed Apples

Dried apples are cooked in sweetened orange juice to produce a real treat. They make a perfect simple side dish for pork as is, but are also good over ice cream for dessert.

9 ounces (250 g) dried apples

1 cup (235 ml) orange juice

1 cup (235 ml) water

½ cup (120 ml) maple syrup

1 tablespoon (15 ml) lemon juice

(continued on page 300)

Coat the inside of a 3-quart (3-L) slow cooker with cooking spray. Place the apples in the slow cooker. Combine the orange juice, water, maple syrup, and lemon juice in a small bowl and pour over. Cover and cook on low for 8 hours, until apples are soft.

Yield: 6 servings

Per serving: 109 calories (2% from fat, 2% from protein, 97% from carbohydrate); 0 g protein; 0 g total fat; 0 g saturated fat; 0 g monounsaturated fat; 0 g polyunsaturated fat; 28 g carbohydrate; 1 g fiber; 20 g sugar; 10 mg phosphorus; 25 mg calcium; 4 mg sodium; 175 mg potassium; 49 IU vitamin A; 0 mg ATE vitamin E; 17 mg vitamin C; 0 mg cholesterol

Tip: These are great warm, right out of the slow cooker, but the leftovers are also good cold.

22

Fix-It-in-15 Desserts and Sweet Things

The slow cooker can also help you with dessert. (If you are like me, there are days when you wish you had one more slow cooker.) There are slow-cooked cakes and fruit recipes here, as well as some that you can put in the oven and bake while you are doing other things. And finally, there is a delightful banana and pineapple frozen dessert that will keep in the freezer until you want it.

Berry Cobbler

Another one of those classic comfort foods, this is a great dessert to make when fresh berries are in season. I probably shouldn't suggest having it with ice cream, but the idea is sure to occur to you even if a don't. It's also good just the way it is or with a little milk poured over it.

1¼ cups (150 g) all-purpose flour, divided

1 cup plus 2 tablespoons (225 g) sugar, divided

1 teaspoon sodium-free baking powder

¼ teaspoon ground cinnamon

¼ cup (63 g) egg substitute, or 1 egg, lightly beaten

¼ cup (60 ml) skim milk

2 tablespoons (30 ml) canola oil

2 cups (250 g) raspberries

2 cups (290 g) blueberries

Coat the inside of a 5-quart (5-L) slow cooker with cooking spray. In a large bowl, combine 1 cup (120 g) of the flour, 2 tablespoons (25 g) of the sugar, the baking powder, and the cinnamon. In a small bowl, combine the egg, milk, and oil; stir into the dry ingredients just until moistened (the batter will be thick). Spread the batter evenly on the bottom of the slow cooker. In a large bowl, combine the remaining ¼ cup (30 g) flour and the remaining 1 cup (200 g) sugar; add the berries and toss to coat. Spread over the batter. Cover and cook on high for 2 to 2½ hours, or until a toothpick inserted into the center comes out clean.

Yield: 8 servings

Per serving: 258 calories (14% from fat, 6% from protein, 80% from carbohydrate); 4 g protein; 4 g total fat; 0 g saturated fat; 2 g monounsaturated fat; 1 g polyunsaturated fat; 53 g carbohydrate; 3 g fiber; 33 g sugar; 95 mg phosphorus; 56 mg calcium; 19 mg sodium; 199 mg potassium; 74 IU vitamin A; 5 mg ATE vitamin E; 12 mg vitamin C; 0 mg cholesterol

Slow-Baked Apples

This is a classic fall dessert. This version is sweetened with brown sugar and contains dried apricots instead of the more common raisins. Put it in the slow cooker and go run your errands (or go to soccer or football practice) and have a delicious, healthy dessert ready for dinner. Serve with granola and caramel topping, if desired.

6 apples, good baking varieties such as Granny Smith, Fuji, or Winesap

2 teaspoons lemon juice

⅓ cup (35 g) chopped pecans

¼ cup (33 g) chopped dried apricots

¼ cup (60 g) packed brown sugar

3 tablespoons (42 g) unsalted butter, melted

¾ teaspoon ground cinnamon

¼ teaspoon nutmeg

2 cups (470 ml) water

Coat the inside of a 6-quart (6-L) slow cooker with cooking spray. Core the apples and peel the top third of each; brush the peeled portions with the lemon juice. Place in the slow cooker. Combine the pecans, apricots, brown sugar, butter, cinnamon, and nutmeg in a bowl. Place a heaping tablespoonful (15 g) of mixture inside each apple. Pour the water around the apples. Cover and cook on low for 3 to 4 hours, or until the apples are tender.

Yield: 6 servings

Per serving: 195 calories (45% from fat, 2% from protein, 53% from carbohydrate); 1 g protein; 10 g total fat; 4 g saturated fat; 4 g monounsaturated fat; 2 g polyunsaturated fat; 28 g carbohydrate; 3 g fiber; 23 g sugar; 37 mg phosphorus; 25 mg calcium; 5 mg sodium; 194 mg potassium; 402 IU vitamin A; 48 mg ATE vitamin E; 7 mg vitamin C; 15 mg cholesterol

Slow Cooker Apple Crisp

Easy to fix and a real family pleaser, this is a recipe that I make often. It's perfect when apples are in season, but you can now get good cooking apples any time of the year. Using granola for the topping makes preparation even easier. Serve with whipped topping, if desired.

4 apples, peeled and sliced, good cooking varieties such as Granny Smith, Fuji, or Winesap

2 cups (480 g) granola

¼ cup (80 g) honey

2 tablespoons (28 g) unsalted butter, melted

1 teaspoon ground cinnamon

½ teaspoon nutmeg

Coat the inside of a 3- to 4-quart (3- to 4-L) slow cooker with cooking spray. In the slow cooker, combine the apples and granola. In a small bowl, combine the honey, butter, cinnamon, and nutmeg; pour over the apple mixture. Cover and cook on low for 6 to 8 hours, or until the apples are tender.

Yield: 6 servings

Per serving: 226 calories (20% from fat, 4% from protein, 76% from carbohydrate); 3 g protein; 5 g total fat; 3 g saturated fat; 2 g monounsaturated fat; 0 g polyunsaturated fat; 45 g carbohydrate; 3 g fiber; 29 g sugar; 87 mg phosphorus; 21 mg calcium; 105 mg sodium; 165 mg potassium; 152 IU vitamin A; 32 mg ATE vitamin E; 4 mg vitamin C; 10 mg cholesterol

Sweet Sparkling Oranges

This make-ahead dessert or breakfast dish will win over even those members of your family who say they don't like oranges. Of course, the almonds and coconut help.

4 oranges

½ cup (100 g) sugar

½ cup (150 g) orange marmalade

1 cup (235 ml) white grape juice

½ cup (120 ml) lemon-lime soda

(continued on page 304)

3 tablespoons (21 g) slivered almonds, toasted

3 tablespoons (15 g) flaked coconut, toasted

Place the orange sections in a large bowl. In a saucepan, combine the sugar and marmalade; cook over medium heat, stirring, until the sugar has dissolved. Remove from the heat. Stir in the grape juice and soda. Pour over the oranges and toss to coat. Cover and refrigerate overnight. Using a slotted spoon, transfer the oranges to a serving dish. Sprinkle with the almonds and coconut and serve.

Yield: 8 servings

Per serving: 194 calories (11% from fat, 4% from protein, 86% from carbohydrate); 2 g protein; 2 g total fat; 1 g saturated fat; 1 g monounsaturated fat; 0 g polyunsaturated fat; 44 g carbohydrate; 3 g fiber; 40 g sugar; 35 mg phosphorus; 57 mg calcium; 14 mg sodium; 246 mg potassium; 222 IU vitamin A; 0 mg ATE vitamin E; 50 mg vitamin C; 0 mg cholesterol

All-Afternoon Fudge Cake

Not all afternoon as in it takes that long to make it, but all afternoon as in it cooks that long. And the result is a delicious, fudgy cake, which is perfect with vanilla ice cream.

1¾ cup (395 g) packed brown sugar, divided

1 cup (120 g) all-purpose flour

6 tablespoons (45 g) cocoa powder, divided

2 teaspoons sodium-free baking powder

½ cup (120 ml) skim milk

2 tablespoons (28 g) unsalted butter, melted

½ teaspoon vanilla extract

1½ cups (263 g) chocolate chips

1¾ cups (411 ml) boiling water

Coat the inside of a 3-quart (3-L) slow cooker with cooking spray. In a small bowl, combine 1 cup (225 g) of the brown sugar, the flour, 3 tablespoons (22 g) of the cocoa, and the baking powder. In another bowl, combine the milk, butter, and vanilla; stir into the dry ingredients just until combined. Spread evenly in the bottom of the slow cooker. Sprinkle with the chocolate chips. In another small bowl, combine the remaining ¾ cup (170 g) brown sugar and the remaining 3 tablespoons (22 g) cocoa; add the boiling water and stir until dissolved. Pour over the batter. Do not stir. Cover and cook on high for 4 to 4½ hours, or until a toothpick inserted near the center of the cake comes out clean.

Yield: 10 servings

Per serving: 360 calories (25% from fat, 5% from protein, 70% from carbohydrate); 4 g protein; 10 g total fat; 5 g saturated fat; 4 g monounsaturated fat; 0 g polyunsaturated fat; 65 g carbohydrate; 2 g fiber; 50 g sugar; 181 mg phosphorus; 149 mg calcium; 45 mg sodium; 414 mg potassium; 140 IU vitamin A; 39 mg ATE vitamin E; 0 mg vitamin C; 12 mg cholesterol

Slow Cooker Lemon Cake

Baking cakes in the slow cooker is not something I had done before starting to think about easier way to prepare home cooked meals. Once I'd tried it I realized what I'd been missing. Cakes such as this delightfully flavored lemon cake with poppy seeds come out moist and perfectly cooked with almost no effort at all.

1¾ cups (210 g) all-purpose flour

½ cup (70 g) cornmeal

1 teaspoon sodium-free baking powder

1 teaspoon sodium-free baking soda

¾ cup (170 g) unsalted butter, at room temperature

1½ cups (300 g) sugar, divided

½ cup (125 g) egg substitute, or 2 eggs

1 cup (230 g) sour cream

½ teaspoon vanilla extract

1 tablespoon (6 g) lemon zest

1 teaspoon poppy seeds

3 tablespoons (45 ml) lemon juice

In a bowl, combine the flour, cornmeal, baking powder, and baking soda. With a mixer, and in another bowl, beat the butter and 1¼ cups (250 g) of the sugar on medium-high speed until smooth. Add the eggs and beat until fluffy, 2 minutes. Add the sour cream, vanilla, lemon zest, and poppy seeds and beat to combine. Reduce the speed to low and slowly incorporate the flour mixture. Place a piece of parchment paper inside a slow cooker, letting the excess come up the sides. Scrape the batter into the slow cooker. Cover and cook on high for about 2½ hours, until set and a toothpick inserted in the center comes out clean. Combine the lemon juice and the remaining ¼ cup (50 g) sugar in a bowl and drizzle evenly over the top of the cake. Holding the parchment paper, transfer the cake to a rack. Let cool for at least 15 minutes.

Yield: 8 servings

Per serving: 489 calories (40% from fat, 5% from protein, 55% from carbohydrate); 7 g protein; 22 g total fat; 13 g saturated fat; 6 g monounsaturated fat; 1 g polyunsaturated fat; 68 g carbohydrate; 2 g fiber; 38 g sugar; 136 mg phosphorus; 84 mg calcium; 41 mg sodium; 214 mg potassium; 721 IU vitamin A; 173 mg ATE vitamin E; 4 mg vitamin C; 58 mg cholesterol

Blackberry Bread Pudding

This fruity bread pudding can be baked ahead of time or while you are eating dinner. The taste is excellent and the preparation time is mostly letting things stand so you aren't tied to the kitchen.

¾ cup (188 g) egg substitute, or 3 eggs, beaten

4 cups (940 ml) nonfat evaporated milk

2 cups (400 g) sugar

(continued on page 306)

1 tablespoon (15 ml) vanilla extract

2 cups (290 g) blackberries

12 slices Low-Sodium French Bread (page 314), cut into 1-inch (2.5-cm) cubes

Preheat the oven to 350°F (180°C, or gas mark 4). Grease a 9 × 13-inch (23 × 33-cm) baking dish. In a large bowl, combine the eggs, milk, sugar, and vanilla. Stir in the blueberries. Stir in the bread cubes; let stand for 15 minutes, or until the bread is softened. Transfer to the prepared baking dish. Bake, uncovered, for 50 to 60 minutes, or until a knife inserted near the center comes out clean. Let stand for 5 minutes before serving.

Yield: 12 servings

Per serving: 360 calories (20% from fat, 12% from protein, 69% from carbohydrate); 11 g protein; 8 g total fat; 4 g saturated fat; 3 g monounsaturated fat; 1 g polyunsaturated fat; 62 g carbohydrate; 2 g fiber; 36 g sugar; 226 mg phosphorus; 253 mg calcium; 119 mg sodium; 363 mg potassium; 403 IU vitamin A; 92 mg ATE vitamin E; 4 mg vitamin C; 25 mg cholesterol

Tip: You can substitute blueberries or strawberries for the blackberries.

Slow Cooker Pumpkin Pie

I admit it's not quite a pie, since it doesn't have a crust. But it tastes the same and has a lot less fat without one. And it cooks all day so you can throw it in the slow cooker in 5 minutes in the morning and have a great dessert ready in the evening.

1 can (15 ounces, or 420 g) pumpkin

12 ounces (355 ml) nonfat evaporated milk

¾ cup (150 g) sugar

½ cup (112 g) Buttermilk Baking Mix (page 27)

½ cup (125 g) egg substitute, or 2 eggs, beaten

2 tablespoons (28 g) unsalted butter, melted

2½ teaspoons pumpkin pie spice

2 teaspoons vanilla extract

Coat the inside of a 3- to 4-quart (3- to 4-L) slow cooker with cooking spray. Combine all the ingredients in a large bowl. Transfer to the slow cooker, cover, and cook on low for 6 to 7 hours or until a toothpick inserted into the center comes out clean.

Yield: 6 servings

Per serving: 297 calories (29% from fat, 11% from protein, 60% from carbohydrate); 8 g protein; 9 g total fat; 5 g saturated fat; 3 g monounsaturated fat; 1 g polyunsaturated fat; 43 g carbohydrate; 2 g fiber; 29 g sugar; 223 mg phosphorus; 201 mg calcium; 104 mg sodium; 411 mg potassium; 11452 IU vitamin A; 94 mg ATE vitamin E; 4 mg vitamin C; 27 mg cholesterol

Granola Bars

These chewy bars go together quickly and make a big batch that you can then use for breakfast or dessert. Sweetened with homey and packed with nuts and raisins in addition to the cereal, they are sure to please.

½ cup (225 g) unsalted butter, softened

1 cup (225 g) packed brown sugar

¼ cup (50 g) granulated sugar

2 tablespoons (40 g) honey

½ teaspoon vanilla extract

½ cup (125 g) egg substitute, or 2 eggs, beaten

1 cup (120 g) all-purpose flour

1 teaspoon ground cinnamon

½ teaspoon sodium-free baking powder

1½ cups (120 g) quick-cooking oats

1¼ cups (32 g) crispy rice cereal

1 cup (110 g) chopped pecans

1 cup (145 g) raisins

Preheat the oven to 350°F (180°C, or gas mark 4). Grease an 8 × 12-inch (20 × 30-cm) baking dish. In a large bowl, cream butter and sugars until light and fluffy. Add the honey, vanilla, and eggs; mix well. Combine the flour, cinnamon, and baking powder in a separate bowl; gradually add to the creamed mixture. Stir in the oats, cereal, nuts, and raisins. Press into the prepared baking pan. Bake for 25 to 30 minutes, or until the top is lightly browned. Cool on a wire rack. Cut into twenty-four 2 × 2-inch (5 × 5-cm) bars.

Yield: 24 servings

Per serving: 182 calories (37% from fat, 6% from protein, 58% from carbohydrate); 3 g protein; 8 g total fat; 3 g saturated fat; 3 g monounsaturated fat; 1 g polyunsaturated fat; 27 g carbohydrate; 1 g fiber; 17 g sugar; 68 mg phosphorus; 28 mg calcium; 27 mg sodium; 158 mg potassium; 161 IU vitamin A; 38 mg ATE vitamin E; 1 mg vitamin C; 10 mg cholesterol

Tip: Substitute chocolate chips for the raisins.

Banana Pineapple Sherbet

Sometimes you want something sweet but not too heavy, after a big meal. This frozen fruity concoction serves that purpose perfectly. And the recipe makes a big batch that can stay in the freezer until needed.

3 cups (705 ml) water

2½ cup (563 g) mashed bananas

1½ cups (300 g) sugar

20 ounces (560 g) crushed pineapple, undrained

6 ounces (170 g) orange juice concentrate, thawed

In a 2-quart (1.8-L) freezer container, combine all the ingredients. Cover and freeze for 5 hours or overnight. Remove from the freezer 15 minutes before serving.

Yield: 12 servings

Per serving: 186 calories (1% from fat, 2% from protein, 97% from carbohydrate); 1 g protein; 0 g total fat; 0 g saturated fat; 0 g monounsaturated fat; 0 g polyunsaturated fat; 48 g carbohydrate; 2 g fiber; 42 g sugar; 22 mg phosphorus; 15 mg calcium; 3 mg sodium; 313 mg potassium; 102 IU vitamin A; 0 mg ATE vitamin E; 27 mg vitamin C; 0 mg cholesterol

23

The Joys of the Bread Machine

Last, but certainly not least, bread. I would have to say that the bread machine is probably the most useful tool or appliance I have had in maintaining a low-sodium lifestyle. Bread is one of those sneaky sodium things. Each slice does not have a *lot*, maybe 200 to 300 mg. But before you know it, if you aren't careful, you've added 1000 mg to your diet in one day.

I got my current bread machine for Christmas five years ago. It was not a terribly expensive model, around $80 at the time, but even so it has a lot of capabilities that I never use. The one nice feature I do like is that it has an automatic dispenser for adding things such as fruit and nuts at the right time. I've made at least one loaf of bread almost every week since I've had it, and many weeks I've made more than one loaf or additional rolls, bagels, or some other bread. If you take that average as one loaf per week and figure that the ingredients are probably at least a dollar cheaper than buying a loaf of commercial bread other than the ones that look and taste like cotton fluff, that is $250 saved over the course of five years, more than three times the cost of the machine. If you calculate the sodium saved at 200 mg per slice, 12 slices per loaf, one loaf per week, that's more than 120,000 mg of sodium that my family did not eat! And that's not even mentioning the wonderful smell and taste of homemade bread.

Making bread in a bread machine is incredibly simple and almost foolproof. You dump the ingredients in, turn it on, and come back a couple of hours later to freshly baked bread. The only other things you may have to do are add other ingredients about 20 minutes into the cycle, if your machine doesn't have the automatic dispenser I mentioned, and check the consistency of the dough about 5 to 7 minutes after you start it. If you are really pressed for time, you can skip that last step, but you do run the risk of ending up with bread that does not have the ideal texture.

Flour from wheat grown in different locations can require variations in the flour-to-water ratio. The time of year you use flour can also affect this ratio; flour tends to be drier and need more water in the winter. The dough should form a smooth ball and not be sticky (too little flour) or lumpy (too little liquid). I've sometimes had to add as much as ¼ cup (30 g) of additional flour or (60 ml) water until it looks right.

All the recipes in this chapter were made using a bread machine and instant yeast, also known as bread machine yeast. If you are using active dry yeast it's best to activate it with warm water as described below. Any of these recipes can also be made without a bread machine. You'll have the same delicious, healthy bread, but you'll have to spend more time mixing, kneading, and shaping. The following general procedures should get you started.

Bread machines generally have you put all the liquid ingredients in, then all the dry, although some do it the other way around. Most keep the yeast separate from the liquid until the kneading. When making bread by hand, however, start with the yeast, liquid, and sugar, then add the other ingredients except the flour, and finally add the flour. Most recipes not designed for a bread machine give you a range of flour; sometimes you need more, sometimes less. So you might want to start with ¼ to ½ cup (30 to 60 g) less than the recipe calls for and then add more until the dough reaches the right consistency.

Start with warm water or whatever liquid the recipe calls for. Around 85°F (29°C) is about right. The idea is to get the liquid warm enough so the yeast grows, but not so warm that it kills it. Mix the wet ingredients and yeast together with a spoon. Stir in the flour until it gets too stiff to stir. Dump it out onto a floured counter and knead until the surface is smooth, adding more flour if the dough is too sticky.

Grease a large bowl. Grease the top of the dough by placing it into the greased bowl, then turning it over so the greased part is on top and the ungreased part is on the bottom. Cover with a cloth and put someplace warm to rise until doubled in size.

When the dough has doubled, punch it down, form into a loaf by kneading and shaping it, then put in a greased loaf pan or on a greased baking sheet. Let rise until almost doubled in size, then place in a preheated 375°F (190°C, or gas mark 5) oven and bake until done, usually when the loaf sounds hollow when tapped on the bottom.

This, of course, is just one way to make bread by hand. It follows the traditional way of doing it. You can find many other methods, including some that reduce the amount of kneading by combining some of the ingredients with a mixer or food processor. Generally speaking, you can use any recipe or method that you like, simply substituting the ingredients.

Old-Time White Bread

If you had a grandmother who made bread, this will remind you of it. This is a great general purpose bread and is a recipe I make often.

4 cups (480 g) bread flour

½ cup (60 g) nonfat dry milk

1½ teaspoons instant yeast

¼ cups (295 ml) water

2 tablespoons (28 g) unsalted butter

1 tablespoon (20 g) honey

Place all of the ingredients into the pan of your machine in the order specified by the manufacturer. Program the machine for the white bread cycle, and press Start.

Yield: 12 servings

Per serving: 199 calories (12% from fat, 14% from protein, 74% from carbohydrate); 7 g protein; 3 g total fat; 1 g saturated fat; 1 g monounsaturated fat; 0 g polyunsaturated fat; 36 g carbohydrate; 1 g fiber; 3 g sugar; 79 mg phosphorus; 43 mg calcium; 18 mg sodium; 105 mg potassium; 127 IU vitamin A; 36 mg ATE vitamin E; 0 mg vitamin C; 6 mg cholesterol

100% Whole Wheat Bread

This recipe makes a fairly firm loaf. The sesame seeds give it a nutty flavor. It's good toasted or for sandwiches.

3½ cups (420 g) whole wheat flour

¼ cup (32 g) sesame seeds

1 tablespoon (6 g) vital wheat gluten

1½ teaspoons instant yeast

¼ cup (80 g) honey

1¼ cups (295 ml) water

2 tablespoons (30 ml) olive oil

Place all the ingredients into the pan of your bread machine in the order specified by the manufacturer. Program the machine for the white bread cycle, and press Start.

Yield: 12 servings

Per serving: 179 calories (21% from fat, 12% from protein, 67% from carbohydrate); 6 g protein; 4 g total fat; 1 g saturated fat; 2 g monounsaturated fat; 1 g polyunsaturated fat; 32 g carbohydrate; 5 g fiber; 6 g sugar; 147 mg phosphorus; 42 mg calcium; 3 mg sodium; 169 mg potassium; 3 IU vitamin A; 0 mg ATE vitamin E; 0 mg vitamin C; 0 mg cholesterol

Nutty Wheat Bread

This loaf features the rich flavors of both wheat and pecans. Try it in a peanut butter sandwich for a real treat.

2 cups (240 g) bread flour

1 cup (120 hg) whole wheat flour

1 cup (110 g) chopped pecans

3 tablespoons (45 g) packed dark brown sugar

2 teaspoons instant yeast

(continued on page 312)

2⅛ cups (270 ml) water

2 tablespoons (28 g) unsalted butter

Place all the ingredients into the pan of your bread machine in the order specified by the manufacturer. Program the machine for the white bread cycle, and press Start.

Yield: 12 servings

Per serving: 210 calories (38% from fat, 10% from protein, 53% from carbohydrate); 5 g protein; 9 g total fat; 2 g saturated fat; 4 g monounsaturated fat; 2 g polyunsaturated fat; 28 g carbohydrate; 3 g fiber; 4 g sugar; 91 mg phosphorus; 15 mg calcium; 2 mg sodium; 115 mg potassium; 66 IU vitamin A; 16 mg ATE vitamin E; 0 mg vitamin C; 5 mg cholesterol

Multigrain Bread

This bread is sweet, with a light color. It makes great sandwiches.

¾ cup (180 ml) skim milk

½ cup (120 ml) water

2 tablespoons (30 ml) canola oil

1½ tablespoons (30 g) honey

2 tablespoons (18 g) raisins

2 tablespoons (30 g) packed dark brown sugar

1½ cups (180 g) bread flour

1¼ cups (150 g) whole wheat flour

¾ cup (90 g) rye flour

2 teaspoons instant yeast

In a blender, blend the milk, water, oil, honey, raisins, and brown sugar. Put this mixture, along with the flours and yeast, into the pan of your bread machine in the order specified by the manufacturer. Program the machine for the white bread cycle, and press Start.

Yield: 12 servings

Per serving: 177 calories (15% from fat, 12% from protein, 74% from carbohydrate); 5 g protein; 3 g total fat; 0 g saturated fat; 1 g monounsaturated fat; 1 g polyunsaturated fat; 33 g carbohydrate; 3 g fiber; 5 g sugar; 100 mg phosphorus; 32 mg calcium; 11 mg sodium; 138 mg potassium; 33 IU vitamin A; 9 mg ATE vitamin E; 0 mg vitamin C; 0 mg cholesterol

Honey Granola Bread

I love this bread toasted, sometimes without anything on it. The sweet taste and crunchy texture are all I really need. But if you want a really special treat, put a little honey on it to bring out the flavor even more.

2⅔ cups (320 g) bread flour

⅓ cup (40 g) whole wheat flour

½ cup (60 g) granola

¼ cup (30 g) nonfat dry milk

2¼ teaspoons instant yeast

1¼ cups (295 ml) water

¼ cup (80 g) honey

1 tablespoon (14 g) unsalted butter

1 teaspoon lemon juice

Place all the ingredients into the pan of your bread machine in the order specified by the manufacturer. Program the machine for the white bread cycle, and press Start.

Yield: 12 servings

Per serving: 172 calories (9% from fat, 12% from protein, 79% from carbohydrate); 5 g protein; 2 g total fat; 1 g saturated fat; 0 g monounsaturated fat; 0 g polyunsaturated fat; 34 g carbohydrate; 1 g fiber; 8 g sugar; 75 mg phosphorus; 26 mg calcium; 23 mg sodium; 97 mg potassium; 64 IU vitamin A; 18 mg ATE vitamin E; 0 mg vitamin C; 3 mg cholesterol

Oatmeal Bread

This tender bread is just slightly sweet. Great for breakfast or for toasting. This is another bread that I make often. It has a flavor that I never get tired of and can be used with any kind of sandwich or meal.

3 cups (360 g) bread flour

1 cup (80 g) rolled oats

3 tablespoons (45 g) packed brown sugar

2 teaspoons instant yeast

2 tablespoons (28 g) unsalted butter

1¼ cups (295 ml) skim milk, lukewarm

¾ cup (110 g) raisins (optional)

Place all the ingredients (except the raisins, if using) into the pan of your bread machine in the order specified by the manufacturer. Program the machine for the white bread cycle, and press Start. Add the raisins at the

beep or about 3 minutes before the end of the second kneading cycle.

Yield: 12 servings

Per serving: 223 calories (12% from fat, 12% from protein, 76% from carbohydrate); 7 g protein; 3 g total fat; 1 g saturated fat; 1 g monounsaturated fat; 0 g polyunsaturated fat; 43 g carbohydrate; 2 g fiber; 10 g sugar; 114 mg phosphorus; 54 mg calcium; 19 mg sodium; 208 mg potassium; 112 IU vitamin A; 31 mg ATE vitamin E; 1 mg vitamin C; 6 mg cholesterol

French Bread

The simple flavor of French bread in an easy-to-make bread machine loaf.

4 cups (480 g) all-purpose flour

2½ teaspoons instant yeast

1½ cups (355 ml) water, at about 105°F (40°C)

Place all the ingredients into the pan of your bread machine in the order specified by the manufacturer. Program the machine for the French bread cycle if available or white bread cycle if not, and press Start.

Yield: 12 servings

Per serving: 154 calories (3% from fat, 12% from protein, 85% from carbohydrate); 5 g protein; 0 g total fat; 0 g saturated fat; 0 g monounsaturated fat; 0 g polyunsaturated fat; 32 g carbohydrate; 1 g fiber; 0 g sugar; 56 mg phosphorus; 7 mg calcium; 2 mg sodium; 61 mg potassium; 0 IU vitamin A; 0 mg ATE vitamin E; 0 mg vitamin C; 0 mg cholesterol

(continued on page 314)

Tip: For a more traditional French loaf process the bread on the dough cycle. When the cycle has finished remove it from the pan, punch it down and shape it into a loaf about 12 inches (30.5 cm) long with tapered ends. Sprinkle a greased baking sheet with cornmeal. Place the loaf on the baking sheet, cover and let rise until doubled, about 25 minutes. With a sharp knife, make diagonal slashes 2 inches (5 cm) apart across the top of loaf. Bake at 375°F (190°C, or gas mark 5) for 25 to 30 minutes or until golden brown.

Italian Bread

Italian seasoning adds flavor to this loaf, which has the dense texture of traditional Italian breads. It's the perfect accompaniment to pasta and other Italian meals. The flavor of the herbs also goes well with salads and soups.

2 cups (240 g) semolina

2 cups (240 g) bread flour

4 teaspoons Italian seasoning

2 teaspoons instant yeast

1¾ cups (415 ml) warm water

2 tablespoons (30 ml) olive oil

1 tablespoon (20 g) honey

Place all the ingredients into the pan of your bread machine in the order specified by the manufacturer. Program the machine for the white bread cycle, light crust setting, and press Start.

Yield: 12 servings

Per serving: 211 calories (13% from fat, 13% from protein, 74% from carbohydrate); 7 g protein;

3 g total fat; 0 g saturated fat; 2 g monounsaturated fat; 1 g polyunsaturated fat; 39 g carbohydrate; 2 g fiber; 2 g sugar; 69 mg phosphorus; 15 mg calcium; 2 mg sodium; 94 mg potassium; 23 IU vitamin A; 0 mg ATE vitamin E; 0 mg vitamin C; 0 mg cholesterol

Tip: Semolina is a hard wheat flour that is often used to make pasta. It can be found in supermarkets that have a specialty grains section.

Almost Sourdough

If you love the taste of sourdough bread, but not the hassle of keeping the starter going, this bread is for you. The vinegar and sour cream give it just enough sourness without being overpowering.

3 cups (360 g) bread flour

1½ tablespoons (20 g) sugar

¼ teaspoon sodium-free baking soda

1¾ teaspoons instant yeast

¾ cup (170 g) sour cream

¾ cup (180 ml) skim milk

1½ tablespoons (22 ml) cider vinegar

All the ingredients should be at room temperature before starting. Place all the ingredients into the pan of your bread machine in the order specified by the manufacturer. Program the machine for the white bread cycle, and press Start.

Yield: 12 servings

Per serving: 157 calories (14% from fat, 14% from protein, 72% from carbohydrate); 5 g protein;

2 g total fat; 1 g saturated fat; 1 g monounsaturated fat; 0 g polyunsaturated fat; 28 g carbohydrate; 1 g fiber; 3 g sugar; 71 mg phosphorus; 41 mg calcium; 14 mg sodium; 91 mg potassium; 88 IU vitamin A; 24 mg ATE vitamin E; 0 mg vitamin C; 6 mg cholesterol

English Muffin Bread

If you want the texture and flavor of English muffins without the work, give this bread a try. It will give you traditional breakfast sandwiches that are both healthier and tastier than the ones you might buy from a fast-food place.

3½ cups (420 g) bread flour

2¼ teaspoons instant yeast

1½ teaspoons sugar

½ teaspoon sodium-free baking powder

1 cup (235 ml) skim milk

½ cup (120 ml) water

2 tablespoons (28 g) unsalted butter

1 teaspoon cider vinegar

Place all the ingredients into the pan of your bread machine in the order specified by the manufacturer. Program the machine for the white bread cycle, and press Start.

Yield: 12 servings

Per serving: 174 calories (14% from fat, 14% from protein, 72% from carbohydrate); 6 g protein; 3 g total fat; 1 g saturated fat; 1 g monounsaturated fat; 0 g polyunsaturated fat; 31 g carbohydrate; 1 g fiber; 1 g sugar; 86 mg phosphorus; 46 mg calcium; 14 mg sodium; 114 mg potassium; 102 IU vitamin A; 28 mg ATE vitamin E; 0 mg vitamin C; 5 mg cholesterol

Herb Bread

The sage and other herbs make this the perfect bread for turkey sandwiches. It is also a good start for making your own stuffing.

3 cups (360 g) bread flour

¼ cup (30 g) nonfat dry milk

1 tablespoon (12 g) sugar

2¼ teaspoons instant yeast

¾ teaspoon celery seed

¾ teaspoon caraway seed

¾ teaspoon crumbled sage

¾ teaspoon nutmeg

1 cup (235 ml) water

¼ cup (62 g) egg substitute, or 1 large egg

1 tablespoon (14 g) unsalted butter

1 teaspoon lemon juice

Place all the ingredients into the pan of your bread machine in the order specified by the manufacturer. Program the machine for white bread cycle, and press Start.

Yield: 12 servings

Per serving: 150 calories (11% from fat, 15% from protein, 74% from carbohydrate); 6 g protein; 2 g total fat; 1 g saturated fat; 0 g monounsaturated fat; 0 g polyunsaturated fat; 27 g carbohydrate; 1 g fiber; 2 g sugar; 65 mg phosphorus; 31 mg calcium; 18 mg sodium; 96 mg potassium; 86 IU vitamin A; 18 mg ATE vitamin E; 0 mg vitamin C; 3 mg cholesterol

Onion Bread

Another great sandwich bread. On the days when I have time, I also like to run this one using the dough cycle and shape it into hamburger rolls.

3¼ cups (390 g) bread flour

1 tablespoon (12 g) instant yeast

2 tablespoons (15 g) nonfat dry milk

2 tablespoons (30 g) packed brown sugar

1 teaspoon freshly ground black pepper

1 teaspoon poppy seeds

½ teaspoon onion powder

1¼ cups (295 ml) water

½ cup (80 g) minced onion

2 tablespoons (28 g) unsalted butter

Place all the ingredients into the pan of your bread machine in the order specified by the manufacturer. Program the machine for the white bread cycle, and press Start.

Yield: 12 servings

Per serving: 170 calories (14% from fat, 12% from protein, 73% from carbohydrate); 5 g protein; 3 g total fat; 1 g saturated fat; 1 g monounsaturated fat; 0 g polyunsaturated fat; 31 g carbohydrate; 1 g fiber; 3 g sugar; 61 mg phosphorus; 24 mg calcium; 7 mg sodium; 92 mg potassium; 77 IU vitamin A; 21 mg ATE vitamin E; 1 mg vitamin C; 5 mg cholesterol

Anadama Bread

Anadama bread is traditional New England bread with cornmeal; it has been around for more than 150 years.

2½ cups (300 g) bread flour

½ cup (60 g) whole wheat flour

⅓ cup (47 g) cornmeal

¼ cup (30 g) nonfat dry milk

2¼ teaspoons instant yeast

1¼ cups (295 ml) water

3 tablespoons (60 g) molasses

2 tablespoons (28 g) unsalted butter

1 teaspoon lemon juice

Place all the ingredients into the pan of your bread machine in the order specified by the manufacturer. Program the machine for the white bread cycle, and press Start.

Yield: 12 servings

Per serving: 174 calories (13% from fat, 12% from protein, 74% from carbohydrate); 5 g protein; 3 g total fat; 1 g saturated fat; 1 g monounsaturated fat; 0 g polyunsaturated fat; 32 g carbohydrate; 2 g fiber; 4 g sugar; 74 mg phosphorus; 36 mg calcium; 12 mg sodium; 172 mg potassium; 102 IU vitamin A; 26 mg ATE vitamin E; 0 mg vitamin C; 5 mg cholesterol

Challah

Challah is slightly sweet egg bread that is often found braided. This version skips that step and produces it directly in the bread machine to make it especially easy.

3 cups (360 g) bread flour

¼ cup (50 g) sugar

1½ teaspoons instant yeast

¾ cup (180 ml) skim milk

½ cup (125 g) egg substitute, or 2 eggs

3 tablespoons (42 g) unsalted butter

Place all the ingredients into the pan of your bread machine in the order specified by the manufacturer. Program the machine for the white bread cycle, light crust setting, and press Start.

Yield: 12 servings

Per serving: 182 calories (19% from fat, 14% from protein, 67% from carbohydrate); 6 g protein; 4 g total fat; 2 g saturated fat; 1 g monounsaturated fat; 1 g polyunsaturated fat; 30 g carbohydrate; 1 g fiber; 4 g sugar; 70 mg phosphorus; 34 mg calcium; 27 mg sodium; 108 mg potassium; 158 IU vitamin A; 33 mg ATE vitamin E; 0 mg vitamin C; 8 mg cholesterol

Golden Fall Bread

This honey-sweetened loaf gets its golden color from mashed sweet potato. It's great for toast and ideal for turkey or chicken sandwiches.

2½ cups (300 g) bread flour

1 cup (120 g) whole wheat flour

1 tablespoon (6 g) vital wheat gluten

2 teaspoons instant yeast

½ teaspoon ground cinnamon

¼ teaspoon nutmeg

¼ teaspoon ground ginger

¾ cup (180 ml) water

½ cup (112 g) mashed sweet potatoes

¼ cup (60 ml) skim milk

¼ cup (55 g) unsalted butter

3 tablespoons (60 g) honey

½ cup (75 g) raisins

½ cup (55 g) chopped pecans

Place all the ingredients except the raisins and nuts into the pan of your bread machine in the order specified by the manufacturer. Program the machine for the white bread cycle, and press Start. Add the raisins and nuts when the beeper goes off, or about 3 minutes before the end of the second kneading cycle.

Yield: 12 servings

Per serving: 246 calories (27% from fat, 9% from protein, 64% from carbohydrate); 5 g protein; 8 g total fat; 3 g saturated fat; 3 g monounsaturated fat; 1 g polyunsaturated fat; 41 g carbohydrate; 3 g fiber; 10 g sugar; 103 mg phosphorus; 28 mg calcium; 10 mg sodium; 198 mg potassium; 2288 IU vitamin A; 35 mg ATE vitamin E; 2 mg vitamin C; 10 mg cholesterol

Potato Rye Bread

Potatoes add extra moistness and fine texture to this flavorful bread. Use it for almost any kind of sandwich from poultry to pork to egg salad.

(continued on page 318)

2¼ cups (270 g) bread flour

¾ cup (90 g) rye flour

1½ tablespoons (20 g) sugar

2¼ teaspoons instant yeast

½ teaspoon freshly ground black pepper

1 tablespoon (7 g) caraway seeds

1 teaspoon dill seeds

1½ cups (355 ml) buttermilk

¾ cup (170 g) mashed potatoes

Place all the ingredients into the pan of your bread machine in the order specified by the manufacturer. Program the machine for the white bread cycle, and press Start.

Yield: 12 servings

Per serving: 154 calories (10% from fat, 14% from protein, 77% from carbohydrate); 5 g protein; 2 g total fat; 0 g saturated fat; 0 g monounsaturated fat; 0 g polyunsaturated fat; 29 g carbohydrate; 2 g fiber; 3 g sugar; 85 mg phosphorus; 52 mg calcium; 38 mg sodium; 141 mg potassium; 40 IU vitamin A; 8 mg ATE vitamin E; 2 mg vitamin C; 2 mg cholesterol

Hummus Bread

If you use commercial hummus, the sodium in this bread is more than most in the book, but still significantly less than commercial breads. I like it using the roasted red pepper hummus, which gives it a great flavor for meat sandwiches.

2 cups (240 g) bread flour

1 cup (120 g) whole wheat flour

⅓ cup (42 g) sesame seeds, toasted

½ teaspoons instant yeast

1½ teaspoons sugar

1 cup (250 g) hummus

¾ cup (180 ml) skim milk

¼ cup (60 ml) oil

¼ cup (62 g) egg substitute, or 1 large egg

Place all the ingredients into the pan of your bread machine in the order specified by the manufacturer. Program the machine for the white bread cycle, and press Start.

Yield: 12 servings

Per serving: 224 calories (35% from fat, 12% from protein, 53% from carbohydrate); 7 g protein; 9 g total fat; 1 g saturated fat; 3 g monounsaturated fat; 4 g polyunsaturated fat; 30 g carbohydrate; 3 g fiber; 1 g sugar; 139 mg phosphorus; 81 mg calcium; 69 mg sodium; 179 mg potassium; 52 IU vitamin A; 9 mg ATE vitamin E; 2 mg vitamin C; 0 mg cholesterol

South American Bread

Similar to breads found in Argentina and other parts of South America, this savory, slightly spicy bread is just what a roast beef sandwich needs.

3 cups (360 g) bread flour

3 tablespoons (21 g) wheat bran

3 tablespoons (30 g) chopped onion

3 tablespoons (12 g) chopped fresh parsley

1 tablespoon (12 g) sugar

¾ teaspoon dried oregano

½ teaspoon minced garlic

⅛ teaspoon cayenne pepper

1 cup (235 ml) water

3 tablespoons (45 ml) olive oil

1½ tablespoons (22 ml) white wine vinegar

1¾ teaspoons instant yeast

Place all the ingredients into the pan of your bread machine in the order specified by the manufacturer. Program the machine for the white bread cycle, and press Start.

Yield: 12 servings

Per serving: 163 calories (22% from fat, 11% from protein, 67% from carbohydrate); 5 g protein; 4 g total fat; 1 g saturated fat; 3 g monounsaturated fat; 1 g polyunsaturated fat; 27 g carbohydrate; 1 g fiber; 1 g sugar; 52 mg phosphorus; 10 mg calcium; 2 mg sodium; 68 mg potassium; 92 IU vitamin A; 0 mg ATE vitamin E; 1 mg vitamin C; 0 mg cholesterol

Tip: You can vary the flavor of this bread by changing the herbs. I like it with ½ teaspoon of cumin added. You can also make it spicier if desired by increasing the cayenne.

Sun-Dried Tomato Bread

This bread has a great flavor for sandwiches (like fresh from the garden tomatoes) and is also good toasted and served with egg dishes for breakfast.

3 cups (360 g) bread flour

¼ cup (25 g) grated Parmesan cheese

2 tablespoons (15 g) nonfat dry milk

1 tablespoon (12 g) sugar

2 teaspoons instant yeast

1 teaspoon dried basil

½ teaspoon freshly ground black pepper

1¼ cups (295 ml) water

2 tablespoons (30 ml) olive oil

2 tablespoons (14 g) chopped oil packed sun-dried tomatoes

1 teaspoon lemon juice

Place all the ingredients into the pan of your bread machine in the order specified by the manufacturer. Program the machine for the white bread cycle, light crust setting, and press Start.

Yield: 12 servings

Per serving: 163 calories (19% from fat, 14% from protein, 67% from carbohydrate); 6 g protein; 3 g total fat; 1 g saturated fat; 2 g monounsaturated fat; 1 g polyunsaturated fat; 27 g carbohydrate; 1 g fiber; 2 g sugar; 66 mg phosphorus; 40 mg calcium; 49 mg sodium; 85 mg potassium; 37 IU vitamin A; 7 mg ATE vitamin E; 1 mg vitamin C; 2 mg cholesterol

Apple Bread

Apples and oatmeal give this bread a lot of flavor and a great texture. It's the kind of bread that you can eat without adding anything, but it's also great with toppings such as honey or apple butter.

(continued on page 320)

1½ cups (180 g) bread flour

1½ cups (120 g) rolled oats

1½ teaspoons instant yeast

½ teaspoon ground cinnamon

1 cup (245 g) unsweetened applesauce

1½ tablespoons (30 g) honey

½ tablespoon vegetable oil

⅓ cup (50 g) diced dried apples

Place all the ingredients except the dried apples into the pan of your bread machine in the order specified by the manufacturer. Program the machine for the fruit bread cycle if available or white bread cycle if not, light crust setting, and press Start. Add the dried apples at the beep or 3 minutes before the end of the second kneading cycle.

Yield: 12 servings

Per serving: 133 calories (10% from fat, 12% from protein, 78% from carbohydrate); 4 g protein; 2 g total fat; 0 g saturated fat; 0 g monounsaturated fat; 1 g polyunsaturated fat; 26 g carbohydrate; 2 g fiber; 6 g sugar; 73 mg phosphorus; 10 mg calcium; 2 mg sodium; 80 mg potassium; 4 IU vitamin A; 0 mg ATE vitamin E; 1 mg vitamin C; 0 mg cholesterol

Banana Nut Bread

Most banana bread is quick bread, raised with baking powder. This yeast version has a subtler flavor that tends to grow on you.

3½ cups (420 g) bread flour

½ cup (55 g) chopped pecans

3 tablespoons (23 g) nonfat dry milk

2 tablespoons (30 g) packed brown sugar

2 teaspoons instant yeast

½ cup (120 ml) water

2 medium bananas, mashed

4 teaspoons unsalted butter

Place all the ingredients into the pan of your bread machine in the order specified by the manufacturer. Program the machine for fruit bread cycle if available or white bread cycle if not, and press Start.

Yield: 12 servings

Per serving: 224 calories (21% from fat, 11% from protein, 68% from carbohydrate); 6 g protein; 5 g total fat; 1 g saturated fat; 2 g monounsaturated fat; 1 g polyunsaturated fat; 38 g carbohydrate; 2 g fiber; 6 g sugar; 77 mg phosphorus; 26 mg calcium; 8 mg sodium; 188 mg potassium; 84 IU vitamin A; 18 mg ATE vitamin E; 2 mg vitamin C; 4 mg cholesterol

Cranberry-Orange Bread

The cranberry-orange flavor of this bread makes it a real hit for breakfast, but it's also perfect for leftover turkey sandwiches. Try it toasted and topped with more of the orange marmalade.

2¾ cups (330 g) bread flour

¼ cup (30 g) nonfat dry milk

2 tablespoons (25 g) sugar

1¾ teaspoons instant yeast

¾ cup (180 ml) water

¼ cup (60 ml) cranberry juice

¼ cup (75 g) orange marmalade

2 tablespoons (28 g) unsalted butter

⅔ cup (100 g) dried cranberries

Place all the ingredients except the cranberries into the pan of your bread machine in the order specified by the manufacturer. Program the machine for the fruit bread cycle if available or white bread cycle if not, and press Start. Add the cranberries at the beep or 3 minutes before the end of the second kneading cycle.

Yield: 12 servings

Per serving: 167 calories (13% from fat, 11% from protein, 76% from carbohydrate); 5 g protein; 2 g total fat; 1 g saturated fat; 1 g monounsaturated fat; 0 g polyunsaturated fat; 32 g carbohydrate; 1 g fiber; 7 g sugar; 54 mg phosphorus; 27 mg calcium; 13 mg sodium; 76 mg potassium; 102 IU vitamin A; 26 mg ATE vitamin E; 2 mg vitamin C; 5 mg cholesterol

Raisin Bread

Raisin bread is one of those classics that everyone likes. To make even more traditional, drizzle a glaze made with ½ cup (60 g) confectioners' sugar and 1 tablespoon (15 ml) water over the top.

2¾ cups (330 g) bread flour

¼ cup (30 g) nonfat dry milk

2 tablespoons (25 g) sugar

1¼ teaspoons instant yeast

1 teaspoon ground cinnamon

1¼ cups (295 ml) water

1 tablespoon (15 ml) vegetable oil

1 cup (145 g) raisins

Place all the ingredients except the raisins into the pan of your bread machine in the order specified by the manufacturer. Program the machine for raisin or fruit bread cycle, and press Start. Add the raisins at the beep or 3 minutes before the end of the second kneading cycle.

Yield: 12 servings

Per serving: 179 calories (9% from fat, 11% from protein, 81% from carbohydrate); 5 g protein; 2 g total fat; 0 g saturated fat; 0 g monounsaturated fat; 1 g polyunsaturated fat; 37 g carbohydrate; 1 g fiber; 11 g sugar; 64 mg phosphorus; 32 mg calcium; 11 mg sodium; 168 mg potassium; 35 IU vitamin A; 10 mg ATE vitamin E; 0 mg vitamin C; 0 mg cholesterol

Rum Raisin Bread

This tasty bread is great for breakfast or snacks. It has a flavor that will remind you of rum raisin ice cream.

3 cups (360 g) bread flour

2 tablespoons (15 g) nonfat dry milk

2 teaspoons instant yeast

2 teaspoons packed brown sugar

¾ cup (180 ml) water

(continued on page 322)

2 tablespoons (30 ml) heavy cream

2 teaspoons unsalted butter

½ teaspoon rum extract

¼ cup (62 g) egg substitute, or 1 large egg

2 tablespoons (30 ml) rum

½ cup (75 g) raisins

Combine the rum and raisins in a small bowl, and set aside to macerate for about 30 minutes. Place all of the ingredients except the rum and raisins into the pan of your bread machine in the order specified by the manufacturer. Program the machine for the raisin or fruit bread cycle, light crust setting, and press Start. Add the rum and raisins at the beep or 3 minutes before the end of the second kneading cycle.

Yield: 12 servings

Per serving: 171 calories (10% from fat, 13% from protein, 76% from carbohydrate); 5 g protein; 2 g total fat; 1 g saturated fat; 0 g monounsaturated fat; 0 g polyunsaturated fat; 32 g carbohydrate; 1 g fiber; 5 g sugar; 63 mg phosphorus; 22 mg calcium; 15 mg sodium; 132 mg potassium; 74 IU vitamin A; 15 mg ATE vitamin E; 0 mg vitamin C; 4 mg cholesterol

Tip: If you prefer to bake without alcohol, substitute water or apple juice for the rum. If desired add ¼ teaspoon of rum extract.

Strawberry Bread

Strawberries and cream cheese flavor this loaf. It will fill the house with a wonderful fruit aroma as it bakes.

3 cups (360 g) bread flour

½ cup (40 g) rolled oats

2 tablespoons (25 g) sugar

2 teaspoons instant yeast

¾ cup (180 ml) skim milk

4 ounces (112 g) cream cheese

⅓ cup (57 g) sliced fresh strawberries

1 tablespoon (14 g) unsalted butter

Place all of the ingredients into the pan of your bread machine in the order specified by the manufacturer. Program for raisin or fruit bread cycle, light crust setting, and press Start.

Yield: 12 servings

Per serving: 197 calories (24% from fat, 13% from protein, 64% from carbohydrate); 6 g protein; 5 g total fat; 3 g saturated fat; 1 g monounsaturated fat; 0 g polyunsaturated fat; 31 g carbohydrate; 1 g fiber; 3 g sugar; 86 mg phosphorus; 38 mg calcium; 38 mg sodium; 108 mg potassium; 191 IU vitamin A; 51 mg ATE vitamin E; 3 mg vitamin C; 13 mg cholesterol

Chocolate Bread

This is a great coffee bread and also good with peanut butter. The chocolate chips tend to melt and make chocolate swirls through the bread.

3½ cups (420 g) bread flour

1½ teaspoons instant yeast

1½ cups (355 ml) water

1½ teaspoons vanilla extract

½ cup (60 g) chopped walnuts

1 cup (175 g) semisweet chocolate chips

Place all the ingredients except the chocolate chips and walnuts into the pan of your bread machine in the order specified by the manufacturer. Program the machine for the raisin or fruit bread cycle bread cycle, and press Start. Add the chocolate chips and walnuts at the beep or 3 minutes before the end of the second kneading cycle.

Yield: 12 servings

Per serving: 254 calories (29% from fat, 11% from protein, 61% from carbohydrate); 7 g protein; 8 g total fat; 2 g saturated fat; 2 g monounsaturated fat; 3 g polyunsaturated fat; 38 g carbohydrate; 2 g fiber; 8 g sugar; 91 mg phosphorus; 38 mg calcium; 13 mg sodium; 124 mg potassium; 26 IU vitamin A; 7 mg ATE vitamin E; 0 mg vitamin C; 3 mg cholesterol

24

Cooking Terms, Weights and Measurements, and Gadgets

Cooking Terms

Confused about a term I used in one of the recipes? Take a look at the list here and see whether there might be an explanation. I've tried to include anything that I thought might raise a question.

Al dente

"To the tooth," in Italian. The pasta is cooked just enough to maintain a firm, chewy texture.

Bake

To cook in the oven. Food is cooked slowly with gentle heat, concentrating the flavor.

Baste

To brush or spoon liquid, fat, or juices over meat during roasting to add flavor and to prevent it from drying out.

Beat

To smooth a mixture by briskly whipping or stirring it with a spoon, fork, wire whisk, rotary beater, or electric mixer.

Blend

To mix or fold two or more ingredients together to obtain equal distribution throughout the mixture.

Boil

To cook food in heated water or other liquid that is bubbling vigorously.

Braise

A cooking technique that requires browning meat in oil or other fat and then cooking slowly in liquid. The effect of braising is to tenderize the meat.

Bread

To coat the food with crumbs (usually with soft or dry bread crumbs), sometimes seasoned.

Broil

To cook food directly under the heat source.

Broth or Stock

A flavorful liquid made by gently cooking meat, seafood, or vegetables (and/or their by-products, such as bones and trimmings) often with herbs and vegetables, in liquid, usually water.

Brown

A quick sautéing, pan/oven broiling, or grilling done either at the beginning or end of meal preparation, often to enhance flavor, texture, or visual appeal.

Brush

Using a pastry brush to coat a food such as meat or bread with melted butter, glaze, or other liquid.

Chop

To cut into irregular pieces.

Coat

To evenly cover food with flour, crumbs, or a batter.

Combine

To blend two or more ingredients into a single mixture.

Core

To remove the inedible center of fruits such as pineapples.

Cream

To beat butter or margarine, with or without sugar, until light and fluffy. This process traps in air bubbles, later used to create height in cookies and cakes.

Cut in

To work margarine or butter into dry ingredients.

Dash

A measure approximately equal to $\frac{1}{16}$ teaspoon.

Deep-Fry

To completely submerge the food in hot oil. It's a quick way to cook some food and, as a result, this method often seems to seal in the flavors of food better than any other technique.

Dice

To cut into cubes.

Direct heat

Heat waves radiate from a source and travel directly to the item being heated with no conductor between them. Examples are grilling, broiling, and toasting.

Dough

Used primarily for cookies and breads. Dough is a mixture of shortening, flour, liquid, and other ingredients that maintains its shape when placed on a flat surface, although it will change shape through the leavening process once baked.

Dredge

To coat lightly and evenly with sugar or flour.

Dumpling

A batter or soft dough, which is formed into small mounds that are then steamed, poached, or simmered.

Dust

To sprinkle food lightly with spices, sugar, or flour for a light coating.

Fold

To cut and mix lightly with a spatula to keep as much air in the mixture as possible.

Fritter

Sweet or savory foods coated or mixed into batter, then deep-fried.

Fry

To cook food in hot oil, usually until a crisp brown crust forms.

Glaze

A liquid that gives an item a shiny surface. Examples are fruit jams that have been heated or chocolate that has been thinned.

Grease

To coat a skillet or baking sheet with a thin layer of oil or butter.

Grill

To cook over the heat source (traditionally over wood coals) in the open air.

Grind

To mechanically cut a food into small pieces.

Hull

To remove the leafy parts of soft fruits such as strawberries or blackberries.

Knead

To work dough with the heels of your hands in a pressing and folding motion until it becomes smooth and elastic.

Marinate

To soak food in aromatic ingredients to add flavor.

Mince

To chop food into tiny, irregular pieces.

Mix

To beat or stir two or more foods together until they are thoroughly combined.

Panfry

To cook in a hot pan with a small amount of hot oil, butter, or other fat, turning the food over once or twice.

Poach

To simmer food in a liquid.

Pot roast

A large piece of meat, usually browned in fat and cooked in a covered pan.

Purée

Food that has been mashed or processed in a blender or food processor.

Reduce

To cook liquids down so that some of the water content evaporates.

Roast

To cook uncovered in the oven.

Sauté

To cook with a small amount of hot oil, butter, or other fat, tossing the food around over high heat.

Sear

To brown a food quickly on all sides using high heat to seal in the juices.

Shred

To cut into fine strips.

Simmer

To cook slowly in a liquid over low heat.

Skim

To remove the surface layer (of impurities, scum, or fat) from liquids such as stocks and jams while cooking. This is usually done with a flat slotted spoon.

Smoke

To expose foods to wood smoke to enhance their flavor and help preserve and/or evenly cook them.

Steam

To cook in steam by suspending foods over boiling water in a steamer or covered pot.

Stew

To cook food in liquid for a long time until tender, usually in a covered pot.

Stir

To mix ingredients with a utensil.

Stir-fry

To cook quickly over high heat with a small amount of oil by constantly stirring. This technique often employs a wok.

Toss

To mix ingredients lightly by lifting and dropping them using two utensils.

Whip

To beat an item to incorporate air, augment volume, and add substance.

Zest

The thin, brightly colored outer part of the rind of citrus fruits. It contains volatile oils, used as a flavoring.

Weights and Measurements

Here is a quick refresher on measurements.

3 teaspoons = 1 tablespoon

2 tablespoons = 1 fluid ounce

4 tablespoons = 2 fluid ounces = ¼ cup

5⅓ tablespoons = 16 teaspoons = ⅓ cup

8 tablespoons = 4 fluid ounces = ½ cup

16 tablespoons = 8 fluid ounces = 1 cup

2 cups = 1 pint

4 cups = 2 pints = 1 quart

16 cups = 8 pints = 4 quarts = 1 gallon

Gadgets

The following are some of the tools that I use in cooking. Some are used very often and some very seldom, but all help make things a little easier or quicker. Why are some things here and others not? No reason, except that most of these are things I considered a little less standard than a stove, an oven, a grill, and a mixer.

Blender

Okay, so everyone has a blender. And it's a handy little tool for blending and puréeing things. I don't really think I need to say any more about that.

Bread Machine

When I went on a low-sodium diet, I discovered that one of the biggest single changes you can make to reduce your sodium intake is to make your own bread. Most commercial bread has well over 100 mg per slice. Many rolls and specialty breads are in the 300 to 400 mg range. A bread machine can reduce the amount of effort required to make your own bread to a manageable level. It takes at most 10 minutes to load it and turn it on. You can even set it on a timer to have your house filled with the aroma of fresh bread when you come home. Even if you're not watching your sodium, there is nothing like the smell of bread baking and the taste right out of the "oven."

Canning Kettle

If you are planning on making large batches of things like pickles and salsa so you don't have to go through the process of making them every couple of weeks, then you are going to need a way to preserve food. Most items can be frozen of course, if that is your preference. But some things just seem to work better in jars. What you need is a kettle big enough to make sure the jars can be covered by water when being processed in a boiling water bath. There are also racks to sit the jars in and special tongs to make lifting them in and out of the water easier. I had a porcelain-covered kettle that I used for this for many years, and it also doubled as a stockpot, before I got the one described below (page 334). It's better for canning than for soup because the relatively thin walls allow the water to heat faster (and the soup to burn).

Deep Fryer

Obviously, if you are watching your fat intake, this should not be one of your most often used appliances. I don't use it nearly as often as I used to, but it still occupies a place in the appliance garage in the corner of the kitchen counter. It's a Fry Daddy, big enough to cook a batch of fries or fish for three or four people at a time.

Food Processor

I'm a real latecomer to the food processor world. It always seemed like a nice thing to have, but something I could easily do without. We bought one to help shred meat and other things for my wife's mother, who was having some difficulty swallowing large chunks of food. I use it now all the time to grind bread into crumbs or chop the peppers and onions that seem to go into at least three meals a week. It's a low-end model that doesn't have the power to grind meat and some of the heavier tasks, but I've discovered it's a real timesaver for a number of things.

Grill

The George Foreman models are the most popular example of this item. My son's girlfriend gave me this for Christmas a few years ago. (And he didn't have the good sense to hang on to her . . . but that's a different story.) I use it fairly often. When we built our house we included a

Jenn-Air cooktop with a built-in grill and for years that was used regularly. It still is for some things; I much prefer the way it does burgers or steak when it's too cold to grill them outside, but it's difficult to clean and doesn't do nearly as nice a job as the Foreman at things like grilled veggies and fish. And the design allows the fat to drain away, giving you a healthier, lower fat meal.

Grinder

Many years ago we bought an Oster Kitchen Center. It was one of those all-in-one things that included a stand mixer, blender (the one we still use), food chopper, and grinder attachment. The grinder was never a big deal that got any use . . . until I started experimenting with sausage recipes. Since then, I've discovered that grinding your own meat can save you both money and fat. Buying a beef or pork roast on sale, trimming it of most fat, and grinding it yourself can give you hamburger or sausage meat that is well over 90 percent lean and still less expensive than the fattier stuff you buy at the store. So now the grinder gets fairly regular use.

Hand Chopper

My daughter got this gem at a Walmart in North Carolina while she was in school there. It was from one of those guys with the podium and the auctioneer's delivery and the extra free gifts if you buy it within the next 10 minutes. Neither of us has ever seen one like it since. The food processor has taken over some of its work, but it still does a great job chopping things such as onions as fine as you could want without liquefying them.

Pasta Maker

I bought this toy after seeing it on a Sunday morning TV infomercial. It's a genuine Ronco/ Popiel "As Seen on TV" special, but try not to hold that against it. Unlike the pasta cutters that merely slice rolled dough into flat noodles, this one mixes the whole mess, then extrudes it through dies with various-shaped holes in them. The recipes say you can use any kind of flour, but I've found that buying the semolina flour that is traditionally used for pasta gives you dough that's easier to work with, as well as better texture and flavor. The characterization of it as a "toy" is pretty accurate. There aren't really any nutritional advantages over store-bought pasta. If you buy the semolina, the cost is probably about the same as some of the more expensive imported pastas. But it's fun to play with, it makes a great conversation piece, and the pasta tastes good.

SaladShooter

We seem to end up with a lot of these gadgets, don't we? This is another one that's been around for a while, but it's still my favorite implement for shredding potatoes for hash browns or cabbage for coleslaw.

Sausage Stuffer

This is really an addition to the Kitchen Center grinder. I found it at an online appliance repair site. It is really just a series of different-sized tubes that fit on the end of the grinder to stuff your ground meat into casings. I do this occasionally to make link sausage, but most of the time I just make patties or bulk sausage.

Slicer

This was a close-out floor model that I bought years ago. Before going on the low-sodium diet, I used to buy deli meat in bulk and slice it myself. Now it's most often used to slice a roast or smoked piece of meat for sandwiches.

Slow Cooker

I've tried to avoid calling it a Crock-Pot, which is a trademark of Rival. Anyway, whatever the brand, no kitchen should be without one.

Smoker

This was another pre-diet purchase that has been used even more since. I started with a Brinkman model that originally used charcoal. Then I bought an add-on electric heat source for it that works a lot better in cold weather. A few years ago the family gave me a fancy MasterChef electric one that seals like an oven and has a thermostat to hold the temperature. Not only do I like the way it does ribs and other traditional smoked foods, but we also use it fairly regularly to smoke a beef or pork roast or turkey breast to use for sandwiches.

Springform Pan

A round, straight-sided pan. The sides are formed into a hoop that can be unclasped and detached from its base.

Steamer (Rice Cooker)

I use this primarily for cooking rice, but it's really a Black & Decker Handy Steamer Plus that does a great job steaming vegetables, too. It does make excellent rice, perfect every time. So I guess the bottom line is that those of you who have trouble making rice like me (probably because like me you can't follow the instructions not to peek) should consider getting one of these or one of the Japanese-style rice cookers.

Stockpot

The key here is to spend the extra money to get a heavy-gauge one (another thing I eventually learned from personal experience). The lighter weight ones will not only dent and not sit level on the stove, but they will also burn just about everything you put in them. Mine also has a heavy glass lid that seals the moisture in well.

Turbo Cooker

Another infomercial sale. It is a large, dome-lidded fry pan with racks that fit inside it. You can buy them at many stores too, but mine is the "Plus" model that has two steamer racks and a timer. It really will cook a whole dinner quickly, "steam frying" the main course and steaming one or two more items. The only bad news is most of the recipes involve additions and changes every few minutes, so even if you only take a half hour to make dinner, you spend that whole time at the stove.

Waffle Maker

I don't use this often, but it makes a nice change of pace for breakfast or dinner.

Wok

A round-bottomed pan popular in Asian cooking.

About the Author

After being diagnosed with congestive heart failure, **Dick Logue** threw himself into the process of creating healthy versions of his favorite recipes. A cook since the age of twelve, he grows his own vegetables, bakes his own bread, and cans a variety of foods at home in La Plata, Maryland. He currently has a website www.lowsodiumcooking.com and weekly online newsletter. He is the author of several cookbooks, including *500 Low-Sodium Recipes*, *500 Low-Cholesterol Recipes*, *500 High-Fiber Recipes*, *500 Low-Glycemic-Index Recipes*, *400 Heart-Healthy Slow Cooker Recipes*, and *500 400-Calorie Recipes*.

Index